PERSONS WITH PROFOUND DISABILITIES

PERSONS WITH PROFOUND DISABILITIES

Issues and Practices

edited by

Fredda Brown, Ph.D.
Institute of Professional Practice
New Haven, Connecticut

and

Donna H. Lehr, Ph.D.
Department of Exceptional Education
University of Wisconsin-Milwaukee

·P A U L· H·
BROOKES
PUBLISHING Cº

Baltimore • London • Toronto • Sydney

Paul H. Brookes Publishing Co.
Post Office Box 10624
Baltimore, Maryland 21285-0624

Typeset by Brushwood Graphics, Inc., Baltimore, Maryland.
Manufactured in the United States of America by
Thomson-Shore, Inc., Dexter, Michigan.

Library of Congress Cataloging in Publication Data
Persons with profound disabilities.

  Includes bibliographies and index.
  1. Rehabilitation—United States.   2. Special education—United
States.   3. Handicapped—Education—United States.   I. Brown,
Fredda.   II. Lehr, Donna H. [DNLM: 1. Community Health Ser-
vices.   2. Education, Special.   3. Handicapped. LC 4015 P467]
HV1553.P48   1989   362.4   88-30468
ISBN 1-55766-015-8

CONTENTS

CONTRIBUTORS

Paul Bates, Ph.D.
Department of Special Education
Southern Illinois University
Carbondale, IL 62901

Fredda Brown, Ph.D.
Institute of Professional Practice
Post Office Box 3469
New Haven, CT 06515

Philippa H. Campbell, Ph.D., OTR/L
Family Child Learning Center
Children's Hospital Medical Center
   of Akron
281 Locust Street
Akron, OH 44308

Rob Davis, M.S.
Institute of Professional Practice
Post Office Box 3469
New Haven, CT 06515

William L.E. Dussault, J.D.
219 East Galer Street
Seattle, WA 98102-3794

Stanley J. Eichner, J.D.
Department of the Attorney General
Civil Rights Division
1 Ashburton Place, 19th Floor
Boston, MA 02108

Ian M. Evans, Ph.D.
Department of Psychology
State University of New York
Binghamton, NY 13901

Diane Eynon, M.A.
Department of Communication Disorders
115 Shevlin Hall
University of Minnesota
Minneapolis, MN 55455

Doug Guess, Ed.D.
Department of Special Education
University of Kansas
Lawrence, KS 66045

Edwin Helmstetter, Ph.D.
Department of Counseling Psychology
Washington State University
Pullman, WA 99164-2131

Jennifer F. Holvoet, Ph.D.
Institute of Logopedics
2400 Jardine Drive
Wichita, KS 67219

Kim Kelly, M.A.
Institute of Professional Practice
Post Office Box 1249
Montpelier, VT 05602

Donna H. Lehr, Ph.D.
Department of Exceptional Education
681 Enderis Hall
University of Wisconsin-Milwaukee
Milwaukee, WI 53201

Mary Jo Noonan, Ph.D.
Department of Special Education
1776 University Avenue, UA 4-5/6
University of Hawaii
Honolulu, HI 96822

Joe Reichle, Ph.D.
Department of Communication Disorders
115 Shevlin Hall
University of Minnesota
Minneapolis, MN 55455

Michael Richards, M.A.
Institute of Professional Practice
Post Office Box 3469
New Haven, CT 06515

Joseph R. Scotti, M.A.
Department of Psychology
State University of New York
Binghamton, NY 13901

Martha E. Snell, Ph.D.
Curry School of Education
Department of Curriculum, Instruction,
    and Special Education
405 Emmet Street
University of Virginia
Charlottesville, VA 22903

Barbara Thompson, Ph.D.
Department of Special Education
University of Kansas
Lawrence, KS 66045

Jennifer York, Ph.D., P.T.
Department of Communication Disorders
115 Shevlin Hall
University of Minnesota
Minneapolis, MN 55455

FOREWORD

In the mid-1970s, the field of special education embarked on an earnest and extensive effort to provide education and treatment to that segment of the population commonly identified as "severely handicapped." This new venture, coupled with a federal mandate and a growing list of dedicated professionals, concerned parents, and social activists, opened the doors to a population of persons with very special needs that had been mostly excluded from the mainstream of community life. Prior to this venture, this was a population that primarily resided in institutions and other segregated settings where active programming was minimal, and removal from society was perceived as both "humane" and economically expedient.

It is acknowledged that far too many persons with severely and profoundly handicapping conditions still reside in segregated environments and quality educational programming is not found in many classrooms. However, given the relatively new focus on the area of severe handicaps, there is reason for pride in what has been accomplished, and optimism for even greater advances to be made in the years to come. The plethora of educational technologies, curricula, and instructional procedures available for students with severe handicaps, accompanied by progressive new social policies and philosophies for including them in the mainstream of society, are likely unparalleled in the history of special education—for any area of exceptionality. Nevertheless, there remains significant and identifiable problems in the success of state-of-the-art practices when applied to those students with the most profoundly, multiply handicapping, and often medically fragile conditions.

It would be less than honest to state, or even imply, that existing educational practices and treatment procedures are truly effective in producing significant developmental changes in those students with the most profound handicaps. In many respects, it can be said that our educational practices throughout the past 15 years have drifted upward to primarily include, so to speak, the most capable members of the population of students referred to as "severely handicapped" and only by inference have the educational needs of students with the most profoundly handicapping conditions been adequately addressed in either the field's published literature, teacher training programs, or classroom practices. In fact, the more recent attention being directed toward these students seems to reflect their increasing numbers in public school programs, coupled with very realistic concerns among teachers and other service providers of just what can and should be done with them in these settings. There is, of course, considerable disagreement as to whether or not, as one teacher was quoted to say, "This is a new wave of students" (c.f.

Thompson & Guess, this volume). Indeed, many professional educators and researchers would prefer to think that this is not a new population of students, and the same instructional technology used with students with "severe handicaps" is equally valid, with modifications for those students with more profoundly and multiply handicapping conditions. This argument is an empirical question that places the burden of proof on those persons advocating for a downward extension and refinement of existing state-of-the-art practices.

However, there appears to be sufficient concern among teachers and other service providers (as also evidenced by the emergence of several subcommittees within The Association for Persons with Severe Handicaps to address the needs of students who are profoundly handicapped and medically fragile) to embark on new educational and treatment directions to either supplement or even replace existing practices for this population of persons with very special needs. These new directions need to address some very fundamental issues pertaining to the pervasiveness of the handicapping conditions experienced by these students, the types of instructional objectives and procedures potentially available and useful for making significant behavioral changes, and, most importantly, a better understanding of quality of life improvements as perceived by both the recipients of the practices as well as those persons who would apply them.

I would submit that the field has tended to underestimate the synergistic influences produced when profound mental retardation (or its apparent manifestation) is accompanied by multiple sensory and motor impairments. These impairments tend to be further accentuated by other medical conditions (e.g., seizures, poor nutrition, reduced oxygen levels, chronic congestion, frequent illnesses) that often influence, in a negative way, even basic alertness and responsiveness. Typical stimulus control objectives and the procedures used to establish them, are, in all likelihood, insufficient to the task—a fact somewhat apparent by the absence of many published studies with students of this type. New instructional procedures will likely need to address ways and methods for improving the overall alertness and responsiveness of these students prior to, or in combination with, current instructional technologies and approaches if appreciable behavioral changes are to be successfully and extensively realized. In doing this, it will be necessary to implement, in its most efficient form, a transdisciplinary team approach that effectively utilizes and incorporates the input and expertise of professionals from a wide disciplinary base including, for example, occupational and physical therapists, nutritionists, respiratory therapists, neurologists, vision and hearing specialists, educators, and computer technology experts. Parents, of course, are also primary to the effectiveness of the transdisciplinary team.

The quality of life issue is probably most apparent when referring to this population of students. The identification of educational objectives, as well as the selection of procedures and technologies to work toward these objectives, are of paramount importance. On the one hand, the existing educational approaches and philosophies are oriented toward first identifying, and then attempting to teach skills that have been selected by others to represent what is perceived as being in the best interest of the student for functional living in integrated environments. Quality of life, as evolved from this perspective, is thus defined as what others would see as their own expectations, standards, and goals—assuming, of course, that, if capable, students with the most profoundly handicapping conditions would choose similar Individualized Education Program (IEP) objectives. It is important to include the active participation of these students in integrated environments because this offers them the greatest opportunity of achieving a better quality of life. Nevertheless, I do speculate that quality of life perceptions for students with profound handicaps might well be quite different from those persons who actively plan for the education and treatment programs for these individuals.

There is a definite need to better view the world from the perspective of individuals with profound handicaps and to "walk in their shoes," so to speak. By doing this, service providers may find that the goals and objectives, no matter how noble, might not be all that important to individuals with profound handicaps if only they could more expressively communicate. For some students with profound handicaps, an excursion to the local grocery store or bowling alley might be considerably less important than a genuine show of affection by others, a reduction in discomfort or pain, or even the discontinuation of (from their point of view) an "intrusive" and not comprehensible training program designed to increase their ability to point to objects or pictures. Indeed, quality of life for persons with profound handicaps might consist of greater opportunities to express, and have acknowledged, their own preferences, likes, and dislikes—even when these expressions conflict with those of attending adults and program planners. From an educational point of view, attempts to improve the quality of life for students with profound handicaps involve the ability to both be led, and to lead.

Being led means that the educator and service provider must better identify desires and needs from their students that relate to how they, as individuals, would like to better control their world. To lead requires educators and service providers to match instructional procedures with opportunities for these students to better express their needs and desires, and then to learn to engage in those skills, activities, and circumstances that have been chosen by them as important. This will require, in this field, a fairly significant change in philosophy for the education and training of students with profound handicaps—a philosophy that allows the student a much greater participation in the identification of what is, or is not to be learned; and a philosophy and orientation that requires others to be much more sensitive to communicative expressions (that are often very subtle) by the student.

It is obvious that work with the population of students identified as profoundly handicapped has just begun. There is yet much to learn from these individuals. However, it is most encouraging that this field is now addressing the educational and training needs of these students, as evidenced by this very book. My respect and admiration for the editors of this book is based both on their professional expertise and their long standing history of interest in providing better educational programs and services to students with the most profoundly handicapping and medically fragile conditions. Similarly, the contributors to this book reflect the best thinking in this area of special education, and their chapters, individually and collectively, should have a major influence on a variety of persons who are looking for new ideas, better methods, and a humane approach to the education and treatment of students with profoundly handicapping conditions. I enthusiastically recommend this book to the field!

Doug Guess, Ed.D.
Department of Special Education
University of Kansas

PREFACE

It is the purpose of this book to present issues and practices as they relate specifically to individuals with profound disabilities. We have met many excellent practitioners who, although thoroughly versed in the literature and practices for people with "severe handicaps," have difficulty when they attempt to apply this knowledge to persons with the most profound disabilities. As the problem is analyzed, we find several sources. First, information relevant to this population is often either assumed under the general label of "severe" or included in the heterogeneous grouping of "severe/profound." It is, therefore, difficult to discern which of the extant research is valid for those persons with profound disabilities. Second, the goals described for individuals with severe disabilities may only, in part, reflect realistic outcomes for persons with profound disabilities. A broader scope of outcomes is necessary to facilitate a realistic and meaningful participation in community life. Third, issues arise in providing services to individuals with profound disabilities that are different than for those individuals with less severe disabilities; however, these issues are not acknowledged in the existing literature.

Many of the concepts and principles developed and implemented for those with less severe disabilities do apply to all individuals with disabilities, regardless of the severity. However, further development is necessary to meaningfully apply these concepts and principles to individuals in this population. We also recognize that issues exist that are unique to this population and must be addressed to understand and meet their needs. We strongly believe that progress can only occur through problem-solving that reflects integration of information across disciplines.

The book begins with a discussion of those unique issues facing professionals in this field. The first chapter of this book is a qualitative research study of teachers' perceptions of who they are serving, and the nature and adequacy of their procedures in meeting the needs of their students. Chapters 2 and 3 present current legal and research issues emerging as services extend to persons with profound disabilities. Considerations related to the identification of meaningful behavioral outcomes are discussed in Chapter 4. A discussion of integration of students with profound disabilities into public schools appears in Chapter 5. The final chapter of the first section of this book presents issues relative to the provision of educational services to students with complex health care needs.

The second section focuses more specifically on practices appropriate for individuals with profound disabilities. Chapters 7 and 8 address the areas of motor and communication development and describe methods for developing these areas within functional contexts. Chapters 9 and 12 provide the reader with descriptions of models for providing preschool and residental programs for young children and adults. Chapter 10, which addresses school-age curriculum, and Chapter 11, which details vocational training, describe the application of current best practices for individuals with severe disabilities to individuals with profound disabilities in each of these areas.

This book is designed to assist professionals in increasing their knowledge and understanding of issues and practices as they relate to individuals with profound disabilites. It will also assist readers in appropriately extending their knowledge of individuals with moderate and severe disabilities to individuals with profound disabilities, and to raise their awareness of the complex issues that emerge in doing so. We feel this book will contribute to the professional development of individuals representing a wide variety of disciplines and interests who are involved in research and service delivery to individuals with profound disabilities.

ACKNOWLEDGMENTS

To the Institute of Professional Practice and the Department of Exceptional Education at the University of Wisconsin-Milwaukee for the support provided during the development of this book.

To Chris, Grayson, Lea, Greg, Jessica, and Geoffrey for understanding why we weren't always there for them.

To Doug Guess for his contribution to our professional development and his encouragement to question what is and what could be.

*To those individuals
with profound disabilities
who have challenged
our beliefs and practices.*

PERSONS WITH PROFOUND DISABILITIES

ISSUES

STUDENTS WHO EXPERIENCE THE MOST PROFOUND DISABILITIES
Teacher Perspectives

Barbara Thompson and Doug Guess

Teachers of students with the most profound disabilities are often confronted with experiences and attitudes not typically experienced by most educators or even most special educators. The following brief "question and answer" section is taken from an initial interview with one of the six teachers who participated in a study conducted by the authors to gain insight into the perspectives of the educators who have daily responsibility for the education of these students.

Question: Tell me Patty, is there a "bottom line" for students with whom you believe we can or cannot successfully work?

Answer: I have had medical professionals suggest that my efforts would be futile. For example, I had a doctor once say that Sam was in a coma. I have to admit this threw me at first. In another case, a doctor told me that Carrie was "brain stem level," and that fluid was accumulating around her brain. I don't think they should say things such as "brain stem level."

Question: Would you explain why you think that, Patty?

Answer: These statements make people not try. We don't know enough about the brain, you just can't say someone is not responding, or isn't learning, or isn't aware. In the case of Sam, I may not be teaching him functional skills, but I am teaching him that there is a world outside of himself and it's a pleasant world and there are things he can do to affect it. After a time, I found that Carrie does show things. She has never shown pleasure, but she is showing displeasure, and an absence of pain. Our job is to allow students to develop to their fullest potential and to be open enough to look for different ways.

Teachers' roles are often not valued by other professionals with whom they work. A significant portion of their school day involves caregiving routines such as changing diapers, feeding, lifting, transferring, and positioning students. The daily routine may also include conducting procedures that are generally viewed as medical in nature and that frequently also involve responding to situations that could be life-threatening. These professionals deal with students who do not appear to respond to them or recognize their presence. Some of their students appear to live in continuous pain, some have conditions that get gradually worse, and a few may even die while in their care.

The following six teachers offer comments about their students, provide positive viewpoints, and exhibit their professional commitment to this field throughout the major part of this chapter. Their experiences and comments emerge as the primary message to those concerned with addressing the needs of students who experience profound disabilities.

Mary Jones teaches in a small town that is part of a special education cooperative. Her six students range in age from 6 to 14. She also works with two infants and their mothers on a weekly basis. Mary team teaches with an instructor of students identified as trainably mentally handicapped. While these students' classrooms are located in a separate building near the regular elementary and high school, they are involved in an integrated school and community training setting for a large part of the school day.

Shelly Price teaches in an urban district. Her classroom is located in a regular elementary building and her five students range in age from 6 to 15. Shelly's classroom is specifically designated for students who experience the most profound multiple handicaps and who have medically fragile conditions.

Rhonda Hall teaches in a large suburban district and has responsibility for eight preschool age students from 3 to 6. This classroom is located in a regular elementary building along with the other district classrooms for students with severe multiple handicaps.

Denise White teaches in a university special education demonstration classroom. She has eight students who range in age from 2 to 5. Her classroom is located in a university building that houses special education demonstration classrooms and faculty from several departments.

Patty Long teaches in a large state residential facility for persons with developmental disabilities. Her students are considered to be too medically fragile to go to the educational facility that is located in a separate building from the living units. Her eight students range in age from 5 to 21, and attend class in a small room near their bedroom and living areas. Students less than 5 and more than 21 years of age sometimes "audit" her classroom.

Ellen Ray also teaches in a large state residential facility for persons with developmental disabilities. Her students are also considered to be too medically fragile to attend classes in the school building that is located elsewhere on the grounds. Therefore, she holds class directly in her students' living unit. Ellen's current class of six students ranges in age from 5 to 21. Older and younger students also "audit" her program.

These teachers care about their students and believe that as teachers they can possibly make a difference in a child's life. They touch upon the discovery of their students' "unique personalities" that sometimes "takes time and sensitivity" to uncover. As Ellen so eloquently explained:

> When I teach, I forget about limitations and think about the students' personalities and get what I can. I forget about the student's handicap and learn to like the child for who he or she is. . . . I look for ways to bring out whatever there is inside of them, to bring out intelligence, if there is a light in there, bring it out, if not, light one. . . . With these students, it is more important to have really good teachers who are creative and innovative.

These six teachers participated in an investigation that sought to describe and interpret experiences and viewpoints of teachers who are responsible for the daily implementation of educational programs for students who experience the most profound multiply handicapping and medically complicated conditions. The research approach employed was based upon methodology described as qualitative, naturalistic, or ethnographic (Bogdan & Biklen, 1982; Glaser & Strauss, 1967; Lincoln & Guba, 1985; Miles & Huberman, 1984; Taylor & Bogdan, 1984). This approach focuses on portraying events, issues, and meaning from the viewpoint of those involved. Qualitative methodology has been advocated for and/or employed by special education researchers who are concerned about children and youth who experience severe handicaps (Ferguson, 1985; Green et al., 1986; Odom & Shuster, 1986; Stainback & Stainback, 1985; Taylor, 1982).

RATIONALE FOR THE INQUIRY

The inquiry was conducted in response to the paucity of literature available to guide policy and practice for students with profound disabilities. The belief that consulting directly with teachers who are perceived as effective and who have had major and sustained responsibility for the educational programs of such students could offer important insights into future research directions and practices was another factor that led to the inquiry. Persons with the most profound multiply handicapping conditions are included in the categorical area of severe multiple handicaps or severe/profound handicaps. This category constitutes an extremely heterogeneous group of individuals with marked differences in functioning due to cognitive, physical, and sensory factors. The United States Department of Education, Bureau of Education for the Handicapped (USOE/BEH, 1974) (now the United States Department of Education, Office of Special Education Program) describes students within this group as children and youth who, "because of the intensity of their physical, mental, or emotional problems or a combination of such problems, need educational, social, psychological, and medical services beyond those which are traditionally offered by regular and special education programs" (RFP 74–10: pp. 2–3).

The considerable range and potential differences of students within this categorical group are illustrated in the American Association for Mental Defiency (AAMD) classification system (Grossman, 1983) and in the criteria for classification within the severe and profound categories. For example, students with profound mental retardation might be able to stand alone by 6 years of age, feed themselves finger food by age 12, and respond to simple directions and put on clothing when they are 15 years old (Grossman, 1977). A student who is ambulatory, has basic self-help skills, and responds to social contact stands in marked contrast to one who has limited to no voluntary muscle control, no apparent response to visual or auditory stimuli, and experiences an array of medical complications. Lorr and Rotatori (1985) point out in their discussion regarding issues of definition surrounding students with severe and profound handicaps that a combination of disabilities is most likely to be found at the severe/profound level. They also stated that students with profound retardation are more likely to experience medical and physical anomalies. Consequently, this group of students presents a significant challenge for professionals during assessment and education.

Rainforth (1982) described students who display the most profound, multiply handicapping conditions as unresponsive individuals who do not demonstrate understanding of daily routines, gestures, or other bases for communication, who show no recognition of significant persons in their environment; who engage in no purposeful movements; and who show minimal response to noise, movement, touch, odors, or other stimuli.

While there is evidence that students who experience the most profound disabilities may require unique procedures, and that educators are becoming frustrated in their efforts to provide appropriate educational programs for these students, there is a paucity of research that provides an empirical base of information from which to develop appropriate procedures. The absence of effective programming practices is apparent in the results of two recent studies. Hotte, Monroe, Philbrook, and Scarlata (1984) compared the differences in gain scores on the Vineland Social Maturity Scale (Doll, 1953) of individuals with profound retardation who resided in a state institution for persons with developmental disabilities, after 3 years of participation in daily 6 hour programming. The subjects were divided into two groups (i.e., low profound, high profound) on the basis of their pretest scores. The individuals in the low profound group gained an average of 1 month on the Vineland Social Maturity Scale, while individuals in the high profound group gained an average of 11 months. The authors conclude that the classification of profound is too broad and suggest that the significant differences among individuals who fall within this classification level need to be considered in establishing programming priorities and needs.

A qualitative study was conducted by Ferguson (1985) to examine the perceptions and views of eight teachers of students with severe multiple handicaps regarding how functional teaching approaches influence curricular decisions.

The functional approach (cf. Sailor & Guess, 1983) is based upon a teacher anticipating a student's future role in society and developing individual programs for the student by examining the requirements for participating in his or her community.

The results of the Ferguson (1985) study reveal that teachers informally divide their students into five groups: 1) "walkers and talkers," 2) "walkers," 3) "behavior kids," 4) "nonambs" or multiply handicapped students who seem aware of their environment but are entrapped by their bodies, and 5) "nonambs" or "extremely multiply profoundly handicapped" students who exhibit few if any responses indicative of voluntary behavior or awareness of the environment. Teachers reported feelings of pessimism about the potential of any approach taken with this final group. According to Ferguson (1985):

> For these students the notion of functional teaching fails utterly. Teachers see no way such students can ever functionally do anything. There are no curricular decisions to be made by teachers because there are no functional alternatives for these students. Educational uncertainty extends to future uncertainty. (p. 58)

An awareness of the needs of these students by national professional organizations is emerging. In February, 1986, the Critical Issues Committee of The Association for Persons with Severe Handicaps formed a subcommittee to identify issues and research needs that address promising practices for this group. The Council for Exceptional Children (CEC) also formed a task force to address issues related to children who are medically fragile and comatose.

Most research and state-of-the-art educational practices developed since the early 1980s have been directed toward children and youth within the severe multiply handicapped classification area who demonstrate higher levels of development than those classified as profoundly handicapped (cf., Bricker & Filler, 1985). Evidence of the paucity of published literature pertaining to individuals with profound handicaps is apparent from the review of literature conducted by Brown, Helmstetter, and Guess (1986). Five journals that published articles pertaining to students with severe handicaps were reviewed in order to examine articles that related to students with profound handicaps for the 5 years of 1980–1984. In the literature, only 49 of the 185 empirical studies specifically addressed individuals with profound handicaps, while the remaining 136 included this group with other populations such as "moderate to profound" or "severe and profound." An analysis of the studies specifically directed toward persons with profound handicaps revealed that 59% were conducted in institutional settings. Only three of the studies were conducted in school settings, and two of those three were in segregated settings. Two studies were conducted in community settings, and no studies were conducted in a home setting. The authors also note that almost all of the studies pertained to either isolated skill development and/or behavioral deceleration programs.

Because there was very little empirical literature to guide policy and practice, it seemed logical and imperative to consult directly with teachers who had been involved in providing daily educational services to students with the most profound multiply handicapping conditions and to employ a qualitative approach in this inquiry. Quantitative methods such as surveys, the collection of demographic data, structured observations, and experimental manipulation of variables are also needed. However, a holistic and interpretative description of the current situation offers important insight for considering issues, policy, and future research directions as well as a basis for interpreting the results of quantitative studies that will, hopefully, be forthcoming. Teachers, support service staff, parents, and other caregivers must be directly consulted if the needs of these students are to be more adequately addressed. If the information and insight that they can offer are not actively sought and seriously considered, it is likely that recommended policy, future training efforts, and educational and treatment programs will have limited use.

PROCEDURES EMPLOYED IN THE INQUIRY

Each of the six teachers invited to participate in this inquiry had held full certification in the severely multiply handicapped classification area, had taught for an average of 5 years with a range of 2–8 years, and had at least 2 years of teaching background with students who experience the most profound disabilities. All were identified as effective by two supervisory or university professionals familiar with their work in the classroom. More specifically, university training personnel and district administrative personnel who had responsibility for programs serving students with severe multiple handicaps were contacted and asked to suggest teachers who, in their opinion, seemed effective in working with students who experience the most profound multiply handicapping and medically complex conditions. They were also asked to suggest teachers who would be able to discuss the possible approaches, needs, and issues concerning the education of these students. Requests for nominations were limited to persons who were working within an approximate distance of 75 miles from the investigators to expedite travel to sites for interviews. The candidates for selection were described as "doing a good job" of programming for students, "innovative and creative" in implementing techniques, holding "positive attitudes" about their students, and acting as strong advocates for their students. Additionally, the selection of the participating teachers was based on an attempt to include professionals who: 1) worked with students of varying age ranges; 2) represented both community and residential settings as well as rural and urban settings; and 3) worked in classrooms specifically designated for students with profound handicaps as well as in classrooms for individuals representing the full range of students with severe multiple handicaps. After the nominations were solicited and demographic variables considered, letters were sent to six teachers inviting them to participate and explaining the investigation. All six teachers accepted the offer.

In the fall of 1986, each participating teacher was individually interviewed twice and given the notes of each interview for review, revision, and validation. After each teacher validated the notes from the particular interview, they were analyzed by the interviewer and an independent reader. A consensus was reached by the interviewers on how to divide the content of the teachers' interview notes into individual units of information or datum. These units were then coded with the participating teacher's number, the page number from the interview document, and the line number on the page. Datum units were then placed on individual cards and a process of sorting and resorting the cards into preliminary categories was conducted until final categories were identified and coded. A document was developed from an analysis of the themes and issues that emerged from the categories of interview data. All six participating teachers were provided with this document and then met as a group to discuss, revise, and/or validate the document's content, interpretations, and conclusions. The participating teachers were first introduced to each other at the group meeting.

The inquiry was directed toward the participating teachers' perceptions of: 1) student characteristics, 2) the nature and adequacy of current practices as well as discrepancies between recommended and current avenues of teaching, 3) the need for additional procedures, and 4) the potential reasons for the inadequacies of current practices. Approximately 30 hours of indepth open-ended interviews were conducted with the participating teachers. The average length of each teacher's first interview was 2½ hours, the average length of their second interview was 1½ hours, and the group meeting was 3 hours in length. Because the interviews were open-ended, the participating teachers were not approached with a set of prearranged questions. While consistent topics were raised and questions posed, each interview was unique in that the focus on the preceding areas was guided by what was important to that individual teacher. In general, the participating teachers presented their opinions and experiences, provided examples relating to student characteristics, related their relevant and successful educational practices, volunteered procedures for management and care, offered information concerning the adequacy of their professional training, and stressed the issues concerning quality of life.

Five major themes emerged from the content of the interview. The themes are directed toward: 1) discussing the characteristics of the students with the most profound disabilities and the meaning of the term "profound"; 2) describing teaching practices and procedures that pertain specifically to these students; 3) identifying the issues of service delivery and roadblocks to integrated environments; 4) highlighting the involvement with families and the special nature of the teacher/parent relationship; and 5) sharing questions, concerns, and feelings about their students and their roles as teachers. The following sections of this chapter address each of these themes.

WHO ARE STUDENTS WITH
THE MOST PROFOUND DISABILITIES?

When asked to describe students with the most profound disabilities, the participating teachers raised issues about the broad meaning and relative nature of this term. They typically discussed the limits of a traditional view of the term "profound," described the characteristics of the students with the most profound handicaps, and provided examples of the relativity of definitions.

A New Group

Teachers see students with the most profound multiply handicapping conditions as different from or a distinct group within the student population that is generally viewed as severely or profoundly disabled. Ellen is responsible for students who, until a few years ago, received no or very limited educational services because of their profound physical and cognitive disabilities as well as serious medical conditions. She described some of her students as being "in a different category than profound," if one compared her students to those identified as profoundly retarded who have been receiving services in most Severely Multiply Handicapped (SMH) classrooms. Ellen noted:

> I now work with 3-year-old students. I thought I would never see a 3-year-old in an institution again, but they are getting younger and more handicapped, because these students used to die. . . . This group needs to be advocated for, this is the new wave.

Denise suggested, "These students are really different from the students we typically think of as students in (SMH) programs, . . . working with these students was like starting in a new field." She feels her training prepared her to work effectively with students with severe disabilities and that she could transfer many of the skills to students who are considered to be trainably mentally retarded, educably mentally retarded, learning disabled, or behavior disordered. However, this group requires a number of additional skills not included in her training program for teaching students with severe disabilities.

Characteristics of Students
with the Most Profound Disabilities

When asked to describe students with the most profound multiply handicapping conditions, all of the participating teachers consistently identified several characteristics. These characteristics include: limited level of awareness, limited response repertoires, no system of communication, and medical complications.

Limited Level of Awareness The limited level of awareness characteristic is primarily based upon cognitive functioning. This term was related to a student's lack of response to stimuli, changes, or persons in his or her environment. Students whom teachers perceive to have the most profound cognitive delays are not viewed as "trapped in their bodies." This is a term reserved for students who do indicate awareness of their environments despite profound physical limitations.

Limited Response Repertoires   The second characteristic, limited response repertoire, is related to physical disabilities. Students are described as having "very limited, if any, voluntary movement." Typically, these students lack voluntary movement and often have interfering abnormal reflexes, aberrant tone, and atypical conditions such as contractures, dislocations, and skeleton deformities.

No System of Communication   The characteristic of having no system of communication relates to both physical and cognitive factors. In general, the participating teachers were in agreement about the absence of a communication system with their students, but expressed differences in opinion in relation to defining what behavior could be considered communicative in its intent. One participating teacher commented that she believed that "human beings have an inherent desire to communicate awareness in some way, . . . either through eye contact, reaching and touching, or a vocalization. This type of communication seems to be missing in many of the students with the most profoundly handicapping conditions." However, another teacher stated that she firmly believed that all persons communicate and that the problem lies in our inability to recognize it. This teacher was concerned about the limited training efforts directed toward recognizing and facilitating communicative intent and the development of alternative systems. She felt that this was a critical area of focus for professionals who worked with students who experience the most profound disabilities.

Medical Complications   Health-related disorders were identified as a highly related or predictable fourth characteristic. Participating teachers were quick to point out that a student with medical problems is not necessarily profoundly disabled; however, a student who is profoundly disabled is more likely to have conditions that are medically complicated and require special procedures.

The participating teachers described many of their students as "frequently ill" and "absent a lot." Conditions most frequently named were serious seizure disorders, chronic respiratory problems, and severe eating disorders with related risks such as vomiting and pneumonia. In addition, these teachers identified severe orthopedic problems (e.g., osteogenesis imperfecta, hip dislocations), apnea, problems with bowel impactions, disorders related to body temperature regulation (e.g., hypothermia), failure to thrive, weight loss, allergies, and immune system disorders.

Profound Is a Relative Term

Teachers view the term "profound" as highly relative and altered by their own experiences, the environment, and the opportunities that are afforded to a student. Ellen made clear distinctions between students who are generally identified as profoundly handicapped. For example, she sees major differences among: 1) students who physicians have classified as "functioning at a brain stem level" and she describes as functioning "below the sensorimotor level"; 2) students for whom you "can stimulate senses and get responses"; 3) students who have "an eye or hand response" and who purposely use such movements as a form of communicating; and 4) students who show evidence of cognitive abilities because of their eye contact and social behavior but "seem trapped in their bodies."

Ellen spoke of a student who had recently been transferred to her classroom and was diagnosed as terminal and physically deteriorating. "His previous teacher had told me, 'I can do no more,' but, he came in at the top of my class; what she sees as low is my high." When asked if this might be an example of the term "relative" used so frequently in Ellen's setting, she responded, "Relative is the big word!"

Patty discussed a different group of students in the same facility and noted that, "I don't think they are profound, although someone else would say they were." She explained that these students could do things like use a callboard or a headstick to signal needs "which are very significant behavior." Shelly told of how her view of a particular group of students in an institutional setting had changed since her experiences with her current students. She had previously perceived these students as being capable of very little, but now she can see that they can really do a lot! Mary also believes that the term "profound" is extremely relative and tied to individual perceptions. She stated:

> Some kids have seemed pretty profoundly handicapped, but after a while they seem less profound. . . . Yet, I see no programming going on for many of these students because people think there isn't much you can do. I just got a little girl who is 6½, very spastic, and supposedly deaf. There were three goals on her IEP [individualized education program] and they were all PT [physical therapy] goals! She was going to school all day for three PT goals. They had her in their very lowest class, I think it was called the sensory integration class. Yet, she is beginning to match picture to objects presented in a functional situation.

While teachers acknowledge that the term "profound" encompasses a broad group of students, they view students with the most profound multiple handicaps very specifically. Furthermore, if a student does not fit the criteria that they use for this group, then they tend to not perceive that student as profoundly disabled. The remaining sections of this chapter are primarily directed to the participating teachers' discussions of students with characteristics that they associate with persons who experience the most profound multiply handicapping conditions. Additionally, several issues and examples are related to students who exhibit some, but not all, of these characteristics.

EMERGENCE OF A CLINICAL
STYLE AND AN ECLECTIC APPROACH

When teachers of children with the most profound multiple handicaps talk about procedures, they place significant emphasis on being "tuned in" to their students. The following comments from the participating teachers illustrate this focus. Ellen reflected that, "Since working with these students, I have experienced a different mental level or attitude. I feel more tuned in to the students and more responsive to their physical and emotional needs." Similarly, Shelly stated that, "They [the students] have so few behaviors that my ability to see changes has increased. The OT [occupational therapist] is always telling me, 'I can see things.' The staff in this classroom are very in tune with these kids."

Essentially, it can be assumed that these teachers are speaking from the perspective of a clinician who relies on sensitive observational skills and intuition in combination with a broad base of information and techniques. This stands in marked contrast to a heavy reliance on an applied behavior analysis perspective and procedures that have dominated this categorical area of special education.

These teachers have not abandoned procedures based upon behavioral approaches. All of these professionals implement data-based measurement and value skills such as those involved in shaping, task analysis, program writing, and effective application of positive reinforcement. However, the participating teachers view these procedures as a small part of a larger array of techniques that come from a wide range of disciplines and theoretical approaches. This becomes apparent when they: 1) describe their goals for students and the techniques that they use to achieve them, 2) identify the predominantly important support professionals, and 3) suggest areas in which they need more information and training. Ultimately, the portrait that emerges from their discussions is one of professionals who are very eclectic in their orientation and clinical in their approach.

Several of the participating teachers discussed colleagues who are, in their view, too heavily invested in applied behavior analysis or "tight operant frameworks" and describe these teachers as "data bound" and "program runners" that are both "rigid" and "inflexible." These participants see such teachers as missing important information because they are more interested in a program and data sheet than in discovering information about a student. For example, Shelly stated that, "You may be looking for one response and they [the students] give you another and it may be just as good or very useful." Ellen noted that, "Their concepts of data are very burdensome to teachers. We need to instill incidental teaching as a way of interaction, . . . seeing what is going on, going with the flow and seeing new skills."

The remainder of this discussion addresses: 1) what these teachers feel are important goals for their students and the procedures that they find effective in achieving them, and 2) the skills that they value and the resources that they need to accomplish their goals.

Goals and Procedures

The teacher's ability to "tune in" to their students is considered to be essential for several reasons. First, a high value is placed on increasing the child's level of awareness and looking for indications that he or she is reacting to environmental input. Next, these teachers search for indications that the student is displaying communicative intent as well as responses that can serve as the basis for developing functional participation. Finally, the participating teachers are deeply concerned with the physical well-being of their students and with picking up on indications that they might be sick, hurt, uncomfortable, or in distress.

Table 1.1 provides a summary of the many procedures, strategies, and techniques described as methods for reaching goals and objectives. Most of these methods are discussed in this section.

Raising the Level of Awareness   All of the participating teachers value their students' change in awareness level. These teachers often search for techniques and procedures that will affect alertness and increase social responsiveness. When they talk about success, these professionals frequently relate it to a change in the alertness or affect of a student.

Table 1.1.   Procedures[a], techniques, and strategies implemented to achieve student goals

Providing systematic sensory stimulation

Providing a high degree of physical contact, including touching, massages, lotion application, holding, rocking, and playful interactions

Providing vestibular stimulation activities (unless contraindicated)

Implementing movement-based techniques derived from van Dijk (1986)

Increasing the effects of responses with materials such as elastic attachments and microswitches

Monitoring the number of staff interactions with students

Implementing feeding procedures that increase nutritional intake

Following positioning, handling, and other therapeutic procedures indicated by the OT and/or PT

Observing subtle responses and conducting movement analyses

Shaping minimal responses into communication and functional participation in activities

Programming for functional sequences

Employing the principle of partial participation

Using age-appropriate materials and activities

Providing changing and varied environments that include community settings

Providing for integrated activities with nondisabled peers

[a]Does not include those procedures specifically related to medical conditions and emergencies.

Each of the participating teachers talked about observing responses such as "eye flutters," "a subtle change in tone," "a subtle change in expression," or anything that suggests that a student is reacting or alerting to some input from the environment. Ultimately, the participating teachers view evidence that shows that the student is aware of his or her environment as an entrance into a world of shared interactions and as the onset of an enhanced quality of life.

When a clear change in alertness and/or affect occurs, most of the participating teachers feel that an important breakthrough has been made. Rhonda explained, "When you get that first smile, it is as exciting as the first one you got from one of your own infants!" Shelly described the first time she took Brian swimming and how he stayed awake all day, ate his entire lunch, and smiled. "He was a completely different kid. His mother offered to pay for the swimming program for the rest of the year if cost ever became an issue."

Ellen pointed out that when students smile and react, people are reinforced for their responses and perceive these students differently. She described a student who was making remarkable progress on gross motor skills ("might even learn to walk"), who still gave no indication that he was aware of anyone or anything around him. To Ellen, increasing this student's level of awareness was more important than reaching criteria on motor programs. Rhonda believes that, "If children can learn to be social, it opens up a whole other world for interactions . . . If children have social skills, they don't see themselves as isolated individuals, they see themselves with other people, with peers, with parents, with other adults." The participating teachers described a number of specific techniques and variables that were primarily related to improving their students' levels or states of awareness and social affect. In general, they addressed procedures related to: 1) increasing stimulation, 2) improving nutrition and health, and 3) introducing stimulating environments.

Increasing Stimulation   Denise indicated that she had found an article on comas that suggested daily systematic full-sensory stimulation that had great relevance to her students. I was thrilled when I read this article; its application to this population is excellent." She now uses many of the techniques and takes data on her students' reactions.

Vestibular stimulation is also viewed as an effective technique by Denise. She indicated that she sees positive changes in tone and increased vocal utterances. Denise believes that if she had known more about these techniques a few years ago she could have helped more students.

Interestingly, Patty indicated that she disliked the term "sensory stimulation" because it implies that children are objects. Patty prefers to think of sensory stimulation as a process of educating students (i.e., providing students with information about their environment).

Because Ellen's students reside in a segregated facility, she is particularly concerned with providing her students with the opportunity of being held and touched. Ellen read an article that noted that death can occur when people do not experience enough human contact. She considers it important to provide these kinds of interactions for her students in the classroom. Ellen also noted that skin breakdowns, which she described as typical for institutionalized children and youth, are not occurring with her students. She attributes this to the holding, touching, massaging, and lotioning that her children receive. Ellen explained that foster grandparents can provide additional opportunities for her students to be handled in this manner.

Patty also commented that she spends a great deal of time holding, rocking, playing, and talking with her students. She believes that they are ignored for a fair portion of their lives and that, therefore, these interactions are essential. Patty also noted that she was alert to and reinforced by any social response that her students might make during these interactions. Rhonda explained that she "played" with her students and that teachers can get a lot out of students by playing with them. She believes that playful interactions are critical to facilitating relaxation and responding.

Improving Nutrition and Health   Denise stated, "When my students eat well, I feel better!" She believes that feeding programs have an important functional value for students and should be given a high priority. Patty wishes she had a video tape of her students before proper feeding procedures were established to denote the increased level of awareness. She talked about John, a former student, who had been placed in the hospital because he had stopped eating, was dehydrated, and experienced kidney failure. His parents had already signed a release for a gastrostomy when she went before his team and asked them to return him to her classroom and to delay the procedure. The team agreed, and she and the paraprofessional staff worked on finding techniques to get him to swallow, as well as increasing his snacks and fluids. John gained 25 pounds during the next several months, and as Patty enthusiastically put it, "the spin off was increased awareness!"

Providing Stimulating Environments   A recurrent theme throughout the participating teachers' interviews was the importance of "places to go" in regard to both quality of life and the increased stimulation that varied environments can offer. Patty likes to take her students to new places (e.g., MacDonalds, the shopping mall) to expose them to different foods, activities, and materials, and to watch their reactions. "It is real reinforcing to see changes!" She believes that one of the most important opportunities that she can provide for her students is the experience of viewing changing, varied, and interesting environments. Patty stated that, "Children who seem to be completely unaware of their environments will surprise you when you get them out of an institution and into interesting and normal settings."

Because the opportunities and settings that are available to these students are limited, the issue of a "place to go" seems to be particularly critical to most of the participating teachers. While the specific settings and conditions seemed to affect how these professionals dealt with this issue, the basic premise remains consistent. The participating teachers value their opportunities to provide their students with a variety of environments, and consider access to stimulating environments an essential component of their students' lives as adults.

While Mary's students' primary classroom is in a building separated from the regular schools, they attend the elementary and high school buildings for a wide range of activities. All of her students receive training in community settings and most receive training in vocational settings. When asked if she thought some of these arrangements and activities would be difficult or impossible for some students, Mary firmly responded, "No, but you sure do see a lot of people who think so! . . . It is more of a challenge, but if we start drawing a line somewhere, it becomes an excuse. No one thought I'd find a job for Janey." Mary enthusiastically reported that access to integrated environments and community-based training provides a curriculum based upon doing something "worthwhile and real" instead of participating in "made-up activities." As Mary states, "Boy, does this make a difference!" She believes that this has not only positively affected her students', but it has also affected the attitude of her parents.

Mary recalled that in a previous classroom, Janey had spent most of her day on a rug in a corner and "did a little bit of van Dijk (1986), some physical therapy, and that was about it." Mary then pointed out that since Janey began going into the community, she had visibly improved. Mary is convinced that something has happened to Janey because of the new and more stimulating environment. "With this student we would go through long dry spells before we got a response, but . . . we are seeing changes."

Denise explained, "It is hard, hard work to go out into the community, but it is worth it." She also expressed dismay about the reality that there was nothing available for students after the age of 21. She firmly believes that her students need places to go during the day, away from their homes or group homes after they leave a school program. While Denise isn't sure how feasible it would be to find jobs for these students, she does believe that they must have different environments and community experiences on a daily basis.

Shelly supports the efforts of her students' parents to organize a post-21-years-of-age program for their children. However, she is doubtful that her students could be involved in work. She noted that, "While a student may only need to have a single response to work, my students don't have even one." She has tried to find ways to take her students into the community despite the fact that their profound disabilities have been used as an excuse for keeping them in the classroom.

Ellen sends her students to the chapel in the institution, invites classes from the school to visit in their unit-based classroom, and would like to move her classroom location away from its living unit location. Both Patty and Ellen take their students into the community for field trips. It was originally difficult to obtain permission from the medical staff to take the students out, but Patty said she was persistent about this matter and eventually convinced staff that it was beneficial. Patty believes that the ultimate goal for her students is to be living and participating in community environments. When asked if she thought that working at a job site would be an appropriate goal for some of her students, she responded that while she wasn't sure if she could find jobs for her students she feels that this could be the goal and that, "We should always try."

Several participating teachers talked about their efforts to increase the stimulation for the students in their classrooms. Concern was expressed with regard to the effects of a deprived social environment that contributed to diminished opportunities for receiving stimulation. These professionals believe that many children and youth with the most profound multiple handicaps are more likely to be ignored because they don't smile, make eye contact, or indicate an awareness that an interaction has been attempted with them.

Denise said, "I'm on the warpath—if I see this [less staff interaction with a certain student] in my room!" In fact, she noted that she had started to take data on the number of interactions that were directed toward specific students so that she could be assured that they would receive as much stimulation as other, more engaging students.

Age-appropriateness is also an issue that arose with regard to increasing stimulation. For example, Ellen feels that using age-appropriate materials and activities with students influences how they are viewed and increases the amount of stimulation that they will receive from others. Ellen believes that there are considerable differences in the responses of classroom staff, parents, support staff, foster grandparents, and unit staff toward her students when their activities, materials, and dress are age-appropriate. All of her students' programs and data sheets are placed in notebooks with designs or pictures on the covers that are typical of the tastes of children and youth of the same age and sex. She found that these notebooks served as a constant reminder to her and the paraprofessional staff that they are working with a young women of 19 years or a 5-year-old boy. She also commented that by giving attention to age-appropriateness, it would provide content about which persons could interact with her students. For example, when 7-year-old Tom began using a computer to develop cause/effect relationships and as a leisure activity, persons began to approach him and talk about his computer, or when the application of makeup became one of 17-year-old Kay's sensory stimulation activities, she began to receive numerous compliments on her appearance.

Establishing Communication and Participation Two closely related goals used by the participating teachers are the establishment of communicative intent and the identification of a single voluntary response that can be used for a wide range of functional responses. Teachers are looking for responses that can serve as the student's way of communicating or indicating needs, preferences, and choices. They are also looking for responses to use as a basis for increasing his or her participation in a wide range of activities. When addressing this topic, they discussed a number of approaches and techniques that are related to: 1) techniques for observing the student in various positions and environments and conducting movement analyses, 2) procedures for increasing the effect of minimal motor responses, 3) movement-based procedures derived from the work of van Dijk (1986), and 4) functional procedures and practice. While increasing awareness is viewed as an essential for quality of life and the future progress of a student, the development of a response or responses is viewed as the key to active and functional participation in the environment.

Utilizing a Response Analysis   Patty indicated that it is important to observe a student in a variety of positions in order to identify a potential movement that can be used to build functional responses. Rhonda also talked about conducting movement analyses and suggests that if you can't find a movement to use, "You shape one." She believes that these students are just like everyone in their responses to success. According to Rhonda, "If you can just find one thing that they can do with one response, you are off to a positive start and other responses are more likely to appear."

Ellen explained that she looks for the highest frequency motor response and the highest frequency sound and tries to determine ways in which to build responses. She described a 5-year-old student whom she "caught running her fingers up and down her gastro tube holder. I got a toy holder and put a doll with a bell around her neck and called her Tinker Bell." After a year of frequent absences due to a series of illnesses, she had a "health breakthrough." During a single week, this student reached the goal of touching her toys. By learning to touch her toys, she then used the same response to reach and touch a panel that activated a tape of music that the staff could tell she liked. According to Ellen, "When I first met this student, I would have said she was not aware of her environment at all; however, I now consider her to be like someone who is trapped in her body."

Increasing Response Effectiveness   Patty believes that one of the most effective techniques that she has ever learned involves attaching elastic to a student's wrist or leg. The elastic is then attached to an object (i.e., toy holder, bar, ceiling). Very minimal movements gain significant effects. With this, the rates of Patty's students' movement have increased rapidly.

Several of the participating teachers discussed having their students use microswitches to activate devices that could provide a variety of effects and allow them to participate in a wide range of activities. While most of these professionals believe that adaptive devices and technology are important to these students, several have indicated that this strategy can be difficult to implement.

Shelly explained that her students don't have enough voluntary movement to activate most switches. Furthermore, they have not seemed very interested in the effects. Patty has found that establishing the use of a switch can take a "very, very long time." What appeared to be an effective, easy device for the student to activate on one day seems to lose its value the next day. Therefore, students have to be given many opportunities to use switches with various devices.

Providing Movement-Based Training Several participating teachers described the application of the van Dijk (1986) techniques when providing movement-based training. While Rhonda found that resonance procedures had been useful in normalizing tone for two of her students, she didn't believe a communication response was established. Mary noted that the van Dijk (1986) procedures were used to teach one of her students to tap to signal that she was ready, and that she now taps when she is ready to work at her community job site.

Making Responses Functional All of the participating teachers stressed the importance of building responses that would result in functional activities and believed that teaching these procedures should be based upon functional sequences and materials. Mary is convinced that since she implemented a community training program, all of her students have improved.

One of Mary's new students, 6-year-old Marge, recently transferred from a sensory integration classroom for students with profound disabilities. Mary explained that Marge was showing progress on a communication board program with her, but not with the speech therapist. The speech therapist used massed trials and materials that were not functional or meaningful to Marge. Mary gave the therapist some of Marge's toys to use for the program, but there was still no progress. Mary noted that when Marge used the communication board to request a toy, the therapist took it away to present the next trial. This resulted in Marge's crying.

Ellen emphasized that students with the most profound disabilities need more intensive instruction on a single objective. In other words, many opportunities to practice responses must be provided for students. She indicated that placing the responses into a functional sequence was very important. Denise agreed with this perspective and indicated that massed trial training was generally very inappropriate.

Ultimately, the development of a response means that needs can be communicated, and the student can partially participate in important environments. For example, Rhonda believes that for these students, a starting point is to teach them at least one voluntary movement that could be used to perform a functional task. Functional tasks might consist of changing their own body position, depressing a button, motioning to have someone help them, or using eye gaze or a pointing response in a nonoral system of communication. Similarly, Mary observed:

> It is important for students who experience the most profound multiple handicaps to participate in something, at least participate, so that they can be a part of their family. We can do quite a bit with one movement. They can partially participate in

quite a bit. It is important to try to find a response that makes the most of what they have.

Ellen indicated, "You are not taking these students toward independence. They are not going to be independent in any skill." She believes that by finding ways to increase awareness and social skills and by shaping functional responses that can be generalized to participation in important multiple environments, teachers are becoming involved in a type of programming that will allow students to affect their quality of life.

Incorporating Physical Well-Being Finally, participating teachers believe that they must be tuned in to the physical state of their students. This focus is directly related to medical conditions and the serious nature of the physical handicaps experienced by students with profound disabilities. These professionals described the importance of attending to cues that might indicate that the student is uncomfortable, ill, injured, or in distress. While attention to these cues can make a significant difference in the student's quality of life, it can also mean the difference between his or her life and death.

Considerable evidence of the sensitivity of these professionals toward their students' physical well-being was offered. For example, at the onset of an interview, Ellen mentioned that Kay, one of Ellen's students, didn't seem to be feeling well, so the activities planned for Kay that morning had been altered. Ellen noted that Kay's menstrual period began and she had diarrhea shortly after their decision to alter her schedule of activities.

Shelly stated that she was able to recognize a pattern that led up to a seizure in her students and could frequently break that pattern and prevent the seizure. She recalled notifying a student's mother about an unusual sound that the student made when he was placed in a sidelier. This student's mother took him to the doctor who discovered that the student had a fractured calcium deposit. Shelly also related an incident in which visitors were observing her as she was working with a student who stopped breathing. Shelly physically manipulated the student until her breathing started again. However, throughout the incident, the observers were never aware that the student had stopped breathing.

Ellen feels that it is critical for teachers to always maintain a constant awareness or alertness to the possibility that a student may be in distress. For example, Ellen always attended to Peter's breathing in order to determine if suctioning was required. She is also very attentive to indications that her students may be either vomiting or choking. Denise mentioned that she recently had to use the Heimlich maneuver on a student when he began to choke. The suctioning equipment in Denise's classroom is checked daily to assure that it is working and ready to use in the case of an emergency. Denise is also alert to her student's other conditions that may lead to constipation, irregular bowel movements, and possible bowel impactions. She also pointed out that if the child is handled or positioned incorrectly, a fracture or painful dislocation could occur.

Positioning skills for the staff are given high priority, and specific precautions and appropriate procedures for each student are stressed.

During Rhonda's interview, she indicated that it is important to monitor seizures carefully. She is concerned that teachers might learn to treat them casually, "because [they] are so used to children seizuring without drastic consequence." Patty is always aware of the temperatures of her students with hypothermic conditions, and is ready to alert the nurse if one of the student's temperature falls below 96 degrees.

In conclusion, the participating teachers view tuning in to their students health and physical needs as an essential part of their work. This involves attention to subtle cues, an awareness of the potential risks associated with various conditions, and a readiness to act if emergencies should arise.

Skills and Information

The point was made in the initial part of this section that teachers of students with the most profound disabilities employ a clinical style and an eclectic approach in their work. This discussion suggested that a heavy or exclusive reliance on applied behavior analysis as a basis for theory and practice is not a characteristic of participating teachers. Evidence of a clinical style and eclectic approach was related to the goals and procedures that they described as important for their students. It is also apparent when they: 1) described the professional skills that facilitated their "tuning in to" students, 2) identified the important support professionals, and 3) suggested the areas in which they need more training and information.

Describing Appropriate Professional Attributes While a wide range of procedures are considered to be essential to working effectively with these students, several basic beliefs about the attributes and skills that allow teachers to use effective procedures emerged from the interviews. First, the participating teachers viewed themselves as hands-on teachers; next, as effective coordinators of information; and finally, as hard working and accountable.

Hands-On Teachers Participating teachers frequently described themselves as hands-on teachers. Their need to have hands-on contact with their students directly relates to the value that these professionals placed on observing and "tuning in to" their students. Rhonda stated, "I wouldn't want someone who preferred to do paper work teaching these kids." Patty explained that she makes decisions and interprets data from the information she gets from her hands-on interactions with her students. Shelly believes that it may be possible to read the child's written program and to look at his or her graph to make program decisions for students who function at higher levels. However, she also feels that it is essential to have hands-on time with her students in order to understand how they are progressing and to provide direction to staff. While Shelly sees the teacher as a coordinator of input and information from a variety of professionals, hands-on contact with her students allows her to use this input effectively.

Rhonda, who teaches preschool students, said, "You have to feel these kids! The more contact, the more information. . . . I have a hard time working with them, unless I'm on the floor."

Effective Coordinators of Information   The participating teachers believe that a wide range of professionals have important information and relevant skills. While these instructors place considerable value on input from other professionals, they believe that it takes a teacher to effectively coordinate the information. They talk about "siphoning information from professionals" and "putting it all together." Ellen explained that, "Ninety percent is watching and constantly assessing and pulling the pieces together, pulling the equipment together, pulling the right people together in order to move forward."

The participating teachers believe that in order to be an effective coordinator, a teacher must have good communication skills and be able to work with a team. They also view the teacher's role in this process as essential and not replaceable by other professionals. Because students with the most profound multiply handicapping conditions frequently need input and techniques from a wider range of disciplines, Patty emphasized that working with these students takes "more training and more knowledge than for any other group of students."

Denise indicated that while professionals from each discipline understand the implications of their particular field for the student, they frequently fail to value the importance of other areas and typically do not understand the importance of integrating techniques and procedures into a meaningful program for a student. She considers a skillful teacher to be one who sees the whole student, is aware of the need for a balanced and functional program, and understands the value of other disciplines.

Hard-Working and Accountable Professionals   It should be noted that all of the participating teachers believed that the data-based measurement of their students' behavior was important. Interestingly, one of the most frequent comments made was that data provided the accountability that instructional programs and procedures were, in fact, being conducted. Several of the participating teachers indicated it would be easier to do very little with students who experience profound disabilities and "to get by with it."

Five of the six participating teachers believed probe data are desirable. Typically, this was related to both the instructor's need to have hands-on interactions with students that allow the teacher to tune in to students responses and to the students' needs for more intensive programming on fewer objectives. With programming on fewer objectives, a representative sample of the students' performance on specific objectives was viewed as acceptable.

Identifying Important Support Professionals   Participating teachers placed a great deal of importance on the skills and knowledge of support staff. They were also very clear about information and skills that they felt were important for teachers of students with profound handicaps to acquire. In many cases, the participating teachers sought this information, developed these skills, and arranged for interactions with support professionals on their own initiative. For example, Shelly called a local hospital and asked if a respiratory therapist would come to her classroom and demonstrate postural drainage procedures. Rhonda arranged numerous in-service meetings by contacting staff from a medical center.

Table 1.2 displays the specific disciplines identified by the participating teachers. It provides evidence of the wide range of disciplines that are perceived as important resources for students with profound disabilities. Table 1.2 indicates the emphasis that is placed on medical procedures and information, as well as the importance of input from a range of health-related professionals. Even so, several of the participating teachers indicated that the development of cooperative team roles with medical professionals, such as nurses, presented new challenges. These teachers described experiences that suggested that their comments, observations, and opinions that related to the health and physical states of their students were perceived to be out of the purview of teachers by some medical professionals.

Ellen, who works in an institutional setting, noted that, "We [teachers in the severely multiply handicapped area] have been trained in role releasing and don't see clear professional boundaries with disciplines like OT and PT, but there is a definite boundary when it comes to nurses and doctors." She talked about how carefully she phrased statements to medical staff so that she could advocate for students without alienating doctors or nurses with whom she works. Ellen also noted that teachers in her setting appeared to become concerned about a student's condition more quickly than the nurses. According to Ellen, this could be, in part, because nurses were more familiar with the medical problems encountered by the student and "we [teachers] don't know what is life threatening."

The participating teachers who work in community settings stated that they encountered difficulties in establishing relationships and communicating with medical personnel. One teacher in a community setting described an expe-

Table 1.2.   Disciplines perceived as critical for team input via direct service and/or consultation

Occupational therapy	Ophthalmology
Physical therapy	Audiology
Neurology	Dietary/nutrition
Respiratory therapy	Nursing
Orthopedics	Rehabilitation engineering
Pharmacology	Communication
Social work	Computer science

rience with a physician who felt that schooling was not appropriate for a student. Most participating teachers who work in community settings said that they did not have direct contact with their students' physicians. Furthermore, one of the teachers indicated that it was difficult to integrate the school nurse into the classroom routine, even though she spent a considerable amount of time in the classroom.

There was some indication that when nurses had established roles in educational settings or on teams concerned with educational planning, cooperative and productive relationships were successfully formed. It is noteworthy to mention that the role of a nurse in Rhonda's school had been established for a period of years. Rhonda described the school nurse as invaluable, able to engage in role release, and very willing to share information and skills. Denise, whose students attend a demonstration classroom in a university facility also placed a great deal of value on the input from the team nurse who has been a member of a special education diagnostic unit for a number of years.

The participating teachers placed very high value on the skills of the occupational and physical therapists. They valued the presence of an occupational and/or physical therapist in the classroom as well as the information and procedures that these disciplines offer. It is interesting to note that teachers placed such great value on these disciplines that can offer them better techniques for executing hands-on procedures with students and for facilitating or developing response repertoires.

Despite the fact that the development of communicative intent and communication systems are perceived as critical for their students, several of the participating teachers had experiences with speech therapists that caused them to view this discipline less positively. In fact, most spoke somewhat wistfully about the need for a speech therapist who had skills that related to their students' needs or an interest in developing such skills.

Important Components of Teacher Training Programs

Table 1.3 lists the content areas and training experiences that the participating teachers felt were inadequate or lacking in their teacher training programs. It also lists those areas and experiences that they believe should be important components of such programs that prepare personnel to teach students with profound disabilities. Several conclusions can be drawn from an inspection of the training areas. First, programs in which these teachers were trained obviously did not adequately address the content that they perceived was needed. Additionally, the disciplines viewed as important and displayed in Table 1.2 directly relate to the training content identified in Table 1.3. Finally, the participating teachers' belief that practicum experiences with these students are essential corresponds to their emphasis on hands-on interactions with those students, as well as to their belief that a number of procedures and techniques can only be learned in a practicum setting.

Table 1.3. Content needing inclusion or increased emphasis in teacher training programs

Informational Content

Child development across all domains

Legal/liability issues and insurance

Current assessment instruments of relevance to this population

Specialized assessment and programming for vision and hearing impairments

Nutrition and implications for planning appropriate diets for this group of students

Medications and their side effects

Specific medical, neurological, and physical conditions predominant in this group

Communicative intent and presymbolic communication

Alternative systems of communication

Preparation for experiencing death and dying

Strategies for effective advocacy

Strategies for working effectively with families

Strategies for working with paraprofessional staff

Strategies for working with personnel in other disciplines

Increased knowledge about the functions of medical and health-related disciplines

Demonstration and/or Skill Training (conducted by qualified personnel)

Practica with students who experience the most profound disabilities

Using microcomputers and adaptive peripherals and assistive devices

Facilitating and shaping communication

Conducting ecological assessments

Positioning, handling, and other therapeutic techniques used by OTs and PTs

Procedures and equipment used in relationship to conditions of concern (e.g., shunts, seizures, constipation and bowel impaction, catheterization, hypothermia, sleep disorders, chronic respiratory disorders and distress, esophageal reflux, aspiration, apnea, allergies, immune system disorders, eating disorders, nasogastric and gastrostomy tube feedings) and first aid and emergency procedures

SEPARATE IS NOT EQUAL

Teachers of students who experience the most profound disabilities are frequently confronted with policy issues and attitudes that directly affect the nature of services afforded their students. These issues can be divided into: 1) policies related to medical conditions and procedures, 2) policies related to homogeneous class grouping, and 3) policies related to integration.

Policies Related to Medical Conditions and Procedures

Policy issues related to medical conditions and procedures typically address which criteria are used to define medically fragile individuals, and who should conduct medical procedures that are required for some students. The participating teachers do not believe that medical conditions should be used as an excuse to deny students who experience profound disabilities the access to services and less restrictive environments. They indicated that they would be willing to conduct routine medical procedures that parents usually conduct in an effort to keep these students in their classrooms. Furthermore, they tend to believe that the ability of a student to tolerate and enjoy classroom experiences is a more important criteria for placement than is a particular condition or need for routine medical procedures.

Ellen talked about a student with severe spasticity who was automatically placed in her class because he had a gastrostomy and tracheostomy, and required frequent suctioning. She advocated for this student to be moved from her class to a classroom in the school facility because he did not have frequent illnesses and had no problems tolerating a 6-hour day. Rhonda explained, "Ten years ago I would have described medically fragile or complicated students differently." "Experience" had altered her view about what constitutes "medically fragile." "Many students who seem very fragile keep bouncing back even after surgery and repeated illness, and many have less problems than you would expect." While professionals from other disciplines taught Rhonda to conduct the procedures that they require, she believes that " . . . the kids have taught me to be comfortable with them, . . . I don't like to see people back off from these kids because they are 'medically fragile.' They [students with medical conditions] need to be handled and played with."

The participating teachers who currently conduct medical procedures talked about their initial fears of providing such services. They also described their anxieties about working with children who required procedures that they had never conducted before. These concerns generally disappeared after the teacher experienced the student and his or her condition. As several of the participating teachers stated, "Experience makes things less scary."

Rhonda described a preschool-age student she had worked with in a private agency. The student had a tracheostomy, a gastrostomy, as well as constant athetoid movements, hearing aids, and visual problems. She required suctioning, and her mother also used a bulb that would force air into her trachea. The student's mother reported that her daughter frequently stopped breathing; therefore the mother never left her side. During the first few days that the child was in Rhonda's class, Rhonda said that she would not move her 3 feet without also moving the suctioning equipment. "I carried the child and my paraprofessional carried the machine whenever we moved her. After about a week, we were moving her freely around the room, and playing with her comfortably." Rhonda recalled that in the 3 years that the little girl was in the program, she had never stopped breathing, but, "We always watched her carefully and kept the bulb nearby." Rhonda also believes that a number of school districts would reject this student on initial contact and put her on a homebound program, "which would be very unfortunate since she profited from being in school. . . . This child loved being there, and was very social."

When asked about specific procedures they are or would be willing to conduct, the participating teachers typically identified giving oral medications, conducting gastrostomy tube feedings, suctioning, and implementing procedures involved with catheterization and colostomy care. They indicated that students who require oxygen should be able to attend school, and tended to express the most concern about inserting nasal tubes because of the risks involved with incorrectly inserting them.

While participating teachers do not devalue the role of the nurse, they perceive routine procedures that parents learn to conduct as feasible for them to administer. All of the teachers indicated that these procedures should be conducted only after training and continued monitoring by the appropriate personnel. Shelly observed that she wasn't sure where school districts, particularly in rural areas, could locate nurses to conduct all of the procedures needed by these students on a daily and routine basis.

Policies Related to Homogeneous Class Grouping

A second policy issue area is related to the practice of creating classrooms that homogeneously group students with the most profound disabilities. These classrooms have a variety of names such as the sensory integration classroom, educational fundamental classroom, therapeutic intervention classroom, and therapeutic classroom.

Lack of clear criteria for placement into these classes is evident. While health-related disorders and medical restrictions are implied by some of the classroom names, the level of cognitive functioning is implied by others. These classes frequently contain students who are remarkably similar. Mary indicated that she was not aware of any specific criteria for placement into her classroom, and while her classroom was called "therapeutic," her students are not medically fragile. However, her students are very profoundly disabled. Interestingly, both of the participating teachers who work in segregated settings noted that attention to medical criteria was becoming a much clearer factor in placement than it had been in the past.

The participating teachers generally favor heterogeneous placement, while recognizing potential problems with this arrangement. Evidence was offered that when a group within a group is created, a rationale for treating them differently is also created. For example, the presence of medical problems has forced some students to remain in the school or facility. Similarly, intellectual levels have been used as the basis for deciding whether the students would or would not benefit from a particular experience that is available to other students identified as severely multiply handicapped.

Teachers of homogeneously grouped students with profound disabilities seem to work harder to justify and get basic services for their students. For example, two participating teachers who work in the residential facility viewed movement toward a 6-hour school day and having an actual classroom apart from the living unit day room as significant accomplishments. Another participating teacher described the care she took to justify activities for her students as an effort to avoid potential restrictions for them.

All of the participating teachers acknowledged their students' need to be around other individuals who could offer important stimulation, and to participate in the activities and experiences generally available in most classrooms. Ellen, who teaches in a living unit area of an institution, added, "That's why I work so hard to get students out of my class." Denise, who has worked in both integrated and segregated settings, said, "I would love to have a range of kids from profoundly disabled to genius level." Rhonda commented, "I don't like to think of our programs as medical programs. It's fun to have a mixture of kids."

In addition to the benefits that a heterogeneous grouping offered to students, several of the participating teachers saw such groupings as important to teachers also. One of the participating teachers suggested that homogeneous grouping could be related to teacher burnout, while another admitted that she missed working with students who function at higher levels.

Contrarily, Patty expressed concern for the safety of her students in a typical SMH or regular education classrooms. Patty indicated that the teacher would need to be very aware of her students' physical and medical needs. Shelly, who teaches in a homogeneous classroom for students with profound handicaps in a regular education building, said that the parents of her students favored this grouping because they were afraid that their children would not receive enough attention in the other SMH's. Shelly believes that there is a reality-basis for their concerns and indicated that she has seen students like hers being ignored in some classrooms. She indicated that it is easy to put the students with the most profound disabilities into an area in the classrooms and then to forget about them while attending to the more active students. In order to keep this from happening, Shelly believes that it would be important to keep the student/teacher ratio low.

Another aspect of homogeneously grouping students with the most profound disabilities emerged from the comments of the three participating teachers who had classrooms that were grouped in this manner. These three professionals commented that the stress level typically associated with students who are active and have behavior problems was very low in their homogeneously grouped classrooms. Shelly noted that these students don't have behavior problems. Consequently, the staff do not feel the effects of stress that are often associated with teaching students with challenging behaviors.

Interestingly, the participating teachers in both community and segregated facilities who received administrative support felt that they had more opportunities to address and change the policy issues that restricted their students. For example, the only participating teacher who was extensively involved in community training commented several times that she had a completely supportive administration. Additionally, the participating teachers who worked in segregated state facilities, whose students experienced the most medically complicated conditions, were able to schedule trips into the community more easily and frequently than the participating teacher who worked in an integrated public school. These professionals who worked in the segregated facilities also described how they affected the policy decisions that related to the treatment and placement of their students by "going before the team"; whereas another participating teacher described a series of strategies that are used to work around the administration, and having to give up on ideas that might have created "waves" that work against her students.

Policies Related to Integration

The third policy issue is related to the availability of integration opportunities. Discussions that addressed integration tended to center around its benefits and overcoming its barriers. Descriptions of the benefits of integration applied to students with severe and profound disabilities, as well as to the regular educational staff, the parents of the nonhandicapped students, and the students in the regular educational classrooms.

Shelly views the presence of her class in the elementary school as an extremely positive situation. She reported that her classroom and students are accepted as part of the program. Students in the regular education classrooms compete for opportunities to come to her room and to take her students to the playground. Shelly also indicated that she has seen a number of touching interactions. For example, Shelly recalled that a nondisabled student who was pushing one of her students around the playground in his wheelchair periodically stopped and wiped saliva from her student's chin. Shelly commented, "No one ever said that his job was to wipe drool, but these students just do those kinds of things." She also noted that even though her students do not talk or indicate that they are aware of any type of communication, the regular education students make her students' time on the playground a very social event by pushing their wheelchairs to different areas of the playground and by periodically stopping and talking to them.

Shelly explained that, "These students [regular education students] accept my students the way they are." She believes they have helped their parents to react the same way. For example, on Parents' Night, the regular education students introduce their parents to Shelly's students by name in the same manner as they introduce their nondisabled friends. Consequently, the parents of students in the regular classrooms at Shelly's school have volunteered their time in Shelly's classroom and contributed in a number of ways, including donating a pet rabbit for her students' observation.

When Denise, a preschool teacher, talked about the benefits of visits from preschool students who were mildly handicapped and at-risk, she emphasized the positive effect that these visits had on both staff and students. "Our kids really notice children who move around, and we need this too, to realize that these children can get into stuff and we should encourage this." She discussed how interesting it was to watch the students interact with her students and described how a small 3-year-old girl from the visiting class liked to help one of her students with profound disabilities by moving her head while saying, "I teach."

The participating teachers revealed that they sometimes experience resistance to integration from their students' parents. While Mary believes that integration into age-appropriate school environments and community-training programs is critical to students with profound disabilities, she also related how the parents of Patty, a student with profound disabilities, initially displayed considerable resistance. After several years of persistent efforts to integrate Patty, her parents' attitude gradually changed. "When I got permission for her involvement at a job site, her [Patty's] mother said, 'I'd be interested in seeing what you can find that she can do.' When I did find something, her Mother said, 'Go for it!' " It is noteworthy to point out that Mary believes that rural communities may present less barriers for integration and community-training because it is easier to approach people you know and who know your students and their families.

The results of this inquiry indicate that one of the most significant barriers to integration is created by segregated facilities and that classrooms in integrated settings, whether homogeneously or heterogeneously grouped, offer considerable opportunity for participation in activities with nonhandicapped peers. While all of the participating teachers valued integration, only the ones who teach in community settings were able to provide examples of consistent and routine interactions between their students and nonhandicapped peers.

Despite the participating teachers' acknowledgment of the undesirable aspects of a segregated residential facility, both Patty and Ellen perceive their roles as valuable and view themselves as internal advocates for a population that has, until recently, been ignored by educators. When asked what would make her teaching situation ideal for her students, Patty answered without hesitation, "Being out of the institution." When asked if she really believed that they would know the difference, she again answered, without hesitation, "They would know the difference." To Patty, an ideal environment for her students would be a loving home with significant others in their lives and the availability of varied, stimulating environments.

Shelly, who once worked in an institutional setting, is not as sure that her students would "know" the difference, but she is sure they are better off living at home and attending school in the community. She is certain that if her students lived in an institution they would experience more distress with regard to basic comfort, care, and acknowledgment of preference. Shelly also stated that she is not sure if one of her students would still be alive if it weren't for his parents' nurturing and care.

In summary, all of the participating teachers saw important benefits to integrated environments for their students. The degree to which they could specifically offer those benefits to their students depended, to the greatest extent, upon where their class was located.

PARENTS AS PARTNERS AND FRIENDS

All six of the participating teachers spent a considerable amount of time talking about the parents of their students. In general, they addressed the importance of exchanging information with parents and the needs for support and assistance that parents experience. The teachers' comments suggested the empathy that they have for the parents of their students when encountering a wide range of difficult decisions and situations. These professionals provided evidence of the teacher/parent relationships that can evolve from a set of common concerns and shared experiences.

Parents are Part of the Team

The participating teachers placed a high value on the information that parents can offer about their children, both through informal interactions and in the development of the IEP. As Denise stated, "There are a lot of professionals who won't ask parents to help or to show them things about their child and this is very sad. . . . " Denise believes that it is important to routinely ask parents to visit with her and to share information.

All of the participating teachers described examples of how parents had provided key information about handling, interacting, stimulating, or reinforcing their child. For example, Valerie, one of Shelly's students, was fed only by the school nurse. Valerie rarely ate all of her meal, frequently choked and gagged, and generally took about 1½ hours to eat. In an effort to improve meal-time procedures for Valerie, Shelly asked Valerie's mother to come to school and show her how she fed Valerie. This demonstration helped Shelly identify effective techniques for feeding her student, and discriminate when she was actually in distress. A large part of the choking and gagging was eliminated by using the mother's technique of telling Valerie to, "Stop that." Shelly now feels confident about feeding her student, and believes that she does a better job than the nurse, in part, because she "took her cues from the mother."

All six of the participating teachers described strategies that enhanced communication and sharing with parents and indicated their intent to be accountable to parents. For example, several of the teachers sent information home to their students' parents on a daily basis and asked the parents to do the same. Denise provides information about fluid intake, solid intake, urinary output, bowel movements, the amount of time the student slept, and seizures. In addition, Denise also lists the individual programs and activities that were conducted and talks about the student's activities of the day. She also includes space on this form for the parent to send information back to her. While Denise gets about a 50% return rate, most of her parents say that they like getting the daily form. Daily contact with parents is less feasible for the teachers in the institutional setting. Both write monthly letters and have occasional telephone contacts with parents and, in several cases, very close relationships have been formed among the teachers and their students' parents.

The IEP represents the primary vehicle for formalizing program direction and identifying student goals and objectives with the child's parents. Participating teachers generally reported positive experiences with their students' parents when developing an IEP; however, several indicated that their students' parents view them as being better able to make appropriate programming decisions and understand their children's wants and needs. Patty described an IEP conference in the institutional setting as being an overwhelming experience due to the number of professionals in attendance and their frequent use of medical terminology. She believes that the nature of these conferences inhibits parent input and involvement.

When parents and teachers agree on IEP goals and objectives, as well as the methods of achieving those goals, parents are likely to perceive teachers as allies. For example, Shelly believes that her students' parents "know their child better than anyone else" and described them as "wonderful." She is extremely impressed with their efforts to find ways to ensure that their children are really treated as a member of the family. When asked to account for the obviously strong and positive nature of her relationship with the parents of her students, Shelly responded, "I ask them, 'What do you want for your child?,' and I mean it. I then work on what they want." Parents see Shelly as their ally in keeping their child in an integrated school setting and appreciate her help in developing a post-21-year-old community program. The parents of Shelly's students repeatedly ask if she will be coming back next year. They constitute Shelly's biggest source of reinforcement. In fact, Shelly had seriously considered transferring to another classroom, but felt that she would be letting the parents of her students down by leaving.

Parents and teachers do not always see eye-to-eye, though. Two participating teachers described interactions with their students' parents that involved differing points of view. Based upon these examples, it appeared that when these parents and teachers did not agree, parents perceived the teachers as adversaries, whereas the teachers tended to interpret parents' behavior as being "overprotective" or "unrealistic." For example, the parents of one of Mary's students originally viewed an attempt to integrate their child into the community and regular school settings as an inappropriate and insensitive act. In this case, the parents' "overprotective" behavior was attributed by Mary to early experiences with medical professionals who had suggested that it was inappropriate for the student to attend school.

Denise indicated that she was concerned about finding the correct way to respond to parents of very young children who have goals that are very discrepant with their child's level of functioning. For example, she discussed one of her students named Billy whose parents had recently asked her how soon it would be before their 4-year-old son would learn to walk and if she would teach him to read Braille. She described Billy as a child with profound disabilities who seizured frequently, had no voluntary movement, and showed very little awareness of his environment. While Denise acknowledged that she was aware of the negative effect of labeling and self-fulfilling prophecies, she believes these questions were clear indications that Billy's parents were not being realistic.

Emotionally Supporting the Parents of Students with Profound Disabilities

According to Rhonda, "Some parents have lived through a lot of fads in programming and are very wise. . . . We all need to have more respect for parents and their needs." The participating teachers view the needs of parents with children who are profoundly disabled as being very important and feel that they have a significant responsibility to acknowledge those needs.

Two of the six participating teachers have access to social workers, and both indicated how valuable such services can be to the parents of children with profound disabilities. They described how effective these professionals had been at finding respite care, locating resources, providing contacts with agencies, and identifying or organizing parent support groups. Interestingly, a distinction was made between social workers who view their role primarily as counselors for parents, and those who are involved in providing parents with critical assistance in obtaining resources.

When a professional social worker is not available, teachers generally perform some of their services, along with their own responsibilities. Shelly commented, "You are the biggest resource these parents have, and they often treat you as their primary resource." She indicated that parents need help locating resources, obtaining financial assistance, and interpreting information from a wide range of professionals. Several years ago, Mary organized and is still responsible for a parent support group that meets on a monthly basis. Patty emphasized, "Parents need to know that a teacher is concerned with more than just what the child does between 8:00 A.M. and 3:00 P.M., and really cares about what happens to the child outside of school." She tells parents that they can call on her at anytime if they have a question or problem. Rhonda also stressed that "sometimes parents just need somebody to listen to them."

The participating teachers also provided insight into the concerns and goals of parents with children who experience the most profound multiple handicaps. Several of the teachers indicated that the parents are most concerned about the role that schooling can play in affecting their child's physical well-being and quality of life. For example, Shelly said that the parents of her students are very interested in programs and procedures that facilitate the physical management of their children so that they can continue to take care of them at home.

Patty explained that many of the parents with whom she has frequent contact are faced with decisions about such things as granting permission for surgery involving significant risks to their child. While these parents are interested in their child's educational program, they are generally more concerned about the medical decisions that they must make and about their child's overall well-being and quality of life in an institutional setting.

When the participating teachers spoke of specific experiences with parents, the intense nature of the supportive interactions that they sometimes have with parents became apparent. Denise talked about providing respite care on the weekends for a child with profound disabilities who seizured constantly and required numerous medical procedures. She described the mother's exhaustion and frustration with the lack of available support services. Denise also related that the mother had discussed her feelings about whether her child would be better off dead than living as she does.

Patty talked about the death of one of her students. The 5-year-old girl was sent to a hospital for surgery soon after being admitted into the institution. The surgery appeared to be successful, however, 2 days later she had cardiac arrest. Patty spent that day and night at the hospital with the child's mother who was informed that her baby was brain dead and that her permission was needed to turn off the life support system. Patty stays in contact with and still sees this mother occasionally. She also related how she had personally arranged for a parent with limited access to transportation to periodically visit her child and spend the day in the classroom. Patty has also driven her students to their homes for weekends when her travel plans took her in a nearby vicinity.

Mary spoke of a long-term relationship she had maintained with the parent of a student who had died, and of the need to continue to be there for parents who have lost their children. She noted that she always invited this mother to the parent group and that this parent continued attending long after her child's death.

While the participating teachers indicated feeling a significant responsibility to respond to the needs of their students' parents, the importance of being nonjudgmental about the decisions that the parents make was consistently stressed. Rhonda believes that many parents feel horrendous guilt because 10 years ago professionals told parents that if they advocated and worked hard enough, their child's functioning level would be significantly improved. She also believes that in the past, professionals lacked sensitivity to the personal needs of parents, frequently failed to take into account the unique nature of each family's situation, and did not consider the problems imposed by limited availability of resources. However, she believes that this is not as true of today's professionals.

All of the participating teachers believed that the parents ultimately make the decision to place their child in an institution when they find that they lack resources and support to continue on their own. They frequently see no other alternatives. Ellen indicated that many of the parents of children with the most profound multiple handicaps place their child in an institution "because, medically, they can't handle it anymore."

IS THIS VALUED WORK?

When asked to identify essential characteristics of those teachers who instruct students with profound disabilities, the participating teachers mentioned attributes such as: hardworking, possessing a sense of humor, organized, flexible, persistent, resourceful, not squeamish about personal care procedures, and trustworthy in a loose supervisory situation. These six teachers also believe that it is essential to be willing to do the same thing over and over again, to be reinforced by small gains, and to be capable of handling setbacks when students get sick and loose ground.

All of the participating teachers were willing to openly share their feelings and to express both the negative and positive aspects of their roles and experiences. While all of these professionals found certain aspects of their role to be unclear or difficult, they did not report the same concerns on a consistent basis. For example, Rhonda feels that there is some confusion about the term "coma" and what environments are most appropriate for children in comas. While she believes that programming and treatment are very important, there is a question in her mind as to whether or not the SMH classroom is an appropriate environment for children who are "truly comatose."

Shelly indicated that while she felt that she was needed, her students' lack of responsiveness made that a more intellectual than emotional response. Shelly's primary source of reinforcement for her efforts came from the parents of her students. She also admitted to feeling frustration about what kind of programs to focus on for her students. Making a shift from students who functioned at higher levels to ones with profound multiple handicaps was and continues to be difficult for Shelly. Interestingly, several of the participating teachers hesitated when asked to relate a success story about a student who experienced the most profound multiply handicapping conditions until they were assured that the success didn't need to involve reaching criterion on a program objective that resulted in an independent skill.

Denise indicated that there were just a lot of things she didn't know. For example, she needed information on the sleep patterns of her students and was concerned about the amount of time some of her students sleep. She was unsure about whether or not she should attempt to wake them up or keep them awake. Denise is also concerned about children who require food and medication and won't stay awake long enough to get anything down, as well as students who have just been given medication and then vomit. She spent a considerable amount of time expressing concern about the judgments that she must make and her need for more information.

Ellen talked about feeling isolated and needing someone to interact with concerning what she was doing in the classroom with her students. "I sometimes feel like I'm begging them [other staff at the institution and professionals in the field] to come and see what we are doing. Most people have no concept of what I do." She indicated that there are still some teachers in the severely multiply handicapped area who can't imagine doing what she is doing now. Ellen wishes that she had more opportunities to discuss her students with others and to "brainstorm" about techniques and ideas.

When prompted to discuss whether they experienced concerns about their students' quality of life, the participating teachers described the distress that they felt for students who constantly appeared to be suffering. The effects of those experiences were visibly apparent when these professionals spoke. They talked about the difficulty of being around and working with a child who is in pain, who cries constantly, or appears to be extremely upset when handled and touched. Patty admitted to always being afraid that she was torturing them. Denise also reported feelings of anger at seeing a child suffer.

These teachers experience a great loss whenever one of their students dies. Ellen talked about organizing a memorial service for one of her students to help herself and her staff deal with the death. Denise described the adverse effects that the presence of a child who was visibly dying had on the day-to-day functioning of her staff. Rhonda talked about the calls that she had received from parents to tell her that their child had died. Patty commented that the death of a child was something that she was not prepared to deal with and stated that it "never gets easier."

Despite the difficult realities of their work, when the participating teachers talked about their roles and their students, primarily positive factors emerged. While all of the teachers noted that they did, in fact, see positive differences in their students, several of them stressed that they may be preventing further complications and regression. Denise explained:

> Some of these children appear to not have made significant changes, however, they are not regressing. It is a terrible thing to see regression. You will see malnutrition, sleeping disorders, bedsores, and increased self-stimulation, if you don't work with these children.

Several of the participating teachers indicated that they liked the "challenge" of their work. Three of them spoke at length about all of the new information related to technology and medicine that was becoming available that might someday make an important difference in their students. Denise pointed out that computer technology had already altered the world for persons with cerebral palsy, and in the future, the outcome would probably be their almost complete independence. She believed that some of these "miracles" might be available for her students as well.

As stated in the beginning of this chapter, the teachers who participated in this inquiry, like their students, believe that they can make a difference, and believe that their students are worth their efforts. Denise expressed anger at hearing professionals say that a child is a "vegetable." "No person is a 'vegetable,' they all do something, they all have human responses." Ellen admitted to sometimes thinking that she was paid too much on those days in which the caregiving routines of her job seemed to dominate her work. However, she commented that she basically knew that her job could only be conducted by a professional educator and that these students required the very best and most resourceful teachers.

Ellen talked about a teacher who had come to her in tears and admitted that she was questioning the purpose of working with her students. She said, "I explained my philosophy to her [the other teacher] and it seemed to help." Ellen's philosophy is, "I'm a person that if you give me someone to work with, I start where they are . . . and try to take these kids as far as they can go." She explained (as all of the participating teachers had) that she has learned to never assume what a student can and cannot do. Ellen expressed the value of her role very specifically by stating:

> The value of a teacher is that there is hope, there is the involvement and attitude about moving on to something else. There is more hope for the parents and the students. There is more hope for quality of life. With a teacher, there is the chance to look forward.

SUMMARY

This chapter reports the results of an investigation that employed qualitative methodology in an attempt to portray the perceptions of six teachers who work with students who experience the most profound multiply handicapping and medically complicated conditions. The investigation was motivated by the belief that consulting with teachers who have had direct and sustained responsibility for the educational programs of these students could offer important insight into future research directions, educational practices, and treatment approaches, as well as insight into the quality and relevance of personnel training programs. Consequently, educators who were considered to be effective and committed teachers of these children and youth were sought as participants of this study and engaged in intensive open-ended nonstructured interviews that were reviewed and validated by each teacher.

An analysis of the interview data makes up the development of categories that emerge into the five primary themes of this chapter. The first theme is directed toward student characteristics and suggests that the participating teachers view students with the most profound disabilities as a specific group within the area of severe multiple disabilities. This then led the professionals to believe that additional information and skills were necessary to teach these students. Student characteristics that were consistently identified by the participating teachers related to the categories of limited level of awareness, limited response repertoires, no system of communication, and the occurrence of medical complications. The term "profound" as it is currently used is described as too broad and relative in meaning.

The second theme indicates that the emergence of a clinical style and an eclectic approach is replacing a heavy or exclusive reliance on an applied behavior analysis perspective, and that these teachers rely on sensitive observational skills and intuition in combination with a broad base of information and techniques. This is apparent from the goals and procedures that are described and directed toward increasing levels of awareness, developing communicative intent, developing a response or responses that can serve as the basis of functional participation, and maintaining and increasing physical well-being of the students. Participating teachers valued skills that facilitated "tuning in" to their students, and the importance of coordinating information and resources that are available from a broad array of disciplines. Additionally, these professionals indicated that many of the techniques and sources of information that they currently value were not components of their university training program.

Another theme is directed toward policy issues and attitudes that result in increased segregation of students on the basis of medical conditions and functioning levels. In summary, these participating teachers valued integrated and varied environments and felt considerable concern about the policy issues that support increased segregation or exclusion.

A fourth theme is directed toward the nature and intensity of interactions with parents. The special relationship that these teachers have developed with parents seems to have emerged from the need to work cooperatively, and to share information of a critical nature, to respond to serious medical and sometimes life-threatening conditions of the students, and to respond to the lack of adequate support systems available to families.

The final theme focuses on the participating teachers' positive and negative feelings regarding their roles and experiences. These professionals openly discussed their responses to caring for children in pain; experiencing the death of a student; the devaluing of their roles by other professionals; and their feeling of confusion, uncertainty, and the lack of information about their students' conditions and related procedures. They also eloquently describe their appreciation for their students as unique and inherently valuable individuals and their view of the critical and important nature of their role as educators.

Ultimately, it must be concluded that the participating teachers share the same values as those currently embraced by professionals and parents who advocate for integrated life-styles for persons with severe disabilities. The underlying and recurrent theme that emerges from the participating teachers' interviews is that their primary goal was to have positive impact on the quality of life of their students. In order to accomplish this, these professionals actively search for strategies, information, and resources that will enhance the functionality and efficacy of procedures and treatment approaches, and raise issues about the environments that should be afforded to their students. To the extent these teachers expressed more, rather than less, fulfillment and enjoyment of their roles and their students, it can be concluded that they believe that they are, in part, achieving their goal. To the extent that they expressed needs for additional information, training, support services, and different opportunities for their students, it can be concluded that these professionals believe that a better quality of life for their students can be obtained.

REFERENCES

Bogdan, R., & Biklen, S. (1982). *Qualitative research for education: An introduction to theory and methods*. Newton, MA: Allyn & Bacon.

Bricker, D., & Filler, J. (Eds.). (1985). *Severe mental retardation: From theory to practice*. Reston, VA: Council for Exceptional Children.

Brown, F., Helmstetter, E., & Guess, D. (1986). *Current best practices with students with profound disabilities: Are there any?* Unpublished manuscript.

Doll, E. (1953). *Measurement of Social Competence*. Chicago: Educational Publishers.

Ferguson, D. (1985). The ideal and the real: The working out of public policy in curricula for severely handicapped students. *Remedial and Special Education, 6,* 52–60.

Glaser, B., & Strauss, A. (1967). *The discovery of grounded theory*. Chicago:Aldine.

Green, C.W., Reid, D.H., McCarn, J.E., Schepis, M.M., Phillips, J.F., & Parsons, M.B. (1986). Naturalistic observations of classrooms serving severely handicapped persons: Establishing evaluative norms. *Applied Research in Mental Retardation, 7,* 37–50.

Grossman, J. (Ed.). (1977). *Manual on terminology and classification in mental retardation*. Washington, DC: American Association on Mental Deficiency.

Grossman, J. (Ed.). (1983). *Classification in mental retardation*. Washington, DC: American Association on Mental Deficiency.

Hotte, R.A., Monroe, H.S., Philbrook, D.L., & Scarlata, R.W. (1984). Programming for persons with profound mental retardation: A three year retrospective study. *Mental Retardation, 22*(2), 75–78.

Lincoln, Y.S., & Guba, E.G. (1985). *Naturalistic inquiry*. Beverly Hills: Sage Publications.

Lorr, C., & Rotatori, A.F. (1985). Who are the severely and profoundly handicapped? In A.F. Rotatori, J.O. Schwenn, & R.A. Fox (Eds.), *Assessing severely and profoundly handicapped individuals* (pp. 38–48). Springfield, IL: Charles C Thomas.

Miles, M.B., & Huberman, A.M. (1984). *Qualitative data analysis: A sourcebook of new methods*. Beverly Hills: Sage Publications.

Odom, S.L., & Shuster, S.K. (1986). Naturalistic inquiry and the assessment of young handicapped children and their families. *Topics in Early Childhood Special Education, 6*(2), 68–82.

Rainforth, B. (1982). Biobehavioral state and orienting: Implications for educating profoundly retarded students. *Journal of The Association of the Severely Handicapped, 6,* 33–37.

Sailor, W., & Guess, D. (1983). *Severely handicapped students: An instructional design*. Boston: Houghton Mifflin.

Stainback, S., & Stainback, W. (1985). Methodological considerations in qualitative research. *Journal of The Association for Persons with Severe Handicaps, 9*(4), 296–303.

Taylor, S.J. (1982). From segregation to integration: Strategies for integrating severely handicapped students in normal and school community settings. *Journal of The Association for the Severely Handicapped, 8,* 42–49.

Taylor, S.J., & Bogdan, R. (1984). *Introduction to qualitative research methods: The search for meaning.* New York: John Wiley & Sons.

United States Department of Education, Bureau of Education for the Handicapped (USOE/BEH). (1974). 21 U.S.C. §1407[7]; 45 C.F.R. §14.1

van Dijk, J. (1986). An educational curriculum for deaf-blind multiply handicapped persons. In D. Ellis (Ed.), *Sensory impairments in mentally handicapped people* (pp. 375–382). San Diego: College-Hill Press.

Is a Policy of Exclusion Based upon Severity of Disability Legally Defensible?

William L. E. Dussault

Is it permissible for an educational agency to deny appropriate educational services to a student who experiences a disability based upon the severity of that person's disability? The initial reaction upon being asked this question should be a resounding negative on both legal and educational grounds. Given the development of federal and state legislative protections for the educational rights of all children with handicaps and the rapidly expanding body of both state and federal court decisions, the issue of exclusion based upon severity of disability should have been put to rest. However, as attention is focused on the educational needs of those children who experience the most severe handicaps, questions of cost-effectiveness and their "ability to benefit" from education continue to surface. Even though the number of people who are raising the issue continues to diminish each year, it is nonetheless important to address their concerns and arguments, and to resolve them without margin for future ambiguity. This chapter addresses the legal basis of the "zero-reject" imperative in special education programs for students who experience severe or profound disabilities.

The History of the Zero-Exclusion Policy

The issue of exclusion based upon severity of disability cannot be understood in a historical vacuum. In order to clearly define the problem, it must be reviewed as part of the development of the public educational system in the United States. The obligation of school districts to provide free and appropriate public education for all handicapped students remains a relatively recent phenomenon. The Education for All Handicapped Children Act (PL 94-142) was enacted on November 29, 1975, and did not become fully effective for children age 3–18, until September 1, 1978.

Public School Education

Public school education from the 17th century to the present time was based upon an evolutionary process from a narrow concept of education that stressed "reading, writing, and arithmetic" to an expanded notion of education that incorporates both broader subject material and more generalized concepts of teaching the process of learning in addition to specific subject areas. Children with disabilities, whether slight or severe, have most often been excluded from those learning opportunities. When it became apparent that certain persons did not make any significant educational progress within the "Three 'R's" curriculum, rather than question the appropriateness of the curriculum, the reaction of early American teachers and principals was to label such persons as incapable of profiting from education (Burgdorf & Bersoff, 1980). Once a child had been determined to be unable to profit from schooling, he or she could, thenceforth, be excluded so that the state's resources could more beneficially be used for those persons that could benefit from educational services.

Special Education

An indirect result of the policy of exclusion was the removal of any incentive for educators to develop programs suited to the needs of children with profound handicaps. Since the teachers did not have to face the problems of teaching such students, there was little reason for developing curricula geared toward their educational needs. Thus, the special educational techniques necessary to assist these children were delayed and consequently reinforced the "unable to be educated" rationale (Burgdorf & Bersoff, 1980). In the early 19th century a few special classes were developed for deaf and hearing impaired children. These classes initially intended to provide assistance for those who were thought to have some capabilities that were impeded by sensory impairments; however, they soon became a "dumping ground" for students who did not fit into or could not manage to succeed in the normal classrooms (Burgdorf & Bersoff, 1980). Ultimately, the creation of these special classrooms at midpoint between total inclusion into the regular classroom or total exclusion from any educational opportunity forced educators to address the problem and to begin designing programs for the needs of handicapped students. However, it must be noted that those students who initially moved into such programs were those with mild handicaps.

As some students showed progress in the newly developing special classrooms, educators began to use the term "educable" to describe them. Those students who could not make it in the special class were denied further access and were deemed to be "uneducable." In 1911, New Jersey became the first state in the United States to legislate special education for students classified as mildly mentally retarded. During the next 20 years, other states followed suit.

As the sophistication of these specialized programs increased, it was demonstrated that students previously thought to be uneducable could actually make advances and become more independent. A new category was created— the "trainable," establishing the continuing dichotomy between the educable and the trainable for many years. Those persons who were considered to be so disabled that they could not benefit from the programs developed for either the educable or trainable were considered to be "subtrainable." It is in the subtrainable population that those persons who were considered to have severe or profound handicaps would normally be found.

Educable, Trainable, and Subtrainable Distinctions

The 1930 White House Conference on Children and Youth adopted the educable/trainable distinction, and recommended that programs be provided for both groups. Programs for those individuals who were labeled trainable developed very slowly over the next 20 years. Programs for the subtrainable were almost nonexistent.

As recently as the late 1960s, the majority of the states had established a legislative scheme that permitted local school districts to educate children with handicaps whom they thought could "benefit from education." This was known as permissive legislation. Mandatory legislation (i.e., legislation that requires local school districts to provide special educational services to all children who are handicapped) was rare.

A distinction was often made in state law between provisions that established permissive state programs for children with disabilities and mandatory attendance laws that allowed school boards or local superintendents to exclude students who were determined to be incapable of benefiting from educational programs. It was often possible for states to point to their progressive and liberal tendencies in establishing special educational programs on the one hand, while on the other hand maintaining an absolute right to exclude those children found to be incapable of benefiting from education under the state's mandatory attendance laws.

Until 1975, the Maine Revised Statutes Annotated (1975) provided that, "The superintendent, school committee or school directors may exclude from the public schools any child whose physical or mental condition makes it *inexpedient* for him to attend" [emphasis supplied].

The New York Education Law (1974) states that:

1) A person included by the provisions of Part I of this Article shall be required to attend upon instruction only if in *proper mental and physical condition.* [emphasis supplied]

2) A person whose mental or physical condition is such that his attendance upon instruction under the provisions of Part I of this Article would endanger the health or safety of himself or of others, or who is *feeble minded to the extent that he is unable to benefit from instruction,* shall not be permitted to attend. . . . " [emphasis supplied]

Many states had enacted provisions similar to that found in the Oregon Laws (1965) of 1947 that continued in effect until 1965:

1) The Boards of Directors of the several school districts of the State of Oregon hereby are authorized and empowered to exclude permanently from the public schools of such district any child or children over ten years of age found to be *mentally unable to benefit* further from the instruction offered in such schools in the manner hereinafter provided. [emphasis supplied]

In the 1960s, as educators demonstrated increasing success in providing programs for those children with more severe handicapping conditions, public demand for increased access grew more strident. As early as 1962, the President's Panel on Mental Retardation (1962) noted the importance of education in establishing an individual's potential for work and self-reliance. The report stated that in some instances a person's:

. . . potential may be so limited that it is insignificant from the standpoint of economic gain. However, it is never insignificant from the standpoint of concern for the welfare and dignity of the individual. The true goal of education and rehabilitation of the handicapped is to help every individual to make the most of his potential for participation in all the affairs of our society, including work, no matter how great or small his potential may be.

The report went on to recommend appropriate educational opportunities for all handicapped children.

In 1971, the C.E.C. Delegate Convention (1971) established as its official position:

Education is the right of all children. The principle of education for all is based on the philosophical premise of democracy that every person is valuable in his own right, and should be afforded equal opportunities to develop his full potential. (p. 1)

Parent advocates, led by the organizational efforts of the National Association for Retarded Citizens (ARC-US), worked effectively to establish a climate at both the state and local level that was receptive to arguments that exclusion of children who are handicapped, regardless of how substantial their disabilities, was not defensible. As the decade of the 1970s opened, great efforts were made to draw a parallel between the civil rights movement that was established by blacks in the late 1950s and 1960s and the ongoing movement to obtain educational rights for children with disabilities.

One important historical factor in the genesis of the right to an appropriate educational opportunity for students who are handicapped is that the movement did not principally originate with educators. As Bates (1976) stated:

> As an educator, I find it somewhat embarrassing that in recent years, attorneys have assumed leadership in obtaining equal educational opportunities for the mentally retarded. For too long, educators have been mere spectators of change awaiting the results of special class legislation, administrative regulations, and right to education lawsuits. Too often we have been in the position of operating after the fact. Our lack of participation has created confusion within the profession and, most tragically, delay in the delivery of services to children. (p. 268)

An awareness of this historical perspective allows for greater understanding of the current reticence that is emanating largely from the established educational community to the extension of full educational opportunities for those individuals who are severely handicapped. There remains a perception that mandatory special educational programs for all children who are handicapped is an obligation that has been imposed upon educators and, in some cases, this is contrary to their professional training, experience, and personal desire.

LEGAL BASIS FOR A ZERO-EXCLUSION POLICY

Initial Policy of Nonintervention in Public School Matters

The traditional stance of the courts in cases involving educational issues has been to adopt a hands-off attitude. In *Watson v. City of Cambridge* (1893), the court was asked to approve the exclusion of a child because he was "too weak minded to derive profit from instruction." The records in the case recited that the child was " . . . troublesome to other children, making unusual noises, pinching others, etc. He is also found unable to take ordinary decent physical care of himself." The court ruled that:

> The management of the schools involves many details; and it is important that a board of public officers, dealing with these details, and having jurisdiction to regulate the internal affairs of the schools, should not be interfered with or have their conduct called in question before another tribunal, so long as they act in good faith within their jurisdiction. (*Watson v. City of Cambridge*, 1893)

In the case of *State ex rel Beattie v. Board of Education of City of Antigo* (1919), a youngster who "has been a crippled and defective child since his birth, [and who has] been afflicted with a form of paralysis which affects his whole physical and nervous make-up" was refused attendance at the local public school under the authority granted by the local school board to supervise the educational program. After a long list of citations, the court held that, "The action of the board in refusing to reinstate the boy seems to have been the result of its best judgment exercised in good faith, and the record discloses no grounds for the interference by courts with its action."

The attitudes of the courts established in these early cases continued as the general rule until the early 1950s. In what was unquestionably the most significant civil rights decision of the century, the United States Supreme Court was called upon to determine the application of the equal protection and due process provisions in the 14th Amendment of the Constitution of the United States to a public educational program that involves "separate but equal" facilities for black students. The Supreme Court, in *Brown v. Board of Education* (1954), stated:

> Today, education is perhaps the most important function of state and local governments. Compulsory school attendance laws and the great expenditures for education both demonstrate our recognition of the importance of education to our democratic society. It is required in the performance of our most basic public responsibilities, even service in the armed forces. It is the very foundation of good citizenship. Today, it is a principal instrument in awakening the child to cultural values, and preparing him for later professional training and in helping him to adjust normally to his environment. In these days, it is doubtful that any child may reasonably be expected to succeed in life if he is denied the opportunity of an education. *Such an opportunity, where the state has undertaken to provide it, is a right which must be made available to all on equal terms.* [emphasis supplied]

While the Court did not determine that there was a federal constitutional "right to education" per se, it did determine that once a state accepted the burden and obligation of providing a public educational program to students within its borders, that education had to be provided to all children, on an equal basis, under the provision of the equal protection and due process provision of the 14th Amendment. The *Brown* (1954) case signaled the end of the courts' general policy of nonintervention into public school matters.

Transition from the Policy of Exclusion

In *Wolf v. Legislature of the State of Utah* (1969), the Utah Court was faced with a policy of exclusion of children with mental retardation having IQs in a range that defined them as trainable. In deciding the case, the Court acknowledged the provisions of the *Utah State Constitution* (1894) that provided for the "establishment and maintenance of a uniform system of public schools, which shall be open to *all* children of the state and be free from sectarian control" [emphasis supplied]. In a brief decision, almost directly paraphrasing the language from the *Brown* (1954) case, the Court found the state's policy of exclusion to be improper. The Court noted that:

> In the instant case, the segregation of the plaintiff children from the public school system has a detrimental effect upon the children as well as their parents. The impact is greater when it has the apparent sanction of the law for the policy of placing these children under the Department of Welfare and segregating them from the educational system can be and probably is usually interpreted as denoting their inferiority, unusualness, uselessness, and incompetency. A sense of inferiority and not belonging affects the motivation of the child to learn.

The Court went on to hold that the children involved were entitled to a free educational program within the framework of the public school systems of the State of Utah. The case has legal significance in two obvious areas: 1) it was a "zero-reject decision—no exceptions or exclusions were made for children who could not "benefit from education"; and 2) by so clearly applying the arguments used and language from the *Brown* (1954) decision in the context of exclusion of children who are handicapped, it set the precedence for the landmark special education cases to follow.

Implementing the Due Process and Equal Protection Provisions

In *Pennsylvania Association for Retarded Children v. Commonwealth of Pennsylvania* (1972) (PARC), the federal district court for the eastern district of Pennsylvania was asked to review the practice of school districts in the state of Pennsylvania of excluding some children with mental retardation between the ages of 6 and 21 from public school opportunities under various state statutes. The statutes authorized exclusion for those children deemed "uneducable" or "untrainable," authorized an indefinite postponement of admission to public school of any child who had not attained a mental age of 5 years, and appeared to excuse any child from compulsory attendance whom a psychologist found unable to "profit therefrom." The Pennsylvania statutes were attacked using the 14th Amendment of the United States Constitution, applying both the due process and equal protection provisions.

In discussing the application of the due process provision the court cited *Wisconsin v. Constantineau* (1971), wherein the United States Supreme Court considered the necessity of a due process hearing prior to stigmatization by the state of any citizen. The Court acknowledged that the stigma of the label of "mental retardation" applied by a school district was substantial and was likened by some parents to a "sentence of death." Such stigmatization could not occur until after constitutionally adequate procedures had been observed.

In reviewing the plaintiffs' equal protection argument, the Court noted that the plaintiffs did not challenge the separation of special classes for children with mental retardation from regular classes or the proper assignment of such children to those classes. The principal argument brought by the plaintiffs was whether the state, having undertaken to provide a public educational program to some children, may deny that education to plaintiffs entirely. The Court, agreeing with the plaintiffs, cited the *Brown* (1954) case and expressed doubts as to the existence of a rational basis that would justify such unequal treatment for children with severe handicaps by school districts.

In the *PARC* (1972) decision, arguments that had previously been primarily legal in nature were coupled with a new, educational assertion that stated that persons with mental retardation are capable of learning, regardless of the severity of their disability. The court noted that:

Without exception, expert opinion indicates that: All mentally retarded persons are capable of benefiting from a program of education and training; that the greatest number of retarded persons, given such education and training, are capable of achieving self-sufficiency and the remaining few, with such education and training, are capable of achieving some degree of self-care; that the earlier such education and training begins, the more thoroughly and more efficiently a mentally retarded person will benefit from it and, whether begun early or not, that a mentally retarded person can benefit at any point in his life and development from a program of education. (Consent Agreement, Paragraph 4)

The unanimous and highly competent professional testimony as to the benefit of education to the plaintiff population with mental retardation was unquestionably of significant benefit in convincing the court to apply the legal rationales put forward by the plaintiffs.

In the Order and Injunction that implemented the *PARC* (1972) Stipulation and Consent Agreement signed by the parties, the court ordered that all of the parties to the suits were directed to not postpone or deny any child with mental retardation the access to a free public educational program and training.

At the same time that the Eastern District Federal Court in Pennsylvania was considering *PARC* (1972), the United States District Court for the District of Columbia was being asked to decide a similar action in *Mills v. Board of Education of the District of Columbia* (1972). The *Mills* (1972) case differed from the *PARC* (1972) case in two important respects. First, it was not decided through the procedure known as a *consent order* (i.e., an agreement signed by all the parties) as was the *PARC* (1972) case. Because the *Mills* (1972) case was decided by a judge subsequent to a trial, it had greater precedental value.

Second, the *Mills* (1972) decision applied to all "exceptional" children within the district, including those who were mentally retarded, emotionally disturbed, physically handicapped, hyperactive, blind, deaf, and speech and learning impaired.

As with *PARC* (1972), one of the prevalent issues in the *Mills* (1972) case was a mandatory attendance provision that allowed for the exclusion of children who were "found to be unable mentally or physically to profit from attendance at school" (Section 31–203, District of Columbia Code). Applying similar analysis as in *PARC* (1972) the court ruled that under the equal protection and the due process provisions of the 14th Amendment of the United States Constitution: "The District of Columbia shall provide each child of school age a free and suitable publicly supported education regardless of the degree of the child's mental, physical or emotional disability or impairment" (Subparagraph 3, Judgment and Decree).

Is There a Federal Constitutional Right to Education?

Shortly after the lower court decisions rendered in *PARC* (1972) and *Mills* (1972), the United States Supreme Court was called upon to review the issue of whether there was a federal constitutional right to education per se. The Supreme Court, in *San Antonio Independent School District v. Rodriguez* (1973), decided that education was not a "fundamental right" included "among the rights afforded explicit protection under our federal Constitution." The issue of education as a fundamental right under state constitutions or laws was brought before the Court in the *Rodriguez* (1973) case (see *Doe v. Board of School Directors of Milwaukee*, 1970; *Reed v. Board of Education*, 1971; and *Wolf v. Legislature of State of Utah*, 1969). The *Rodriguez* (1973) decision raised questions as to the standards that had to be applied to the equal protection provision analysis for establishing a right to educational opportunity for all children who are handicapped.

Traditionally, the United States Supreme Court has applied two levels of review in "equal protection" cases depending upon the constitutional importance of the rights involved or the category of the class of individuals who are seeking protection under the act. The two tests are labeled the "strict scrutiny or compelling justification" test or the more lenient "reasonable or rational basis" test. Plaintiffs in both the *PARC* (1972) and the *Mills* (1972) cases had argued a "strict scrutiny" test on the basis that education was both a "fundamental interest" and that children with handicaps were part of an "inherently suspect category." The *Rodriguez* (1973) case rejected the theory that education was a "fundamental interest" as it was not specifically protected as a federal constitutional right per se (for more information, see Wald, 1973). As indicated, the "fundamental" nature of a right to an educational program under a *state* constitution was not addressed.

The *PARC* (1972) and *Mills* (1972) cases appeared to determine that the denial of education to children with mental retardation violated the "rational basis" test; however, neither decision was focused directly on the issue. While the *PARC* (1972) and *Mills* (1972) cases gave advocates for children with disabilities strong rhetoric to use and further fueled the public outcry for mandation of educational programs for persons with handicaps, the *Rodriguez* (1973) case, by denying a constitutional basis to the right to education, allowed for further litigation on the underlying issue of the "constitutionality" of the right to education for children who are handicapped. While the *Rodriguez* (1973) case involved nonhandicapped children, the implications for children with handicaps were clear. States needed only to provide a minimal justification for excluding children from public schools, instead of the higher justification required when fundamental interests are involved (Brakel, Parry, & Weiner, 1985).

Emphasis in Obtaining Special Education Shifts

At this time, much of the emphasis in obtaining the right to special education for all children who are handicapped, regardless of the severity of their disability, shifted from the courts to the state legislatures and Congress. By approximately 1975, all of the 50 state legislatures had already passed or were actively considering mandatory special education laws. In addition, the federal government was actively involved in the drafting and passage of PL 93-380 and PL 94-142.

Virtually all of the new state laws enacted as a result of the efforts of parents and parent advocacy organizations on behalf of children with handicaps incorporated provisions that required the education of all children with handicaps. The federal act (PL 94-142), while not, by strict interpretation, a mandatory law that all states were required to follow (they were required to follow PL 94-142 only if they wanted federal financial assistance), provided that a state had to demonstrate in its state plan that it would assure that:

> (C) All children residing in the state who are handicapped, *regardless of the severity of their handicap*, and who are in need of special education and related services, are identified, located, and evaluated, and that a practical method is developed and implemented to determine what children are currently receiving needed special education and related services and what children are not currently receiving special education and related services. [emphasis supplied]

A similar provision was incorporated into PL 94-142, at Section 20 U.S.C. Section 1414(a)(1)(C)(ii), that emphasized that children should be identified, located, evaluated, and served, "regardless of the severity of their handicap." This was carried out in the federal regulations implementing the act.

PL 94-142 thus confirmed the decisions in both the *PARC* (1972) and *Mills* (1972) cases that stated that "all" children who are handicapped should have a right to free and appropriate public education. Parallel state acts seemed to give the same explicit direction. This should have put to rest any claim that children with severe or profound handicaps could continue to be excluded.

Interpreting PL 94-142

The United States Supreme Court, in the *Board of Education of the Hendrick Hudson Central School District v. Rowley* (1982), was given the first opportunity to interpret the provisions and meaning of PL 94-142. In that case, the Court carefully reviewed the legislative history and basis for the act. At Footnote 5 of the opinion, the Court specifically noted that, "In addition to covering a wide variety of handicapping conditions, the Act requires special educational services for children *regardless of the severity of their handicap*" [emphasis supplied].

The Court cited various sections of PL 94-142 for its basis. The Court also cited the *Mills* (1972) and the *PARC* (1972) cases, noting the significant role they played in the development of the federal act. At Footnote 23 of the opinion, the Court stated that, "We thus view these references in the legislative history as evidence of Congress' intention that the services provided handicapped children be educationally beneficial, *whatever the nature or severity of their handicap*" [emphasis supplied].

The decision, taken as a whole, clearly requires access to appropriate educational services for all children who are handicapped, regardless of the severity of their disability. Moreover, the Court ruled that the educational program to which the children are entitled is to provide them with an educational benefit, the amount to be determined on a case-by-case basis.

Further support for a "zero reject policy" can be found in the U.S. Supreme Court's January, 1988 decision in the case of *Bill Honig, California Superintendent of Public Instruction v. John Doe and Jack Smith* (1988). Justice Brennan, writing a 6–2 majority opinion concerning a school district's unilateral disciplinary action against students with severe behavior problems, carefully outlined the history and congressional intent behind PL 94-142. He noted the relationship of the *Brown* (1954) civil rights rationale of education to the right to appropriate special education for children with handicaps.

In discussing school district exclusionary practices, the Supreme Court's opinion noted congressional intent as follows:

> Congress attacked such exclusionary practices in a variety of ways. It required participating States to educate *ALL* disabled children, regardless of the severity of their disabilities, 20 U.S.C. Section 1412(2)(C), and included within the definition of "handicapped" those children with serious emotional disturbances. (Section 1401[1]) [emphasis supplied]

The Supreme Court's opinion reinforces earlier statements made by Justice Rehnquist in Footnote 5 of the *Board of Education of the Hendrick Hudson Central School District* (1982) decision and explicitly emphasised the inclusion of ALL children under the protection of PL 94-142 regardless of the severity of the child's disability.

Rational Basis Test

Two cases decided in 1976 and 1980, respectively, have left a cloud of concern, especially for parents and professionals dealing with those persons defined as profoundly handicapped. The first case, *Cuyahoga County Association for Retarded Children and Adults v. Essex* (U.S.D., N.D. Ohio) (1976), challenged Ohio's present School Attendance Act of the Ohio Revised Code at § 3321.03 that authorized an exception to compulsory attendance for children who have been determined to be "incapable of profiting substantially from further instruction." The parent/plaintiffs used the same arguments as in both the *PARC* (1972) and the *Mills* (1972) cases that stated that exclusion violated both the equal protection and due process provisions of the 14th Amendment to the United States Constitution.

For the first time, a federal district court had available decisions from the Supreme Court in both *Brown v. Board of Education* (1954) and *San Antonio v. Rodriguez* (1973), clarifying the Supreme Court's position on the "right" to education as it relates to the 14th Amendment. With a long list of supporting citations, the district court adopted the "rational basis" test. In the *Cuyahoga* (1976) case, the Court noted that:

> In order to invalidate a classification (as a basis for different treatment) under the "rational basis" test, it must be shown that it is arbitrary, does not rest upon some ground of difference having a fair and substantial relation to the object of the legislation, or that no state of facts exists which would reasonably support a legitimate state interest therein.

After a careful review of the Ohio statutes, the court determined that the basis for exclusion of students with profound handicaps from the system was the students' incapability of profiting from further instruction. The court specifically held that: "Such a classification is sufficient to meet the rational basis test." In so holding, the court ruled that the state agency had a "rational" justification for treating students with mental retardation who fell into the severe or profound disability categories differently than other children, and as such, the equal protection provision was not violated. This holding was in direct contradiction to the holdings of both the *PARC* (1972) and the *Mills* (1972) cases.

The court did note that the procedures for classifying the children used in Ohio were inadequate and, thus, violated the due process provisions of the 14th Amendment of the Constitution. The court stated that in order to exclude children under the statutory provisions, a more protective procedure would have to be established. Finally, and perhaps most importantly, at Footnote 7 at the end of the decision, the court observed that PL 94-142 had just become effective at the federal level. The court indicated that if the state of Ohio accepted federal money pursuant to the new act, the issue of exclusion would become moot because of the federal act's requirements that all children had to be included in the state's educational program. Subsequently, the State of Ohio amended its legislation and did accept funds under the federal act, significantly reducing the importance of the *Cuyahoga* (1976) decision.

Care versus Education

The second decision authorizing the exclusion of persons who are "profoundly retarded" from mandatory state educational programs is *Levine v. State of New Jersey Department of Institutions and Agencies* (July, 1980). This case involved a claim by the parents of two school-age children identified as profoundly retarded who resided in state institutions for persons with mental retardation. The state of New Jersey was attempting to collect the cost of the institutional care and maintenance of the students from the parents. The parents contended that they should be allotted a credit for the cost of the public school education the children should have received as guaranteed by the education clause of the New Jersey State Constitution.

In analyzing the *Levine* (1980) case, the court first reviewed the purposes of the education clause contained in the New Jersey State Constitution, noting that " . . . the essential purpose of which is to maximize public education so that citizens may function politically, economically, and socially in a democratic society (p. 236, Decision).

The court then took great pains to acknowledge society's obligation to provide for the "care" of persons with mental retardation, distinguishing the concept of "care" from "education." A long list of citations and articles supporting a broad interpretation of the concept of "education" was acknowledged by the court and then disregarded with no clear justification or explanation. The conclusion reached by the court was that the services provided to the children of plaintiffs was properly characterized as "care," rather than "education," which would have been protected under the state's constitutional educational clause.

The Court stated that:

> The sad fact endures that there is a category of mentally disabled children so severely impaired as to be unable to absorb or benefit from education. It is neither realistic nor meaningful to equate the type of care and habilitation which such children require for their health and survival with "education" in the sense that that term is used in the constitution. (p. 237, Opinion)

The court then went on to review the New Jersey statutory procedure of defining educable, trainable, and subtrainable children, noting that children who are subtrainable are those who have overall IQ levels of less than 24, and whose mental deficiencies do not bring them even to the level of children with mental retardation who are trainable. The court held that the plaintiffs, as the parents of subtrainable children, were not constitutionally entitled to have their children's institutional care provided free of charge at public expense. The decision was based upon the distinction between "care," to which there was no constitutional entitlement, and "education," which was required to be provided under the educational clause of the New Jersey State Constitution. The court was either not presented with or was not convinced of the evidence that the services provided to those children who were characterized as being "profoundly retarded" and qualified for state approved "education." It is unknown whether this arose because of a failure to present sufficient expert testimony or an underlying ignorance or prejudice on the part of the court.

The court then considered equal protection arguments applicable to children classified as having profound handicaps. The court was able to support the different classification because of the fact that the children were receiving "care" rather than "education" and that it was the care issue that placed them in a different class, not the degree of their disabilities.

Accordingly, the "equality" of treatment protected under the Constitution was to be evaluated against other children in "care" settings rather than children in "educational" settings. No inequality was found.

The court also applied the "rational basis" test, noting that there was not a fundamental right to "care" that was similar to the fundamental right to "education" that existed under the New Jersey State Constitution. The court also concluded that persons "afflicted with mental impairments" did not constitute a "suspect class" in the constitutional sense; notwithstanding the court's citation of numerous articles supporting that position. While the court did indicate that such individuals might appear, on some grounds, to qualify, it concluded that a "suspect class" was not created. The court could not offer any legal or factual basis for this conclusion.

It should be noted that this was a decision of the New Jersey State Supreme Court and not a federal district court. The issue of application of federal laws, such as PL 93-112, Rehabilitation Act of 1973, § 504 and PL 94-142, Education of All Handicapped Children Act of 1975, was addressed only at the end of the decision. In a very confusing two pages, the court acknowledged that it was not capable of applying the federal laws and regulations to the New Jersey state system. It stated: "All of these questions embrace a very complex subject matter which is most appropriately the concern of governmental specialists" (p. 245). The case was then remanded to an administrative tribunal to determine the application of the federal laws and regulations.

While it is not generally useful to cite dissenting opinions by judges in disagreement with the majority, Justice Pashman (Pashman, 1980), in opening his dissenting opinion, made pertinent statements. Part of those statements are as follows:

> Today the majority brands a group of children as uneducable and unfit citizens because it mistakenly believes the legislature has done so. By its unquestioning deference to an imagined legislative intention, the majority has completely abdicated its fundamental responsibility of constitutional judicial review. The majority leaves these children to the dubious protection of what it calls "humanitarian and compassionate instincts" and what *others would call political expediency*. This result diminishes more than our state's constitution's guarantee of education; it diminishes the meaning of our common humanity. For it is by education that each of us, including the plaintiffs, attains the full measure of the humanity that we possess. (p. 247, Decision) [emphasis added]

The *Levine* (1980) decision has very limited applicability for several reasons. First, as previously indicated, it is a state supreme court decision and not a federal district court case. Second, it is based upon a highly questionable factual distinction between the concepts of "care" and "education." As illustrated by the early portions of this chapter, distinctions based upon severity between students with mental retardation no longer have broad professional acceptance in the educational community. Finally, it avoids any discussion of the federal laws that apply to the provision of services to persons with disabilities, including federal discrimination provisions for persons who are handicapped (PL 93-112, Rehabilitation Act of 1973; PL 98-527, Developmental Disabilities

Act Amendments of 1984; and PL 94-142, Education for All Handicapped Children Act of 1975).

The court's constitutional analysis may also be faulty as illustrated by the following points. First, in order to avoid the equal protection arguments applicable to the state constitution's educational provision, the court had to characterize the services received by the children who were defined as being profoundly handicapped as "care" rather than "education." Second, the court applied a "rational basis" test to the equal protection analysis.

Equal Protection Concerns

The United States Supreme Court offers guidance, in addition to the aforementioned material, to determine the appropriate test to be applied in equal protection concerns related to persons with disabilities. In *City of Clayburn v. The Clayburn Living Center* (1985), the United States Supreme Court was asked to apply equal protection arguments to the action taken by the town council of the City of Clayburn in denying a zoning application filed by the Clayburn Living Center, a group home for persons with mental retardation. In divided opinions, the Court reviewed the case with a historical application of the "strict scrutiny" and "rational basis" tests applicable to equal protection analysis. In its majority opinion, the Court stated that it was applying a "rational basis" test to review the action taken by the City of Clayburn against the individuals with handicaps who would be residing in the group home. Based upon the application of the "rational basis" test, the Court found that the city's action violated equal protection. However, as accurately pointed out by the concurring opinion of Justices Marshall, Brennan, and Blackmun, the level of scrutiny applied by the Court to the city's action in denying the housing application was not the level of scrutiny pertinent to a "rational basis" approach. The Court's actual procedure was that used in a "strict scrutiny" case. The result of the *City of Clayburn* case is that the Supreme Court has announced that it will apply a "rational basis" approach but has implemented that approach through a "strict scrutiny" analysis. The implications of this procedure for future decisions are unclear. However. should the Court apply the same method of scrutiny to cases involving education of children who are profoundly handicapped, it is reasonable to predict that significantly different treatment, based solely upon the diagnosis or degree of mental retardation, would be found to be in violation of the equal protection provision of the 14th Amendment of the United States Constitution.

SUMMARY

This chapter discusses the initial question of whether or not it is permissible for an educational agency to deny services to children who are labeled as profoundly disabled based upon the severity of the child's disability. It should be clear at this point that if the educational agency accepts federal funds originating from PL 94-142, then such a denial would be in violation of the act. It is also very likely that even if an educational agency is not receiving federal funds for special education, a denial of educational services would likely violate state constitutional provisions and equal protection provisions of the 14th Amendment of the United States Constitution. Finally, if appropriate procedures are not used in such a denial, the due process provisions of the 14th Amendment would be violated as determined in the *Cuyahoga* (1976) case. The legal basis of the Zero Exclusion Policy is well established. It is now time to dismiss the arguments about whether education for children with profound handicaps should occur, and concentrate instead on how educational programs can be developed for those children.

REFERENCES

Bates, P. (1976). The right to an appropriate free public education: Reaction comment. In M. Kindred, J. Cohen, D. Penrod, & T. Shaffer (Eds.), *The mentally retarded citizen and the law* (pp. 251–270). New York: Macmillan.

Bill Honig, California Superintendent of Public Instruction v. John Doe and Jack Smith, 98 LE 2d 686, 108 S. Ct. 592 (Jan., 1988).

Board of Education of the Hendrick Hudson Central School District v. Rowley, 458 U.S. 187 (1982).

Brakel, S.J., Parry, J., & Weiner, B.A. (Eds.). (1985). *The mentally disabled and the law* (3rd ed.). Chicago, IL: American Bar Foundation.

Brown V. Board of Education, 347 U.S. 483, 493, 74 S.Ct. 686, 691, 98 L. Ed. 873, (1954).

Burgdorf, R.L., Jr., & Bersoff, D.N. (1980). Equal educational opportunity. In. R.L. Burgdorf (Ed.), *The legal rights of handicapped persons: Cases, materials, and text* (pp. 53–315). Baltimore: Paul H. Brookes Publishing Co.

C.E.C. Delegate Convention. (1971, April). Basic commitments and responsibilities to exceptional children. *Exceptional Children*, 181–187.

City of Clayburn v. The Clayburn Living Center, 105 S. Ct. 3249 (1985).

Cuyahoga County Association for Retarded Children and Adults v. Essex, 411 F. Supp. 46 (N.D. Ohio 1976).

Doe v. Board of School Directors of Milwaukee, No. 377770 C.C.D. (Milwaukee Cir. Court, Civ. Div., Wisc., 1970).

Fourteenth Amendment of the United States Constitution (Equal protection and due process provisions), Subparagraph 3, Judgment and Decree (1868).

Levine v. State of New Jersey Department of Institutions and Agencies, 84 NJ 234, 418 A. 2d 229 (1980).

Maine Revised Statutes Annotated, Title 20, §911, deleted by Ch. 510 §21, 1975.

Mills v. Board of Education of the District of Columbia, 348 F. Supp. 866 (D.D.C. 1972).

New Jersey State Constitution, Art. VIII, §4, para. 1 (1947).

New York Education Law, Title 4, Art. 65, §3208, derived from the Education Law of 1910, §624 as amended by Ch. 191, §11 (1974).

Oregon Laws, Ch. 463, S.B. 98 (1947), repealed by Ch. 100, §456 (1965).

Pashman, J. (1980). *Levine v. State of New Jersey Department of Institutions and Agencies Decisions*, 84 NJ 234, 418 A. 2d 229.

Pennsylvania Association for Retarded Children v. Commonwealth of Pennsylvania, 334 F. Supp. 1257 (E.D. Pa. 1971).

Pennsylvania Association for Retarded Children v. Commonwealth of Pennsylvania, 343 F. Supp. 279 (E.D. Pa. 1972).

President's Panel on Mental Retardation. (1962, October). *Report to the President: A proposed program for national action to combat mental retardation* (Leonard W. Mayo, Chairman). Washington, DC: Author.

Public Law 93-112, *Rehabilitation Act of 1973*, §504, 1973.

Public Law 93-380, *Education of the Handicapped Act Amendments of 1974*, 20 U.S.C. §§1401-1461, 1973.

Public Law 94-142, *Education for All Handicapped Children Act of 1975*, 20 U.S.C. §§1401-1461, 1975.

Reed v. Board of Education, 453 F. 2d 238 (2d Cir. 1971).

San Antonio Independent School District v. Rodriquez, 93 S. Ct. 1278 (1973).

School Attendance Act. Ohio Revised Code, §3321.03 (1976).

State ex rel Beattie v. Board of Education of City of Antigo, 169 Wisc. 231, 172 N.W. 153, (1919).

Utah State Constitution, Art. 10, Ch. 138, §1, 28 Stat. at Large 107 (July 16, 1894).

Wald, P.M. (1973). The right to education. In B.J. Ennis, P. Friedman, & B. Gitlin (Eds.), *Legal rights of the mentally handicapped* (Vol. 2, pp. 831–955). New York: Practicing Law Institute.

Watson v. City of Cambridge, 157 Mass. 561, 32 N.E. 864 (1893).

White House Conference on Children and Youth. (1930).

Wisconsin v. Constantineau, 400 U.S. 433, 91 S. Ct. 507, 27 L. Ed. 2d 515 (1971).

Wolf v. Legislature of the State of Utah, Civil No. 182646 (Salt Lake County, 3rd Judicial District Court, Utah, Jan. 8, 1969).

RESEARCH ON PERSONS LABELED PROFOUNDLY RETARDED

Issues and Ideas

Jennifer F. Holvoet

(3)

Maslow (1954) has stated that "The proper place for a scientist is in the midst of the unknown, the chaotic, the dimly seen, the unmanageable, the mysterious, the not-yet-well-phrased" (p. 15). If this is so, the area of profound retardation, the processes that cause it, the ways it can be prevented or ameliorated, the techniques for habilitating those who are profoundly retarded, and the effects that these persons have on others and on society itself should be of interest to research scientists. However, at this time there are many procedural and ethical issues that appear to be hampering the development of a systematic research focus.

Though research is conducted that is of importance to this population, its developments are scattered throughout the journals of many different professions. It is as though there is a huge jigsaw puzzle that no one has ever seen in its entirety, and as though the people who are putting it together are scattered across the world with their own separate part of the puzzle. Furthermore, these scientists do not know who possesses the missing information for the puzzle or which parts are still undefined. Because no one has ever seen this completed research puzzle, many scientists do not recognize the significance of their work as an important part of the overall puzzle of profound retardation. Instead, many researchers may see their studies simply as pieces of other puzzles such as learning theory, cognitive development, physical development, behavioral sciences, or neuroscience.

If valuable research is to be conducted in the area of profound retardation, then some direction must be determined, different parts of the puzzle must be defined, and the parts must be pulled together across professional lines.

This chapter explores some of the procedural and ethical issues that need to be recognized, some of which need to be resolved before a systematic research focus can be attained. This chapter offers a brief overview of some of the research areas that are currently being explored and pinpoints some areas that might be worthy of future research.

PROCEDURAL AND ETHICAL ISSUES

Some important procedural and ethical issues that impinge on research efforts in the area of profound retardation are: homogeneity, diagnostic labeling, informed consent and other regulations, communication among professionals, and paradoxical attitudes of persons in the "helping" profession.

Homogeneity

A central premise of research is that information derived from the individuals being studied can be used with other persons who bear the same label or have similar characteristics. This presupposes that there is some type of homogeneity among persons with profound disabilities. If homogeneity cannot be demonstrated, then previously untried procedures used to improve a patient's or student's condition must be considered to be experimental treatment, rather than research. This is not to deny that rigorous research methods could be used to establish whether the experimental treatment is effective with this particular person, but rather to emphasize that the results could not accurately be called research.

Thus, for research to be conducted in the area of profound retardation, there must be a general agreement that persons who are labeled profoundly handicapped are homogeneous, at least with respect to the trait or characteristic that is being investigated.

Persons with profound retardation comprise approximately 1%–3% of the world's population (Mercer, 1973). They may be defined in terms of their performance on standardized tests of intelligence and adaptive ability. Thus, one could say that persons with profound disabilities hold in common the inability to demonstrate most of the types of skills that standardized tests measure. If this were used as the only criterion, then this population would indeed be homogeneous. This population could also be defined in terms of characteristics shared by a majority of its members. Rainforth (1982), for example, describes these persons as those:

> . . . whom are virtually unresponsive in the teaching situation. These unresponsive students do not demonstrate understanding of daily routines, gestures, or other bases for communication, although they may grimace or groan with discomfort. They show no recognition of even significant persons in their lives. They may

sit or grasp objects but they engage in no purposeful movement. They demonstrate little if any observable response to noise, movement, touch, odors, or other stimuli. When compared to normal children, these students frequently lack the abilities even newborn infants possess. (p. 33)

A grouping based on what a child does not demonstrate is a tenuous basis for assuming the persons with profound disabilities are homogeneous since it is not clear whether these deficits are due to a lack of opportunity, teaching, or ability. Nonetheless, it must be recognized that anthropologists have conducted research on populations that are probably as diverse as the population of persons with profound retardation (e.g., Australian aborigines, "street people") and that most research on other handicapping conditions has been based on the assumption that the finding of similar characteristics, even if they are deficits, constitutes homogeneity until it is demonstrated to be otherwise. It should also be noted that every population can be broken into subgroups and that research on the larger populations is sometimes the only way of deducing important but not easily discriminable subgroups. This has happened in the areas of autism, hyperactivity (attention deficit disorder [ADD]), and self-injurious behavior.

In this author's opinion, it makes some sense to assume some homogeneity in this population for the purposes of initial research; however, detailed subject description should be a part of all reports in order to evaluate whether the group needs to be broken down further.

Diagnostic Labeling

Providing a diagnostic label for a person whose behavior or skills differs from the norm has been a point of controversy since the 1970s. Proponents of labels feel that they facilitate treatment by promoting grouping of persons with similar characteristics, providing a rallying point for advocacy efforts, and enhancing the probability of research efforts on specific problems. Certainly the demand for homogeneity in research populations leads the researcher to value labels. The scientist must be able to describe how the members of the population being studied are alike. If subgroups are found that react differently to certain treatments or that exhibit slightly different sets of characteristics, then it is likely that researchers will invent new labels to distinguish these subgroups. The process of labeling is a very basic part of research because it facilitates communication among professionals.

Professionals opposing diagnostic labels believe that while they may be helpful to the researcher, they may be harmful to the person who is being labeled. They believe that labels contribute to deviance by creating a "self-fulfilling prophecy." In other words, the opponents believe that once a person is labeled "mentally retarded," others will treat that person in a much different way than they would someone who is labeled normal. This differing treatment (e.g., low expectation, fewer pressures to conform, less exposure to different situations) can actually ensure that the person will continue to show the characteristics of his or her labeled population. In addition, the label can take on a life of its own and rob the person of essential humanity. For example, parents of a newborn with an intestinal obstruction may make a much different decision about whether surgery should be performed if they are told that the child is "mentally retarded" than they would make if they were told that the infant was "normal in every other respect."

There have been numerous empirical studies, some showing the negative consequences (cf. Hobbs, 1975) and others, the positive effects (cf. Seitz & Geske, 1976) of diagnostic labeling of the behavior of others and the subsequent effects of that behavior on the child. Currently, it appears that labels may have more negative effects on certain types of individuals than on others. Fernald and Gettys (1980), in a review of this area, conclude that:

> Labels are likely to be the most damaging when the child, his parents or teacher were not previously aware that the child was deviant, because the label might become a self-fulfilling prophecy. Labels are most likely to be helpful when people were greatly bothered by the child's behavior but were unaware of what caused it. (p. 232)

Professionals interested in the area of profound retardation need to address the issue of labeling carefully. It certainly appears that consolidating research from the many different disciplines that have information relevant to profound retardation (e.g., medicine, psychology, speech, physical therapy, education, genetics, neurology, biochemistry) would be facilitated if reliable diagnostic labels were used. If the opponents of labeling become too vociferous, research efforts could be damaged or slowed. However, an unthinking use of labels, especially during discussions of research findings with the general public, could also have some very negative effects. There is always the danger that the diagnostic label could lead people to believe that these persons are incapable of learning and, thus, deny research and therapeutic services to these individuals. Being able to label one group may also open the door to the labeling of other groups who could suffer negative consequences from it. For example, if it is allowable to label a person profoundly retarded, some might view it permissible to label another person profoundly mentally ill. Thus, if labeling is allowed in order to promote studies and advocacy issues, research persons in these areas have a strong obligation to use the labels in the most judicious and nonharmful manner possible.

Informed Consent and Other Regulations

A third procedural issue relates to whether current governmental regulations such as those related to informed consent are so stringent that they preclude certain types of research with persons who are profoundly handicapped.

Current guidelines for research using human subjects require informed consent from participants before the research study can be conducted (Federal

Register, 1981; National Commission for the Protection of Human Subjects of Biomedical and Behavioral Research, 1977). Within these consent procedures is also the proviso that the subject has the right to discontinue being a part of the study at any time. Informed consent has three essential elements (Lowe & Alexander, 1981): 1) communication of adequate information, 2) a subject capable of understanding it, and 3) a subject who voluntarily decides to become a part of a study after being told what is to be done and why.

Given the pervasive difficulties that persons with profound retardation display in the areas of receptive communication, expressive communication, self-awareness, and cognitive skills, it seems quite clear that it would be difficult to achieve informed consent from members of this population. Thus, if research is to be conducted with this group, a way around this procedural issue must be found.

It should be pointed out that the major purpose of informed consent is not to protect the subjects from harm as many laypersons suppose. Subject protection is the responsibility of the investigator and the peer review processes (Lowe & Alexander, 1981). Rather, the purpose of informed consent is to respect the person's status as a human being by ensuring that he or she has the right of choice. Certainly, informed consent is not the only way to ensure that a subject's personhood is respected. This author and several other ethicists and researchers (Cleland, 1979; Kane, Robbins, & Stanley, 1982; Lowe & Alexander, 1981) feel that informed consent is not so all-important that without it research opportunities for those populations who may be most in need of its potential benefits must be denied. Lowe and Alexander (1981) state that:

> In our opinion, society should demonstrate its concern for such people [people who clearly could never give informed consent] by devising means to permit research while still providing them with adequate protection, rather than allowing the unavailability of informed consent to prevent research that may ultimately help the subjects themselves or others with the same disorder. (p. 117)

Some researchers have used parental consent to allow those persons who are unable to give informed consent (e.g., infants, persons with severe or profound retardation, persons with severe mental illness) to participate in research. Although this is a common practice, its appropriateness and legality are controversial (Keith-Spiegel, 1983; Lewis, McCollum, Schwartz, & Grunt, 1969). One argument against parental consent is that a parent's interests may not be a reflection of the child's interests. Another argument is that parental consent opens the doors for abuse of the informed consent regulation with other populations. For example, it is unclear exactly where to draw the line between persons with mental retardation who could give informed consent and those who could not.

It has also been suggested that using impartial advocates as opposed to obtaining parental consent could be done in various stages of research being conducted with subjects who could not give informed consent (Pryce, 1978). This may, or may not, be a viable avenue; however, it appears to have the same problems as parental consent.

Also clouding the issue of consent is the fact that persons who are profoundly retarded may be less able than nonhandicapped or less handicapped persons to express a desire to stop participating in a study. If a person with a profound handicap cries, tantrums, or is self-abusive during the study and these behaviors are, in some degree, a normal part of the student's repertoire, these behaviors may not be regarded as expressions of dissatisfaction about what is being done to, or required of, him or her. In fact, these responses may be explained by some researchers as characteristic responses to the experimental procedure (e.g., an extinction burst). However, if the child's rights are being protected by an advocate, but the advocate is unaware that this child's behavior repertoire includes behaviors like these, the advocate might have the child released from the research on the basis of discomfort or unhappiness that actually has no basis in fact. If research is to be conducted with human subjects who are profoundly retarded, it is important that "informed consent" become more than a procedural step. Researchers must look behind the paperwork and the rote aspects of the procedure and ensure that the intent of the regulation (i.e., showing respect for the participant by allowing as much choice as possible) is met.

Communications among Professionals

Another serious procedural issue revolves around professional communication. The question can be asked, "Are professionals who are interested in the area of profound retardation accumulating and communicating information in a way that promotes systematic interdisciplinary research?"

In the initial stages of investigating any new area, there are usually isolated groups of people who are working on some aspects of the problem. However, regardless of how innovative or well-designed these investigations are, it is unlikely that great strides will be made until the different investigators and theorists come together and begin to systematically map out the subtopics and the relationships among the subtopics that need to be investigated. Research in the area of profound retardation currently appears to be at the isolated, individualistic level. It is unlikely that research with an individualistic focus will expand into large-scale effort that would produce widespread results until: 1) there is more communication with persons who are trying to deal with problems related to profound retardation on a day-to-day basis, 2) there is open communication of the results of innovative therapies without regard to scientific rigor, 3) there is both an acceptance and method for reporting negative results as well as successful outcomes and, 4) one or more scientists decide to correlate information across several disciplines in an attempt to obtain an overall picture of the issue. Once these factors occur and the project reaches financial stability, specific research foci can be designated and groups of scientists can then begin to look into each of these areas in depth.

An example of how this process works is well illustrated by the Acquired Immune Deficiency Syndrome (AIDS) research. In the late 1970s, little was known about AIDS; however, through communications in journal articles and at medical symposiums, several physicians discovered that they had patients with the same symptomology. This problem was quite serious because all of these physicians' patients were dying. The doctors, upon discovering the common ground, began to communicate among themselves. There were no formal studies run, just passing of information about what seemed to be working or what they were trying and why. As more publicity was generated, more and more physicians became part of this communication network and researchers became interested in the problem. The researchers took the information generated by the practitioners and developed theories and studies. The practitioners and researchers began to collaborate, passing on their tales of failure as well as success. Initially, most of the effort focused on treatment, but it soon became clear that finding a treatment might depend on an understanding of the cause. Investigators in the areas of sociology (who gets the disease), immunology (how is the disease related to what is already known about the immune system), and serology (how does the disease develop) became interested and each group contributed their knowledge. Prevention was another important subtopic of interest and researchers in epidemilogy, health education, and vaccine production became a part of the total research picture.

In spite of the diversity of professionals investigating AIDS, the field was still small enough that the researchers were aware of one another and interested in each other's findings. Thus, from attempts to treat, encouragement of innovative therapies, open communication between practioners, development of theories, research based upon the most promising theories, and continued communication between many disciplines, research into the AIDS virus has grown in a systematic approach with well-defined objectives.

The science of profound retardation is in the early stages of attempting to treat, just as AIDS research was when it first began to address the problem. There are really no documented "best-practices" for the treatment of persons with profound disabilities. Everything teachers, parents, or therapists do with persons from this population is experimental. Certainly the steps they choose to take are based upon procedures that they have implemented with persons with similar characteristics. However, until the results of these treatments are solicited across disciplines and communication among these persons is facilitated and utilized by research scientists to develop specific research foci, the field will continue to be disorganized and without direction. Professionals must carefully examine current practices in journals and in professional symposia and conventions to be sure that opportunity for developing systematic research still exists. Professionals must see if their demands for scientific rigor cut off communication from persons who directly care for individuals and who are trying new and different procedures; whether their persistence in only publicizing successful treatments leads to a false sense of security; and whether current symposia, conventions, publications, and professional behavior encourage divergent and interdisciplinary thinking. Lastly, professionals must recognize that successful research does not come from scattered individual studies in disconnected areas; but rather, it comes from concerted efforts to build a "big picture" together.

Paradoxical Attitudes

There is a basic paradox in the attitudes of professionals who deal with persons who are handicapped. This paradox will have a significant effect upon what type of research is conducted. Professionals value persons with disabilities regardless of the severity of their handicaps. This belief that persons, even with profound disabilities, have value has most recently manifested itself in the outrage expressed by professionals, parents, and advocacy groups when they learned that some members of the medical profession were denying treatment to certain infants with handicaps based upon the premise that these children would have a poor "quality of life" and were better off dead (cf., TASH Resolution, 1983). However, valuing an individual implies that there is respect for that individual. Downie and Telfer (1980) declare that respect implies "an active sympathy with their [the valued person's] projects. . . . Sometimes this requires us to give positive assistance, to make another person's ends our own ends, and sometimes it means standing back and allowing them to do what they want" (p. 38). Furthermore, the attitude of respect requires a recognition that the other person may have values that may differ significantly from that of the professional, and, thus, aims and needs may also vary (Downie, 1985). One thing is clear as professionals think about persons (or even objects) that they truly value—they do not try to change these persons (or things) into something else.

Although many interventionists profess to value the individual with handicaps (and this author believes that this is done sincerely), people in the helping professions paradoxically support two efforts that are almost diametrically opposed to "valuing." One of these efforts is the support of screening programs and efforts to prevent handicapping conditions. As noted by Wikler (1980):

> It takes considerable rhetorical agility to urge the public to support screening programs so as to prevent the conception of handicapped individuals while at the same time insisting that full respect be paid to such developmentally disabled adults as are already among us. (p. 2)

Some professionals have already begun to see this paradox and are actively withdrawing their support from screening and prenatal diagnosis.

The second paradoxical effort has received far less attention. This effort deals with helping professions, especially those concerned with special education, therapy, and behavior change, that have as a main goal changing the behavior or skills of the person with handicaps. Not only is the focus on change, but it is on changing persons with handicaps to be more like "normal" people. This is not a new phenomenon; however, it is one that has seemingly increased in strength as the ideas of community-based education, community-based vocational training, functional skill training, and social validation procedures have been increasingly promoted by professional groups and parent organizations. The benefit that persons with handicaps derive from education is increasingly being equated with the acquisition of skills that will allow the individual to function more independently (albeit, in many cases, with only partial participation or with less than fully developed skills) in vocational, community, and home settings.

If research is to focus on devising successful methods of teaching "functional skills," then it is important to determine just what are functional skills (Brown, Helmstetter, & Guess, 1986). Does a functional skill or behavior provide an outcome that is meaningful to the person who is disabled or to others in the environment? The current push for social validity suggests that researchers are currently putting more emphasis on outcomes that are meaningful to others. This trend is not new. Cleland (1979) noted that:

> . . . at gut level we know that even if we teach the ambulatory profoundly mentally retarded to deposit their body wastes in the proper "bank," such a self-help skill addresses only a lower order need, *and* one that they themselves, could they articulate their desires, might reckon a rather silly waste of time. While few could deny the importance of sanitation practices, this writer would venture that we teach toileting with great zeal principally to serve our own ingrained social overlearnings. (p. 39)

The normalization viewpoint may also cause professionals to punish or try to eradicate some behaviors that society views as unacceptable but that may be quite pleasant to the individual or effective in gaining his or her desired ends (i.e., behaviors that are functional for that individual). For example, there is little doubt that rumination is a very unpleasant looking and unusual behavior, but such behavior can be much more effective in ending tasks that he or she does not wish to perform than the more socially acceptable verbalization, "I don't want to do this anymore!". Given that it may take 3 or more years to teach the child to be able to perform a more socially acceptable behavior (or a simpler form of it), and that it may be a less effective tool for getting what the child wants, teachers are put in the position of eliminating behaviors that are already functional and replacing them with those that are less functional, though more acceptable. Given the state of the art of education for persons with profound handicaps (e.g., professionals still don't know how to teach them very fast or very well), continuing to eliminate such socially unacceptable behaviors without being able to replace them with equally functional skills could leave the "educated" person with profound retardation worse off than before he or she was "helped." Many people might argue that eliminating the rumination would be functional because more people would be willing to come into contact with the child, thus expanding the child's opportunities to interact with others and learn new skills. But, if the child must be dehumanized in order to eliminate the rumination, then what? Does the focus on changing the child lead to behaviors that are diametrically opposed to valuing the person as an individual, with needs and desires of his or her own?

The paradox described above lies at the heart of all research that is conducted because where scientists choose to focus their efforts depends upon what they really believe. If professionals believe that to be happy and have a good quality of life, a person must be able to partake in the rituals of job, housework, shopping, keeping oneself neat and clean, and taking care not to offend others, then research efforts must focus on ways to achieve these goals and/or on prevention of handicapping conditions if these prevent even partial attainment of these goals. If professionals believe that other things make up a quality and pleasant life, then research efforts should focus on delineating what these things are, whether persons who are handicapped currently have these things, and if not, how such things could be attained. In such research, professionals may find that research needs to focus on the ways society should and could be altered to accommodate the needs of individuals who are disabled, rather than on ways to teach these individuals could adapt to society (cf. Blatt & Biklen, 1986; Gold, 1972).

If, however, researchers and "helping" professionals wish to stand behind the value of these individuals, *as they are*, not as they wish to change them to be, then research might need to focus more on what type of impact these individuals may have on others, how persons with profound handicaps develop the skills they do, and what needs their current behaviors fulfill. From the answers to these questions, services might evolve that are very different in nature from present intervention efforts.

CURRENT AND FUTURE RESEARCH EFFORTS

The two major research efforts in the field of profound retardation are in the areas of biomedical research and research in habilitation and education. The types of research conducted in these two areas do not focus on the same questions or work from a similar set of values. The biomedical research focuses primarily on prevention. The habilitation work focuses on changing the individual who is handicapped so that he or she can become better integrated into society. The profound retardation field would probably be better served if researchers in the two areas could jointly formulate questions and research projects.

Biomedical Research

Biomedical research that is applicable to the field of profound retardation can be divided into three large subgroups. First, there is research that seeks to define the symptoms and causes of particular syndromes in the hope that these types of information will lead to specific treatments. The gene mapping (determining exactly which genes on a chromosome are responsible for a particular trait) techniques used with syndromes such as "Fragile-X" and Lesch-Nyhan are examples of this type of research. Currently, most of this research is still at the level of determining syndromes and etiology; however, there is hope that continued research will indeed lead to effective treatments. Opponents of this type of research point to the fact that increasing the ability to identify syndromes through techniques such as amniocentesis and gene mapping in the absence of proven treatments has led to a program of prevention through abortion. Aside from the moral issues surrounding abortion, there are very realistic fears that the ease of prevention in this manner may lead researchers astray from the goal of developing therapies, since abortion is less expensive and far more simple than developing innovative therapeutics.

A second area of research, behavioral neuroscience, looks at the processes of growth in the developing central nervous system and examines exactly how the central nervous system works. It is possible that progress in behavioral neuroscience will lead to treatments that will allow professionals to affect development that is going awry or to induce the nervous system to compensate for developmental deviations. The work by Kastin and Sandman (1983) that investigates the role of peptides in mental retardation, the research by West and Del Cerro (1976) that maps the migration of cerebellar Purkinje cells, the study by Rosenzweig and Bennett (1976) on the role that environmental enrichment can play in actually modifying the central nervous system, and the field work of neurologists (Bjorklund, Johansson, Stenevi, & Svendgaard, 1975; Lynch, 1983) who are studying axonal regeneration, are all examples of biomedical research efforts that may benefit mankind by preventing or ameliorating certain handicapping conditions. One of the drawbacks of such research is that it is slow and expensive. It is basic research and as such is often ignored or seen as not useful to those individuals who must deal with persons who are handicapped on a day-to-day basis. Furthermore, such research presently depends on experiments conducted with live animals. Whether such research is seen as valuable enough to override the concerns of those persons who are opposed to the use of living creatures as subjects will be fought out in the political arena.

The third area of research seeks to develop drugs, surgery, transplants, or implants that will compensate for, or replace, damaged and missing structures, hormones, and enzymes. One type of research being conducted in this area that has led to much controversy is genetic engineering. Genetic engineering refers to techniques whereby the genetic material from one organism is combined with that of another organism in order to produce a selected trait (Kegley, 1985). When genetic engineering is performed on the germ-cells (e.g., a sperm, an egg), the desirable trait can be passed on to the next generation. This technique, combined with the development of gene mapping, *in vitro* fertilization (i.e., fertilization of an egg outside the mother's body), and successful pregnancies resulting from the implantation of an egg that was fertilized *in vitro,* has given researchers the technology needed to prevent certain handicapping conditions. Biomedical research is now at a point where it will soon be possible to remove eggs and sperm from two potential parents, examine them to see if there are any known defects, replace the defective material, fertilize the egg, and implant it with the realistic expectation that the end result will be a healthy child (Laura, 1985). Although this scenario is full of promises, many are still fearful of such a process.

There are many concerned scientists and laypersons forming alliances to put pressure on politicians to call a moratorium on genetic engineering and similar research. Objections to such genetic tinkering can be put forth on the grounds of safety (i.e., what are the long-term ramifications of these techniques?), on moral and religious grounds (i.e., should researchers play God?), and on ethical grounds. Even if genetic engineering is used for the purposes of preventing serious handicapping conditions, it will still raise many issues that should be of concern to professionals who are interested in persons with handicaps. Laura (1985) lists three of these issues: 1) utilization of these techniques presupposes that handicaps are a sign of inferiority and should be prevented; 2) the more able researchers are to prevent handicaps, the less likely society is to be tolerant of those that exist, and will continue to exist since these techniques will not prevent mutations or handicaps caused by prenatal or perinatal factors; and 3) the questions of what defects are, and what defects will be eliminated, depends on who is doing the defining and the eliminating. This being the case, it is entirely possible that progressively more and more traits would come to be regarded as defects.

Similar controversies surround the areas of organ transplantation, fetal surgery, and drug therapy. With this era of new techniques such controversial issues must be addressed.

Research in Habilitation and Education

Research in habilitation and education is necessary if students with handicaps are to continue to increase their skills, improve their motor functioning, and gain control of their environments. For the most complete information, research efforts must look at all parts of the habilitation/education paradigm, including: 1) researching the developmental process and how it progresses in persons with profound retardation, 2) determining the degree to which an adapted environment is necessary to help the child gain and maintain functional skills, 3) deciding whether the break down of skills into smaller segments is a necessary and useful strategy, 4) pinpointing the types of behaviors that are common among persons with profound retardation and the possible functions that these behaviors might serve, 5) determining the types of stimuli that motivate or capture the attention of persons who are profoundly retarded, 6) establishing methodologies that are effective in teaching new skills to this population, and 7) applying accurate and useful measurement systems that help determine whether change in the desired direction is occurring.

Developmental Process   Research into the typical developmental processes of persons with profound retardation would be of great interest and could serve to direct other research efforts. Just as Gold and Barclay's research (1973) showing that students with severe handicaps generated typical learning curves when acquiring a new skill (although the skill was learned at a far slower rate), gave impetus to the demand for vocational education for persons with mental retardation, so might information about the development and learning of this population serve as a guide for assessment and services. It has been said that persons who are handicapped may develop skills in sequences quite different from those developmental sequences delineated for nonhandicapped persons. The relationship between the skills may also be quite different (Brown, 1987). However, with the exception of research conducted by Guess, Rues, Warren, and Lyon (1980), there appears to have been very little research done in this area since the late 1970s.

Enabling Environmental Factors   The effect of the environment on the development of behavior has been recognized and investigated in varying ways since professionals began using behavior analysis as a rehabilitation tool. The search for the most enabling environment appears to have been split into three different categories. Some investigators have focused on the effects of certain aspects of the environment upon the child's spontaneous behavior. Examples of this type of work include: Hutt and Viazey's (1966) research into the effects of group size on the peer interactions of autistic children, and Walker et al. (1985) work on the effects of structured leisure activities on the maladaptive behaviors of institutionalized adults. Another group of investigators has looked at the feasibility of designing adaptive environments that are more easily manipulated than "normal" environments. For example, Sayre and McKelvey (1983) designed an environment for persons who are profoundly handicapped where simple movements would activate lights, noises, toys, and other stimulating events. The furniture was adapted so that it was less likely to produce destructive behavior and more likely to elicit exploration. This environment, although quite effective in encouraging exploration and interaction among the subjects, was quite different from the living environments of nonhandicapped persons. Thus, this research was critisized by Hutchins and Renzaglia (1983) who felt that this environment was so artificial that it hindered the participants from ever achieving a less restrictive environment, and that the cost of such adaptations was so high that the cost-benefit ratio could not be defended. Sayre and McKelvey (1983) responded to this criticism as follows:

> First of all, just what is "normalization"? Are we to work for the appearance of environmental normality (e.g., the living room looks like mine at home) or should we concentrate on the essence of what society at large considers a "normal" life-

style? We would like to suggest that such an essence is made of two terms . . . autonomy and choice. (p. 72)

The last group of researchers investigating enabling environments has been concentrating on whether community environments are intrinsically more enabling than more restrictive environments. Research of this type is exemplified by the work of Sokol-Kesslu, Conroy, Feinstein, Lemanowicz, and McGubbin (1983) who used matched subjects to measure the differences in adaptive and maladaptive behaviors in clients who were institutionalized and those who lived in group homes.

Task Analysis Breaking skills down into their component parts for training (i.e., task analysis), has proven to be a successful strategy in improving the learning for many persons in the handicapped populations. For example, if a child with mental retardation has difficulty learning to brush his teeth, breaking the skill down and teaching each step separately can make the child's learning more effective. It is possible that more refined and detailed task analyses would be useful in educating persons with profound handicaps.

In the area of communication, for example, current efforts to teach individuals with profound retardation have resulted, at best, in increasing the number of vocalizations, repeated failures in shaping these vocalizations into verbalizations, or the learning of utterances that can only be elicited under very specific conditions. It is not clear whether this failure is because professionals have not broken these skills down enough, whether they have not paid enough attention to eliciting stimuli, or whether such efforts are doomed to failure and the time would be better spent learning the lexicon of persons with profound handicaps. It appears that research could help answer these questions. Those who wish to pursue a more refined task analysis might begin by exploring the implications of some of the infant communication research. For example, Langlois, Baken, and Wilder (1980) have investigated prespeech respiratory behavior during an infant's first year of life. These researchers noted that an infant must learn special breathing patterns to support vocalization, and that these are significantly different from breathing patterns that simply sustain life. They noted that breathing patterns that simply sustain life do not allow the infant to store enough air to make either a long or low-pitched vocalization. However, crying seems to incorporate a breathing pattern that is much closer to a speech pattern and, thus, may serve two important functions: 1) signaling another to take care of his or her needs, and 2) establishing a breathing pattern conducive to speech at a time when there is likely to be someone around who might shape speech sounds.

Another area of infant research that might lead to new insights into the skills that need to be taught if vocalizations are to be shaped into verbalizations deals with the temporal regularity of prespeech vocalizations. These studies (e.g., Delack, 1975; Laufer, 1978, 1980; Oller, 1979) indicate that the duration and spacing of vocalizations and protosyllable utterances are extremely important in the development of verbalization. The fact that temporal regularity seems to be programmed by the central nervous system may give some insights into why it has been so difficult to shape the vocalizations of individuals who are profoundly handicapped into verbalizations. In habilitative efforts, it may be of as much importance to reinforce appropriate temporal patterns as it is to focus on shaping the vocalizations toward recognizable protosyllables and syllables.

Those persons who lean toward the theory that a better analysis of eliciting stimuli might prove productive in enhancing spontaneous speech might use research on caregiver-infant interactions as a starting place. Several studies (Stern, 1974; Stern, Beebe, Jaffe, & Bennett, 1977; Stern & Gibbon, 1979) have illustrated the importance of the temporal aspects of maintaining mother-infant social interactions. Since many children with profound handicaps are essentially nonresponsive, it is probable that caregiver-child interactions are curtailed since the caregiver is not reinforced for using typical interactive patterns. Similar studies between persons with profound handicaps and significant others in their environment might be deemed valuable in providing leads into non-traditional, spontaneous communications that occur and lead to new directions in habilitative efforts. Work in this area has already begun with persons who are deaf-blind (Siegel-Causey & Guess, in press).

Behavior and Its Functions Valuable information might be gleaned from studies conducted in the behavior analytic tradition where spontaneous behaviors are observed and the antecedent and consequent events are recorded and analyzed to determine if there are consistent relationships. Although this information can be used to build more effective teaching programs, it is an equally valuable tool for determining the functions of behavior. The following studies are examples of this type of research. One is the study conducted by Favell, McGimsey, and Schell (1982) that indicated that sensory reinforcement was the underlying reason for certain self-stimulatory and self-injurious acts, and that by providing alternative activities that stimulated the same senses, the reinforcement could, in fact, reduce the maladaptive behavior. The second study deals with the function of self-injurious behavior. This study was conducted by Iwata, Dorsey, Slifer, Bauman, and Richman (1982). These investigators conclusively showed that self-injurious behavior could have at least three different functions. They also illustrated that it was possible to determine which function the behavior had for a particular student. Although both of these examples focus on maladaptive behavior, there is no reason that similar research could not be conducted on spontaneous adaptive behavior.

Motivation and Attention The difficulty in teaching persons with profound retardation lies, in part, in the fact that many of these individuals seem unresponsive to typical instructional materials and reinforcers. Whether this nonresponsiveness is a direct result of nervous system damage, of learned helplessness, or of poor choices of materials and reinforcers is not clear. Research that looks at each of these alternatives and specific remediation methods would be valuable.

One such area of research has been proposed by Rainforth (1982). She suggests that studying the biobehavioral state cycles of children who are profoundly handicapped with varying behavioral characteristics would: 1) help identify the quiet, alert state (i.e., a condition associated with learning in infants) in persons in whom it may be difficult to recognize; 2) help identify patterns of neurological organization and disorganization and how these differ from the patterns seen in nonhandicapped infants; and 3) allow researchers to study the influence of different stimuli upon the biobehavioral state of persons with unusual neurological organization patterns.

Similarly, studies such as those detailing the effect of body contact and vestibular-proprioceptive stimulation on the visual alerting of premature infants (Gregg, Haffner, & Korner, 1976; Korner, 1979; Korner & Thoman, 1970) are instructive both in their findings that might be applicable to persons with profound retardation, and in the thorough and sensitive way they analyzed vestibular-proprioceptive stimulation in an attempt to develop a system that would be maximally effective without overwhelming the immature nervous system of the fragile organism. For example, when Korner (1979) studied the effect of waterbed motion on apnea (i.e., not breathing) episodes experienced by preterm infants, the following aspects of motion were analyzed in terms of their possible effect on the newborn: the direction of the oscillations, the intensity of oscillations (i.e., size of the wave and rise time), the regularity and temporal patterns of the motion, the length of time that the stimulation should be applied, and the similarities of the stimulation with what the infant might be experiencing if he or she were still in utero. Similar attention to all of the variables that make up the types of stimulation presented to individuals who are profoundly handicapped must be the norm, rather than the exception, if appropriate modes of promoting attention and neurological organization are to be determined. This is especially true if the child is to respond in the best manner possible to complex, natural environments.

Perception of contingency relationships is another research area that may be critical to providing better educational services to persons with profound handicaps. Learning depends upon the individual being able to see relationships between events (i.e., when A happens, then B happens). Behaviorists have proposed that perfect contingencies (i.e., when A happens B inevitably occurs) enhance learning by making the relationship between the events easier to perceive. Contingency relationships can be modified by having the consequence fail to occur on some occasions after the first event takes place (i.e., intermittent reinforcement) or by having the "consequence" occur independently of the response (i.e., noncontingent reinforcement). Researchers such as Seligman (1975) and Watson (1979) have shown conclusively that when an individual fails to perceive a contingency between his or her behavior and some recurrent stimulation, then the ability to perceive contingencies in later situations will be impaired even if the relationship is then perfectly contingent and obvious.

It appears likely that persons with profound handicaps receive frequent intermittent and noncontingent reinforcement because of the nature of their disabilities. For example, the deficits in responsiveness, communication, and social skills make it more likely that others will provide for them and stimulate them noncontingently. The damaged motor and perceptual systems that often accompany profound retardation also make it likely that attempts to do things will "pay off" only intermittently. If these suppositions are true, then the research cited above leads researchers to predict that these individuals would have difficulty perceiving contingency relationships. Further research could be conducted to examine how to make response-contingency relationships more perfect for these children and whether doing so at an early age makes a difference in their abilities to focus on, and learn from, the environment.

Research on the effects of different types of stimulation and potentially reinforcing events needs to continue. The presence of central nervous system damage in many persons who are profoundly handicapped may have an effect on the types of stimulation that are perceived as most pleasant or meaningful. These persons may be more sensitive to olfactory, tactile, and vestibular-proprioceptive stimuli since these are more primitive senses that are of relevance in utero. In nonhandicapped infants, the vestibular system develops and matures early during fetal life ($9\frac{1}{2}$ weeks); therefore, this system may be more intact than the visual and taste systems that develop relatively later. Similarly, the olfactory system is hidden deep within the brain, making it somewhat less open to assault or damage during the later stages of pregnancy and birth. Knowing which systems are the most relevant and functional to the person with profound handicaps may help researchers to decide which environments might be best at any given time for catching the child's attention and providing interesting feedback. For example, repeated visits to a bakery shop might be more motivating than visits to a video arcade to a child who is more sensitive to odors than to auditory or visual stimulation.

Innovative Methodologies   Research must continue in its effort to develop procedures and methods that result in learning and a better life for persons diagnosed as profoundly retarded. Current research efforts that are attempting to devise effective, nonaversive techniques for decreasing maladaptive behavior should be continued. Similarly, new techniques for developing communication, motor, leisure, and social skills should continue and be expanded.

Measurement Systems   With persons who are profoundly handicapped, there may be a need to develop measurement systems that are more sophisticated technologically and that allow researchers to measure discrete, physiological responses. Unfortunately, the use of such methodologies requires some type of trade-off between the desire to keep the child in as natural a state as possible and the need for systems that can provide various types of information that may make the child's interaction with natural environments more productive.

Current reliance on measurement systems that depend strictly on an observer visually or auditorally monitoring voluntary responses results in a significant disadvantage when it comes to studying and teaching persons with profound retardation. Many measurement systems designed for infant research have relied on physiological measurement. It is possible that similar measurement techniques would enhance the effectiveness of habilitation and education with persons with profound retardation.

One such system that seems particularly applicable to persons with profound retardation is the use of the habituation paradigm to study perception and discrimination. This paradigm depends upon an apparent physiological mechanism that allows persons to be more sensitive to novel stimuli than to familiar stimuli (Sokolov, 1963). The research was conducted on infants' cognitive development and discrimination. In this study, the researcher presents one stimulus (e.g., the mother's face) for several trials. Initially, the child looks at the stimulus fairly steadily, but as it is repeated, he or she becomes "habituated" and pays less attention. At this point, the researcher presents a different stimulus (e.g., a stranger's face). If the child looks at this stimulus longer than he did the last few presentations of the habituated stimulus, the child has demonstrated discrimination between those two stimuli. Naturally, appropriate control procedures are necessary to support the inference of discrimination (See Cohen & Gelber, 1975, for a detailed description of appropriate control procedures.)

This paradigm has been used with infants to study the discrimination of shape (Cooke, Birch, & Griffiths, 1986), the concept of same versus different (Caron & Caron, 1981), and the discrimination of vocal sounds (Walker-Andrews, 1983), to mention just a few areas. Switzky, Woolsey-Hill, and Quoss (1979) demonstrated the utility of the habituation paradigm with children who were nonverbal, and profoundly handicapped, giving researchers a tool that could be used to measure the acquisition of receptive language, concepts, and perception in children who are nonverbal and motorically handicapped. Unfortunately, researchers and practitioners have not built on this initial effort.

Sonographic and spectographic analysis might be a valuable tool for persons interested in shaping vocalizations, since these types of technology could give quick and very accurate feedback to the practitioner on whether a vocalization is close, in all dimensions, to the desired sound. It would certainly be more precise than relying on the human ear. Many studies have already been conducted using these tools to analyze the cries of nonhandicapped infants and infants with various disabilities for diagnostic purposes (cf. Karelitz, Karelitz,

& Rosenfeld, 1960; Michelsson & Wasz-Hockert, 1980). However, little research has been conducted to determine if such analyses could enhance therapeutic efforts.

If research is to use sophisticated and expensive tools for measurement, there must be some hope that the information can be used by practitioners. Whether society will support the use of such tools in educational settings and whether professionals will find ways to use such tools to enhance training in natural environments remains to be seen; however, current trends are not encouraging.

SUMMARY

Research efforts in the area of profound retardation have been diverse and fragmented. There are many reasons for this. Some of these are procedural and ethical issues such as questions of homogeneity, the appropriateness of labeling, rules regulating the way in which research is to be conducted with human subjects, and the effect of culturally ingrained beliefs on the delivery of human services. If a systematic research focus is to be attained for persons with profound retardation, then some of these issues will need to be resolved. It appears that if research is to be done with this population, much of it will be conducted in the areas of biomedical and habilitation and education research. These areas are discussed and suggestions are offered in an effort to produce current research efforts that serve as models or starting points for research that is related to individuals with profound retardation.

REFERENCES

Björklund, A., Johansson, B., Stenevi, U., & Svendgaard, N. (1975). Reestablishment of functional connections by regenerating central adrenergic and cholenergic axons. *Nature* (London), 253, 446–448.

Blatt, B., & Biklen D. (1986). Ethics. In J. Wortis (Ed.), *Mental retardation and developmental disabilities* (Vol. XIV, pp. 109–134). New York: Elsevier/North Holland.

Brown, F. (1987). Meaningful assessment of people with severe and profound handicaps. In M.E. Snell (Ed.), *Systematic instruction of persons with severe handicaps* (pp. 39–63). Columbus, OH: Charles E. Merrill.

Brown F., Helmstetter, E., & Guess, D. (1986). *Current best practices with students with profound disabilities: Are there any?* Unpublished manuscript, Institute of Professional Practice, New Haven, CT.

Caron, A., & Caron, R. (1981). Processing of relational information as an index of infant risk. In S. Friedman & M. Sigman (Eds.), *Preterm birth and psychological development* (pp. 219–240). New York: Academic Press.

Cleland, C. (1979). *The profoundly mentally retarded.* Englewood Cliffs, NJ: Prentice-Hall.

Cohen, L.B., & Gelber, E.R. (1975). Infant visual memory. In L.B. Cohen & P. Salapatek (Eds.), *Infant perception: From sensation to cognition* (Vol. 1, pp. 347–403). New York: Academic Press.

Cooke, M., Birch, R., & Griffiths, K. (1986). Discrimination between solid forms in early infancy. *Infant Behavior and Development, 9,* 189–202.

Delack, J.B. (1975). *Prosodic features of infant speech: The first year of life.* Paper presented at the Eighth International Congress of Phonetic Sciences, Leeds, England.

Downie, R.S. (1985). Ambivalence of attitude toward the mentally retarded. In R.S. Laura & A.F. Ashman (Eds.), *Moral issues in mental retardation* (pp. 29–42). Dover, NH: Croom Helm.

Downie, R.S., & Telfer, E. (1980). *Caring and curing: A philosophy of medicine and social work.* London: Methuen.

Favell, J.E., McGimsey, J.F., & Schell, R.M. (1982). Treatment of self-injury by providing alternate sensory activities. *Analysis and Intervention in Developmental Disabilities, 2*(3), 83–104.

Federal Register. (January 26, 1981). *Final regulations amending basic HHS policy for the protection of human research subjects.* Washington, DC: Department of Health and Human Services.

Fernald, C.D., & Gettys, L. (1980). Diagnostic labels and perceptions of children's behavior. *Journal of Clinical Child Psychology, 9*(3), 229–233.

Gold, M.W. (1972). *An adaptive behavior: Who needs it?* (rev. paper). Chicago: Proceedings of the National Association of Superintendents of Public Residential Facilities Region V Interaction Workshop on Community Living for Institutionalized Retardates.

Gold, M.W., & Barclay, C.R. (1973). The learning of difficult visual discriminations by the moderately and severely retarded. *Mental Retardation, 11*(2), 9–11.

Gregg, C.L., Haffner, M.E., & Korner, A.F. (1976). The relative efficacy of vestibular-proprioceptive stimulation and the upright position in enhancing visual pursuit in neonates. *Child Development, 47,* 309–314.

Guess, D., Rues, J., Warren, S., & Lyon, S. (1980). *Quantitative assessment of motor and sensory/motor acquisition in handicapped and nonhandicapped infants and young children: Volume 1: Assessment procedures for selected developmental milestones.* Lawrence: University of Kansas, Early Childhood Handicapped Institute. (ECI Document No. 255)

Hobbs, N. (1975). *The futures of children.* San Francisco: Jossey-Bass.

Hutchins, M.P., & Renzaglia, A. (1983). Environmental considerations for severely handicapped individuals: The needs and the questions. *Exceptional Education Quarterly, 4*(2), 67–71.

Hutt, C., & Viazey, J.M. (1966). Differential effects of group density on social behavior. *Nature, 209,* 1371–1372.

Iwata, B.A., Dorsey, M.F., Slifer, K.J., Bauman, K.E., & Richman, G.S. (1982). Toward a functional analysis of self-injury. *Analysis and Intervention in Developmental Disabilities, 2*(3), 3–20.

Kane, J.M., Robbins, L.L., & Stanley, B. (1982). Psychiatric research. In R.A. Greenwald, M.K. Ryan, & J.E. Mulvihill (Eds.), *Human subjects research: A handbook for institutional review boards* (pp. 193–205). New York: Plenum.

Karelitz, S., Karelitz, R.F., & Rosenfeld, L.S. (1960). Infants' vocalizations and their significance. In P.W. Bowman & H.V. Mautner (Eds.), *Mental retardation* (pp. 439–446). New York: Grune & Stratton.

Kastin, A.J., & Sandman, C.A. (1983). Possible role of peptides in mental retardation. In F.J. Menolascino, R. Neman, & J.A. Stark (Eds.), *Curative aspects of mental retardation: Biomedical and behavioral advances* (pp. 147–164). Baltimore: Paul H. Brookes Publishing Co.

Kegley, J.A. (1985). Genetics and mental retardation. In R.S. Laura & A.F. Ashman (Eds.), *Moral issues in mental retardation* (pp. 161–183). Dover, NH: Croom Helm.

Keith-Spiegel, P. (1983). Children and consent to participate in research. In G.B. Melton, G.P. Koocher, & M.J. Saks (Eds.), *Children's competence to consent* (pp. 179–211). New York: Plenum.

Korner, A.F. (1979). Maternal rhythms and waterbeds: A form of intervention with premature infants. In E.B. Thoman (Ed.), *Origin of the infant's social responsiveness* (pp. 95–124). Hillsdale, NJ: Laurence Erlbaum Associates.

Korner, A.F., & Thoman, E.B. (1970). Visual alertness in neonates as evoked by maternal care. *Journal of Experimental Psychology, 10,* 67–78.

Korner, A.F., & Thoman, E.B. (1972). The relative efficacy of contact and vestibular stimulation in soothing neonates. *Child Development, 43*(2), 443–453.

Langlois, A., Baken, R.J., & Wilder, C.N. (1980). Pre-speech respiratory behavior during the first year of life. In T. Murray & J. Murray (Eds.), *Infant communication: Cry and early speech* (pp. 56–105). Houston, TX: College-Hill Press.

Laufer, M.Z. (1978). Infant voice. *The seventh symposium on care of the professional voice, Part II: Life span changes in the human voice* (pp. 13–22). New York: The Voice Foundation.

Laufer, M.Z. (1980). Temporal regularity in prespeech. In T. Murray & J. Murray (Eds.), *Infant communication: Cry and early speech* (pp. 284–309). San Diego, CA: College-Hill Press.

Laura, R.S. (1985). Mental retardation and genetic engineering. In R.S. Laura & A.F. Ashman (Eds.), *Moral issues in mental retardation* (pp. 185–207). Dover, NH: Croom Helm.

Lewis, M., McCollum, A.T., Schwartz, A.H., & Grunt, J.A. (1969). Informed consent in pediatric research. *Children, 16,* 143–148.

Lowe, C.U., & Alexander, D.F. (1981). Informed consent and the rights of research subjects. In H. Wechsler, R. Lamont-Havers, & G. Cahill, Jr. (Eds.), *The social context of medical research* (pp. 97–126). Cambridge, MS: Ballinger.

Lynch, G. (1983). The cell biology of neuronal plasticity: Implications for mental retardation. In F.J. Menolascino, R. Neman, & J.A. Stark (Eds.), *Curative aspects of mental retardation: Biomedical and behavioral advances* (pp. 99–109). Baltimore: Paul H. Brookes Publishing Co.

Maslow, A.H. (1954). *Motivation and personality.* New York: Harper & Row.

Mercer, J. (1973). The myth of 3% prevalence. In G. Tarjan, R. Eyman, & C. Meyer (Eds.), *Sociobehavioral studies in mental retardation* (pp. 1–18). Washington, DC: American Association on Mental Deficiency.

Michelsson, K., & Wasz-Höckert, O. (1980). The value of cry analysis in neonatology and early infancy. In T. Murray & J. Murray (Eds.), *Infant communication: Cry and early speech* (pp. 152–182). San Diego, CA: College-Hill Press.

National Commission for the Protection of Human Subjects of Biomedical and Behavioral Research. (1977). *Research involving children* (DHHS Publication No. OS 77–004). Washington, DC: Department of Health, Education, and Welfare.

Oller, D.K. (1979). Syllable timing in Spanish, English and Finnish. *Amsterdam studies in theory and history of linguistic science IV* (Vol. 9). Amsterdam: John-Benjamins B.V.

Pryce, I.G. (1978). Clinical research upon mentally ill subjects who cannot give informed consent. *British Journal of Psychiatry, 133,* 366–369.

Rainforth, B. (1982). Biobehavior state and orienting: Implications for educating profoundly retarded students. *Journal of The Association for Persons with Severe Handicaps, 6*(4), 33–37.

Rosenzweig, M.R., & Bennett, E.L. (1976). Enriched environments: Facts, factors, and fantasies. In L. Petrinovich & J.L. McGaugh (Eds.), *Knowing, thinking, and believing* (pp. 179–213). New York: Plenum.

Sayre, T.H., & McKelvey, J.B. (1983). A response to Hutchins and Renzaglia. *Exceptional Education Quarterly, 4*(2), 72–74.

Seitz, S., & Geske, D. (1976). Mothers' and graduate trainees' judgements of children: Some effects of labeling. *American Journal of Mental Deficiency, 81,* 362–370.

Seligman, M.E. (1975). *Helplessness: On depression, development and death.* San Francisco: W.H. Freeman.

Siegel-Causey, E., & Guess, D. (in press). *Enhancing nonsymbolic communication interactions among learners with severe disabilities.* Baltimore: Paul H. Brookes Publishing Co.

Sokol-Kesslu, L.E., Conroy, J.W., Feinstein, C.S., Lemanowicz, J.A., & McGubbin, M. (1983). Developmental progress in institutional and community settings. *Journal of The Association for Persons with Severe Handicaps, 8*(3), 43–47.

Sokolov, E.N. (1963). *Perception and the conditioned reflex.* New York: Macmillan.

Stern, D.N. (1974). Mother and infant at play. In M. Lewis & L. Rosenblum (Eds.), *The effect of the infant on the caregiver: The origin of behavior series (Vol. 1, pp. 187–214).* New York: John Wiley & Sons.

Stern, D.N., Beebe, B., Jaffe, J., & Bennett, S.L. (1977). The infant's stimulus world during social interaction: A study of caregiver behaviors with particular reference to repetition and timing. In H.R. Schaffer (Ed.), *Studies on interaction in infancy* (pp. 177–202). New York: Academic Press.

Stern, D.N., & Gibbon, J. (1979). Temporal expectancies of social behaviors in mother-infant play. In E.B. Thoman (Ed.), *Origins of the infant's social responsiveness* (pp. 409–430). Hillsdale, NJ: Lawrence Erlbaum Associates.

Switzky, H.N., Woolsey-Hill, J., & Quoss, T. (1979). Habituation of visual fixation responses: An assessment to measure visual sensory-perceptual-cognitive processes in nonverbal profoundly handicapped children in the classroom. *AAESPH Review, 4,* 136–147.

TASH Resolution. (1983). The Association for the Severely Handicapped: Policy statement of the Critical Issues Committee. Newsletter 9, June 1, 1.

Walker, G.R., McLaren, K.P., & Bonaventura, S. (1985). Changing places: A look at some of the realities of institutional behavior management. *Mental Retardation, 23*(2), 79–81.

Walker-Andrews, A.S. (1983). Discrimination of vocal expressions by young infants. *Infant Behavior and Development, 6,* 491–498.

Watson, J.S. (1979). Perception of contingency as a determinant of social responsiveness. In E.B. Thoman (Ed.), *Origins of the infant's social responsiveness.* Hillsdale, NJ: Laurence Erlbaum Associates.

West, M.J., & Del Cerro, M. (1976). Early formation of synapses in the molecular layer of the fetal heart cerebellum. *Journal of Comparative Neurology, 165,* 137–160.

Wikler, D. (1980). *Ethical issues in programming for developmentally disabled adults.* Paper presented at the Central Conference for University Training Programs in Developmental Disabilities, Illinois.

DEFINING MEANINGFUL OUTCOMES FOR PERSONS WITH PROFOUND DISABILITIES

(4)

Ian M. Evans and Joseph R. Scotti

The rights of persons with profound and multiple disabilities to receive high-quality habilitative services have clear moral, legal, and pragmatic foundations. These foundations have been well-documented throughout this book. One of the fundamental principles underlying such rights is the separation of the intrinsic worth of an individual from the apparent or anticipated value of that person's actions to society. By definition, individuals with profound mental retardation will make little, if any, direct contribution to society through their behavior (i.e., labor, intellect, artistic talents). This statement is not unduly pessimistic since the premise is that such individuals are valued in other ways. However, it does have important implications for the evaluation of services and programs because judgments that are made concerning program quality must ultimately be based upon the perceived value of the behavioral outcomes that are achieved (Evans & Brown, 1986). Thus, even if services do not need to be justified on the basis of their behavioral benefits to the intended recipient, discriminating valuable programs from less successful ones will require careful specification of the types of outcomes that are meaningful. Such evaluation criteria not only influence judgments about the program, but also determine program direction and thrust. The goals and objectives of any educational service are derived from assumptions regarding the outcomes that are seen as desirable for the population being served.

Portions of this chapter were based on work supported by Cooperative Agreement # G0083C0040, "School Span Assessment Needs for Children with Handicaps," from the United States Department of Education, Special Education Programs. The opinions expressed herein do not necessarily reflect the position or policy of the United States Department of Education and no official endorsement should be inferred.

In this chapter, the behavioral outcomes for persons with profound disabilities that have been reported in the literature are discussed. The authors examine the explicit and implicit criteria that are used to judge the meaningfulness of these outcomes. As these criteria extend beyond (and in some cases away from) the recent professional preoccupation with functionality, a conceptual framework for judging the meaningfulness of outcomes that encompasses dimensions of behavior other than generally recognized skills is developed. Finally, problems in outcome evaluation are related to "educational validity" (Voeltz & Evans, 1983) concerns. The veridical measurement of an outcome and the value placed upon it are very different. The latter is based upon prior social expectations with the satisfaction for certain outcomes resting on the match between those expected and those achieved (Evans, 1985b). These expectations are discussed in relation to how they arise in those who are involved with services for persons with profound disabilities and how they may be shaped in constructive directions.

It is worth asking, at this point, whether the assessment of program outcomes for persons categorized as profoundly disabled does, or should, represent a set of concerns different from those pertinent to individuals with severe but less debilitating handicaps. Special issues on this topic are discussed in this chapter. In addition, the dangers, particularly for societal expectations, of stressing the extreme limitations in adaptive functioning that individuals who are profoundly handicapped experience are also discussed. Advocates for persons with profound retardation are often caught in the classic bind of simultaneously articulating the deficits or differences that characterize this particular group of individuals. Ideologically, many professional insist that there are no qualitative differences in handicapping conditions (that, indeed, even the use of such a term is inappropriate). Following this reasoning, the standards, expectations, and criteria that have emerged in the field for persons who are "moderately" and "severely" handicapped apply perhaps equally to those who are the most profoundly disabled. The authors offer an explanation as to why this optimistic viewpoint, if it is to gain serious acceptance, needs to be translated so that skill deficiencies can be recognized and constructively defined without fostering a deficit orientation or overly negative expectations.

PAST OUTCOME MEASURES

Conditioning Measures

Behavior modification grew to its prominent position partly by demonstrating that the basic principles of learning that had been explored in the animal laboratory, also applied to human behavior. Therefore, it is not surprising that some, if not all, of the earlier investigations of behavior modification were carried out on subjects who were very handicapped in order to demonstrate the generality of principles, rather than to design habilitative programs. A typical example of this strategy is the early paper by Fuller (1949) who reinforced vertical arm movements in an individual described as "vegetative." Fuller used sweet warm milk squirted into the person's mouth as a reinforcer. Further examples of this approach are seen in the works of Rice and his colleagues (Rice, 1968; Rice & McDaniel, 1966; Rice, McDaniel, Stallings, & Gatz, 1967) who employed such operant responses as arm raising, pulling on a metal ring, and moving the head into midline. (Also see the works of Deiker & Bruno, 1976; Kuhlenbeck, Szekely, & Spuler, 1964; and Piper & McKinnon, 1969.)

Obviously, in these studies the dependent measures (i.e., the form of the response and its properties) were selected for the experimenter's convenience and in accordance with the traditions of the operant laboratory. Very often, this meant that the measured outcome was a change in the rate of some simple motor response. There was no attempt to establish a new form of behavior nor any concern that repetition of the motor response might not be a natural or typical activity for the person. The classical conditioning paradigm has also been used to demonstrate the applicability of basic laws of animal-learning to human subjects that lack elaborate verbal or cognitive repertoires, such as infants, patients who were in a coma, or people with profound mental retardation. In a sense, the classical conditioning paradigm has always been a strategy for communicating with nonverbal subjects; with any reliable conditioned reflex as an indicator, it is possible to test the limits of what a subject can perceive, discriminate, remember, and so forth. Except for some applications such as audiometry, the potential of the classical conditioning paradigm for exploring the cognitive capacities of individuals with limited expressive performance repertoires has never really been adequately explored and developed. Therefore, the behavioral outcomes of early operant or classical conditioning studies were, in themselves, trivial. However, studies of this kind lent credence to the modifiability of behavior in persons with profound mental retardation who were at that time still being labeled as "uneducable" and incapable of learning even simple contingencies. Rice's (1968) study led him to conclude that, "does not is not equal to cannot" (p. 301). This is an important concept for raising professional optimism and expectations as it places the responsibility upon the professional for designing creative procedures and equipment that will allow individuals who are profoundly disabled to fully accomplish acts that they are capable of performing.

It should be noted that individuals who are profoundly disabled are an extremely heterogeneous group with a wide variety of neurological and other organic defects. Thus, an interesting outcome of the operant conditioning research with this population of individuals has been the finding that they, perhaps, do not follow the exact same "laws" of conditioning that intact, nonorganically damaged persons follow. As Landesman-Dwyer and Sackett (1978) point out, this statement should not be taken to imply that their behavior is chaotic or otherwise unresponsive to environmental contingencies. The previously noted operant research attests to the contrary. However, the professional must be aware that persons with profound disabilities may require extensive shaping and training procedures, that acquisition curves are likely to be atypical, and that such phenomena as "spontaneous extinction" may occur (Landesman-Dwyer & Sackett, 1978; Rice & McDaniel, 1966). Hypothetically, neurological differences that would result in these conditioning differences would ultimately be definable in terms of damage to specific brain areas. For example, "spontaneous extinction" may be related to a memory recall deficit. Alternately, such behavioral differences may be the result of much more diffuse processes. Ultimately, such findings could have a direct effect upon the choice of behavioral outcomes and their likelihood of success.

Variation in Excess Behavior

While the early studies based upon behavioral principles generally ignored the meaningfulness of the behaviors to be conditioned, this became a less prominent practice when the focus of the treatment was on the reduction or elimination of an inappropriate behavior. In these intervention programs, the target behavior was selected because it was deemed undesirable in some way, and, thus, reductions or deceleration of that behavior would be, ipso facto, valuable. Thus, the efficacy of the intervention could be determined entirely from observing a reduction in the target behavior relative to its pretreatment rate. It is now widely recognized that this is a naive assumption (Voeltz & Evans, 1983; Wolf, 1978). Given the extensive discussions on this topic, the authors will not repeat all the various arguments; however, there are some that are especially relevant to programmatic outcomes for individuals who have profound disabilities.

One of the more obvious difficulties with evaluating interventions that deal with excess behaviors is whether the most serious or detrimental behavior was targeted in the first place. Persons with profound handicaps might be expected to have a number of inappropriate behaviors so that reduction in one or two of them might not be as significant as a reduction in one of the others. The seriousness of a behavior is itself a social judgment, except perhaps in some of the more obvious cases where the behavior is causing immediate physical harm to the individual or to other persons. Thus, clinicians need to consider whether the reduction in the excess target behavior(s) actually had secondary positive outcomes for the client. For instance, did the reduction in the inappropriate behavior lead to greater social opportunities or a less restrictive living arrangement? These are what might be referred to as the ripple effects of the reduction in a negative target behavior (Evans, 1985a). The positive benefits of the intervention should continue even though the formal intervention has ended.

A second obvious difficulty with judging a treatment program by the reduction of an excess behavior is of special significance to clients who have very

limited behavioral repertoires. It would not be considered particularly successful if a negative behavior, regardless of its apparent deleteriousness to the individual, were reduced and no positive alternative was taught that could take its
place. This concern is based upon the assumption that excess behaviors always
have some sort of reciprocal positive alternative behavior. This leads to the
third concern—that if negative behaviors have positive alternative forms, it
means that the negative behaviors must have a function that is not inappropriate. Thus, the negative behaviors may have some meaningful function for the
individual and the question arises whether these behaviors may be indicative of
other negative circumstances. One interpretation of a high level of negative
behaviors is that there is something wrong with the treatment program or the
environmental arrangement in general, rather than that there is something
wrong with the client. A related interpretation is that the negative behaviors
reflect the lack of more positive skills that have the same function, and, thus
again, are revealing of deficits in the program (Durand, 1982).

Change of State Measures

There is a tendency, when thinking of the behavioral assessment of skills or
deficits, to view behavior change in terms of specific acts or operants. However,
in assessing clinical treatment outcomes for nonhandicapped persons, it would
be just as common to obtain measures that reflect emotional states. Of course,
emotional states (e.g., happiness, depression, anxiety) are often inferred from
verbal self-report. This would not be possible with persons with profound disabilities. However, there are many other possible indices of emotion, such as
facial expression, willingness to approach or avoid a situation, activity level, or
physiological measures such as heart rate, blood pressure, or galvanic skin response. Unfortunately, there are few examples of these kinds of outcome measures used as indices of the effect of a program on individuals who are profoundly handicapped. The percentage of time spent in which one's facial
expression is judged (e.g., neutral, happy, angry) would not be a very difficult
measure to obtain.

   One interesting outcome measure might be what in other contexts has
been called "engaged time." Engaged time means the amount of time an individual spends continuously involved in the activity that he or she is expected to
be performing. Thus, if the expectation was that the person was ostensibly in a
leisure/recreational activity, then engaged time would be the percentage of time
that the person is participating with enjoyment. The authors have often noted
persons with profound disabilities in leisure situations, such as watching television, where there was no evidence that the individual was really participating
(e.g., complaints if the channel was changed or the television was turned off,
laughter at humorous situations, visual attentiveness to the television set).

   In rehabilitation settings where there is a need to ensure that the persons
who are severely injured do not spend excessive amounts of time in bed, out-

come measures have been developed in which the important index is percentage of time that the patient is up and about (Parris Stephens, Norris-Baker, & Willems, 1984). This type of measure could easily be adapted to the present purpose. The closest example of this being conducted is the very interesting study by Landesman-Dwyer and Sackett (1978). In this study, the intervention was to provide additional levels of stimulation to nonambulatory individuals in an institutional setting. The intervention was relatively simple and involved an "enriched" situation with toys and mobiles. The clients were physically positioned in such a way that they could be in contact with the visually enhanced environment. One of the outcome measures was a change of state measure— the percentage of time awake during normal waking hours. Lagged sequential observations (i.e., discovering the events that regularly follow the target event at different intervals of time) had previously indicated that the sleep/wake pattern of these clients was abnormal. Instead of being awake for a long period of time during the day and asleep for most of the night, these individuals were sleeping and waking repeatedly over short periods of time. The outcome analysis revealed that the result of the stimulation program was a more normalized cycle of sleeping and waking, specifically, longer periods of wakefulness following the "enriched" activity period.

Another useful dimension of behavior change that does not require a priori specification of a defined type of response is *behavioral complexity*. Originally described by Landesman-Dwyer and Sackett (1978), behavioral complexity can be defined simply as the proportion of different behaviors observed to occur within a specified time interval. Of course, whether such behavioral complexity is really beneficial depends upon validating criteria that clients exhibiting complexity are better off than those who do not display such variability. Unlike the other change of state measures mentioned, there are no obvious normative comparisons by which to judge. If a client exhibits a wide variety of maladaptive behaviors, such behavioral complexity is likely to be judged undesirable. However, even this situation may be more desirable than total inactivity, especially since it provides strong evidence that the individual is responsive to differences in his or her environment. Nevertheless, in contrast to the prolonged periods of inactivity that are often observed in persons with profound mental retardation, behavioral complexity can be reasonably thought of as indicating a more active state or, at least, a state more interactive with the environment. Indeed, Landesman-Dwyer and Sackett (1978) found that those individuals with disabilities in their study who exhibited higher degrees of behavioral complexity also showed marked increases in environmental contacts, looking behavior, and vertical head movements. They also fell asleep less frequently after exposure to a play situation and exhibited fewer fixed action sequences (i.e., invariant idiosyncratic behavioral sequences thought to be reflexive in nature). Along similar lines, LaMendola, Zaharia, and O'Brien (1987), in their evaluation of a caregiving modality known as "foundation care" (i.e., care that involves health, nourishment, nurturance, stimulation, and exploration), reported that the measure of behavioral complexity differentiated their program from the outcome of a traditional Intermediate Care Facility.

Norm-Referenced Tests

For a person to acquire useful behaviors, certain "cognitive" processes must be present: motor coordination, sensory integration, perceptual processes, and memory. Therefore, it would be useful to have some general idea of possible deficits of persons with profound handicaps in these areas. This would allow the necessary compensations in the teaching approach to be made, just as one would adapt a situation for someone who was blind. Unfortunately, there are no independent measures of these capacities and processes as there are for sensory acuity. The nearest approximations are neuropsychological tests, since these are designed to determine whether a more basic process is still intact after an injury or suspected injury to the brain. Thus far, there are only a few examples of neuropsychological tests being used constructively with persons having profound physical and intellectual impairments; however, it would seem to be a promising area. For instance, after different types of injury to the brain, immediate memory is greatly impaired such that a patient would not be able to remember having just seen someone or what was just said to him. Clearly, this is a very debilitating loss and it is not known if similar difficulties are experienced by persons whose severe handicap is developmental in nature. Furthermore, since the etiology of profound disability is often attributable to specific types of injury to the brain and its development, tests designed to investigate such injuries would seem to have promise.

Much more commonly used, needless to say, are intelligence tests; however, such tests are developed in the absence of any particular theory of intelligence. They are ad hoc tests, loosely covering certain cognitive areas and may involve reasoning, comprehension of language, and numerical concepts that almost always require a number of cognitive processes for performance. The items of these tests are included on the basis of age norms, demonstrating that they range in level of difficulty. The easier items are thus, by design, appropriate for younger children and so the anomaly of adults with profound handicaps being compared to these young infants has resulted. One possible advantage of the standardized test is its reliability. If a test is repeated by another examiner at another time, differences in the obtained score are attributable to improvement, or deterioration, in the client's behavior.

REFINEMENTS IN BEHAVIORAL OUTCOME MEASURES

Function versus Form

One of the most important distinctions in contemporary behavior theory for analyzing meaningful behavior is that of function versus form (White, 1980). Many very different behaviors can have the same function. For example, if the function of walking is to get from the cafeteria to the work site, pressing a switch on a motorized wheelchair is an equally successful alternative form of behavior. However, if the function is to get exercise, then an alternative form might be an aerobic activity performed prone on a mat. This useful concept allows one to think of functional behaviors, those that achieve a critical effect, regardless of the complexity of the form used to achieve that effect.

An example of this approach has been provided by Green, Canipe, Way, and Reid (1986). These authors defined an activity as functional if it met the criteria for a given class or domain. For instance, a behavior in the self-help domain would be considered to be functional if it achieved a critical effect that would otherwise have to be performed by someone else, such as putting on one's jacket. A communicative behavior was considered functional if it could be performed at least weekly outside of the classroom. Thus, a functional communication skill might involve teaching the student to nod his or her head "yes" in response to questions; however, teaching the student to point to a picture of Santa Claus would not be a functional skill (Green et al., 1986). These examples effectively illustrate that behaviors that are functional are not necessarily complex as well. An interesting twist has been added to this analysis by Reid and his colleagues (cf., Reid et al., 1985) by defining some materials as functional, namely "those objects that would be used to complete a given activity in a nonclassroom setting." These researchers studied the effects of introducing functional tasks and materials into the classroom, improving the physical environment to encourage interaction between the student and the educational context, and providing staff supervision to support their positive efforts. The dependent variables included the overall time that the students were on task (i.e., engaged in an assigned activity); the time that the students spent interacting in some way with staff members; and, when on task, whether or not that task performed by the student was functional. This last category, as the focus of the program, showed large improvements, but other positive behavioral category increased as well. Some students were able to learn how to use adaptive equipment to stuff decorative pillows for which they earned a small monetary stipend. To quote Green et al. (1986):

> Perhaps the most significant outcome of this investigation is optimism regarding the nature of educational services that can be provided to individuals who have profound mental and physical impairments. As expressed by the classroom staff, it was no more difficult to involve their students in meaningful tasks such as activating a cassette recorder or opening a food container than it was to use their more typical tasks such as stacking plastic blocks or putting pegs in pegboards. (p. 169)

In many contexts, of course, the form of a behavior that is going to be functional is controlled by the physical requirements of the environment. However, when the class of behaviors has a leisure function, there is a seemingly infinite variety of effective forms since the objective or critical effect is to "have fun." A similar point can be made about social behaviors. If a set number of functions that are served by social behaviors could be defined, then a variety of successful ways of achieving those functions could be determined. This is the approach adopted by Meyer and her colleagues (Meyer et al., 1983) in developing a new measure of social skills. The initial task in the development of their instrument was to define a limited number of social goals that are achieved by a wide variety of social skills. For example, there are many social behaviors that are designed to gain entry into a social situation or access to a social interaction (e.g., approaching a group of other children and asking to play, calling a friend to wangle an invitation to a party). Other discrete functions of social skills are such things as providing positive feedback to others, accepting negative feedback and modifying one's behavior accordingly, and exiting or terminating a social interaction.

Having defined 11 such functions, Meyer and her coworkers (Meyer et al., 1983) then described different levels of complexity or sophistication in achieving functions that were not simply related to age. The lower levels typically did not involve elaborate verbal operations, the planning of future events, or other "cognitive" elements. However, even the lowest level of complexity would produce the critical effect, just as would the more complex behaviors. To illustrate, consider the function of *initiating* a social interaction. Eye contact, a brief smile, or holding out a desirable toy might well be the kinds of first level behaviors that will successfully induce a peer to come over and engage in an interaction. Notice that these behaviors are not just appropriate for young children. Adults initiate social interactions in much the same way. Perhaps an adult would not hold out a toy, but there are comparable ways of initiating a social exchange, such as offering a magazine to the passenger sitting next to you on a plane. Of course, these lower level behaviors are not as sophisticated as other ways of initiating interactions, such as telephoning someone and arranging to meet him or her for lunch, but they may be equally as effective. This approach is conceptually quite different from one that scales social behavior according to age norms for typical content activities. Furthermore, this approach helps to define simple, but effective, versions of more complex behaviors.

Component Model of Functional Competence

A tactic similar to that of Meyer et al. (1983) was followed by Evans, Brown, Weed, Spry, and Owen (1987) and Brown, Evans, Weed, and Owen (1987) in the development of an outcome assessment inventory that would veridically represent the degree to which a student with handicaps had actually mastered the everyday skills required for daily living. The unit of analysis selected was that of a routine—an activity that has a distinct beginning and end, and that achieves a critical effect. Routines can be clustered into three broad domains: personal management, the activities that are necessary to maintain and care for oneself in society (e.g., washing, dressing, shopping, budgeting money); leisure, activities that are done for their own sake, for enjoyment (e.g., hobbies, play, group sports); work, those activities that are required by others (e.g., attending school, performing a job). In the leisure domain, substitution of any acceptable activity that has a recreational function is possible; however, in the personal management domain, it is important to perform specific routines. For example, in dressing, there are simpler forms of the behavior (i.e., some clothes do not require zipping, tying, buttoning, or worrying about color coordination) but not simpler levels. Therefore, rather than trying to establish different levels of the same function, these authors proposed a way of breaking down complex routines into units or components that are independently meaningful.

The key feature of this approach is that the core components (i.e., the actual activities needed by the individual in order to achieve the critical effect of the routine) are not subdivided into steps, as they are in a traditional task analysis. It is presumed that in order to be competent in a routine, all of the steps would be necessary. In other words, there would be no particular advantage for the individual to be able to do four of the nine core steps of a routine, since without all nine he or she could not successfully achieve the critical effect. However, there are other components, in addition to the core physical actions, that are necessary for the successful completion of a routine. These would have some independent advantage to the individual. For example, all activities require some kind of preparation (e.g., assembling materials, getting the workspace ready) and termination (e.g., ending the activity, putting things away, returning the environment to its previous state). Although the particular actions involved in preparing (e.g., getting the bread and peanut butter) and terminating (e.g., closing the bread bag, wiping the table) are routine specific, the general principle is that these types of actions need to be done and are common across routines. Therefore, it is likely that the ability to do these two components would generalize across routines (Evans, Weed, Brown, & Weld, in press). The authors would argue that if a person was unable to perform the core of a routine, but could carry out the prepare or terminate components independently, this would constitute a more meaningful contribution to the completion of the routine than being able to do one or two steps of the core that alone could not achieve the critical effect.

Meaningful participation in a routine can be accomplished through the component of *initiation*. For individuals with the most profound disabilities, independently performing the initiation component of a routine may be all that is possible. Such an individual providing a signal that he needs to be toileted would generally be preferred over the complete lack of any component of the toileting routine. If a hand signal or the pushing of a buzzer results in being assisted to the toilet and having clean, dry clothing, then the critical effect has been achieved as a result of that person's action. Initiating can be performed without the rest of the routine necessarily following independently. Initiating means starting a routine at the appropriate time and place, or indicating to others that there is a want or need to perform the routine. Examples of this include the aforementioned toileting scenario, handwashing when noticing one's hands are dirty, telling someone that it is time to leave, or indicating a desire to watch television. Obviously, an individual who is profoundly handicapped would have more appropriate interaction with the environment if he or she could initiate routines, even though he or she were completely physically dependent upon some other person to actually perform the routine. In an important sense, the routine then belongs to that individual, even though he or she cannot perform the actions independently. The individual is then the *initiator* of the event. Very often for persons with profound disabilities, the routines are initiated by the caregiver and so become that person's routines. If the caregiver initiates bathing for someone who is profoundly disabled, the routine is then a work routine for that person, not a personal management routine for the person with the handicap. Thus, the caregiving relationship moves from being that of helper or assistant to that of controller. It negatively influences the kinds of attitudes held by professional caregivers as well as the social relationship between the provider and the recipient of care. The perspective presented places the initiation and control of events with the client, and it can have profound effects upon the relationship between clients and caregivers.

Motor Measures

Previously in this chapter, some of the early operant conditioning studies were mentioned that employed simple motoric responses. It was noted that these initial studies were not habilitative in nature; rather, they were investigations of the conditionability of subjects who had profound disabilities. However, more recently, such simple motor responses have become the targets of habilitation research and have been viewed as desirable outcomes. For example, Murphy and Doughty (1977) reported their successful attempt to establish controlled arm movements in seven individuals who were nonambulatory, profoundly mentally retarded, and multiply handicapped. The movements that they established included pulling down on a rope and pushing on a panel. While these responses are reminiscent of the earlier operant studies, Murphy and Doughty (1977) specifically targeted these responses because of their usefulness in preparing these individuals for other, more meaningful activities requiring the manipulation of objects. Through a gradual procedure of shaping higher response frequencies and increasing the response demands (i.e., through the use of heavier weights and longer session durations), the individuals came to reliably produce these simple motor movements. The immediate benefits included the prevention of muscle atrophy and improved muscle tone and strength. These are meaningful outcomes in themselves, in addition to being possible precursors to more complex behaviors.

Landesman-Dwyer and Sackett (1978) employed simple motor responses as the outcome measures in their comprehensive analysis of persons who were nonambulatory, profoundly mentally retarded. These responses included increases in general activity levels, behavioral complexity, eye movements, head and facial movements, trunk and limb movements, and vocalizations. These were the specific behavioral outcome measures that they employed to assess the effects of their experimental treatment. None of these responses were intentionally prompted, shaped, or reinforced. They were, instead, the outcome of providing environmental stimulation at a higher level than that which individuals received in their ongoing ward situations. The increases in these behaviors suggest an increased level of engagement with, and responsiveness to, the environment. These alone might be deemed desirable goals. However, one may argue that individuals must be exhibiting some minimum level of activity in order for their behaviors to be gradually shaped into even more meaningful and complex behaviors.

The motor skill deficits of persons with profound disabilities vary greatly, ranging from those individuals who are nonambulatory and exhibit severe contractures to those who are partially or fully ambulatory and may exhibit a few rudimentary skills. An attempt to cover the range of motor skills that would comprise meaningful outcomes for this heterogeneous group is beyond the scope of this chapter. However, there is an approach that reduces even the most complex behaviors into their component elements in a manner somewhat different from traditional task analysis. This approach breaks motor movements into the elements that comprise a *movement cycle*. The six basic elements of a movement cycle include reach, point, touch, grasp, place, and release, with the additional elements of pull, push, shake, squeeze, tap, and twist being added as the task demands increase (Pollard, 1984). The desired outcome in this approach is to independently increase the frequency of each motor element and then combine them into a complete movement cycle. Such a cycle can be tailored to motor skills at various levels of complexity, such as putting on a shirt, brushing teeth, or making contact with a nearby toy. Depending upon the level of disability, the elements themselves or the complete movement cycle (i.e., skill) might be viewed as the desired outcome.

A meaningful outcome associated with motoric responses is that of endurance. Certainly it can be agreed that the aerobic status of persons with profound disabilities worsens rapidly from individuals who are ambulatory to those who are nonambulatory and bedridden. Regardless of the complexity of the response selected, from riding an exercise bicycle (Weber & Thaeler, 1987) to simple trunk, head, and arm movements (Burch, Clegg, & Bailey, 1987; Dewson & Whiteley, 1987; Murphy & Doughty, 1977), persons with profound disabilities do not show acceptable levels of endurance for general physical exercise. This may be chosen as an outcome measure, with its ensuing aerobic benefits and improvements in muscle tone and strength. It is suggested that even simple arm movements in persons with the most severe disabilities can be gradually shaped to frequencies and durations that would provide some physical benefits (Murphy & Doughty, 1977).

Finally, one may consider eye movements under the area of motor measures. Clearly, for any individual to learn from contingencies, he or she must be in contact with environmental stimuli. Some type of orienting response must occur, such as eye movements directed at certain visual stimuli. "Looking" is just one example of a precurrent behavior, defined by Skinner (1953) as a behavior that brings people into initial contact with stimuli, thereby creating the opportunity to respond to those stimuli and meet the consequences. In persons with the most profound physical disabilities, eye orientations may be one of the more competent behavioral responses available, assuming adequate vision. Sighted individuals are not likely to reach for and grasp objects unless they first direct their gaze upon those objects. Stella and Etzel (1986) have demonstrated in nonhandicapped preschool children that eye orientations are under stimulus control and can provide evidence that discrimination learning has occurred. The technology currently exists that enables professionals to monitor eye movements electronically and to use this output with simple programs on personal computers. Such technology makes eye orientation and movement a potentiallly important outcome for even individuals with the most disabling handicaps. This is not to suggest a return to the days of "eye contact" and "attention span" programs, but the functional use of eye movements. Some examples of this may include rolling the eyes up to indicate "yes" and down to indicate "no"; indicating preferences by directing eye gaze upon the object of choice; or, with the aid of special goggles and a computer, turning battery operated toys on and off or producing words and images on the computer screen. The limit here, as elsewhere, is on the inventiveness of the professional caregiver. (See Chapter 7 this volume, for a further discussion of the functional relationship among motor skills and other domains.)

Quality of Life as Effective Behavior

The most basic common denominator for defining "quality of life" would appear to be an individual's possession of a repertoire of *effective behaviors*. Effective behaviors are those that produce an effect upon the environment, most importantly, the social environment in the case of human beings. These behaviors must be modifiable, in turn, by the environment (i.e., they must be responsive to the contingencies of reinforcement). This definition would cut across all levels of behavioral functioning, such that the presence of effective behaviors indicates some degree of quality to a life, with variations existing among individuals in terms of the form and quantity of those behaviors. Thus, one outcome measure for quality of life would be an individual's ability to produce change in the persons around him or her.

Persons who are profoundly disabled do not possess very many effective behaviors. Some individuals perhaps do not possess any such behaviors. Meanwhile, other persons may possess extensive repertoires of effective behaviors that have come to be viewed as excessive and are targeted for deceleration (i.e., self-injurious behavior that might be functioning to attain interactions from others). Persons with profound disabilities may be able to smile, laugh, and move a limb, but unless these responses produce environmental change and are in turn modifiable, they are not effective behaviors.

The first level of effective behavior is simply that of behavior engagement. Defined by McWilliam, Trivette, and Dunst (1985) as the amount of time spent interacting with the environment, behavior engagement sets the occasion for learning (cf. Favell & Risley, 1984). It is suggested that behavior engagement is a sensitive, reliable, and useful measure since the degree of engagement appears to be a function of environmental parameters, such as the physical arrangement of a setting, access to materials, instructional methods, and severity and nature of handicapping condition (cf. McWilliam et al., 1985). The work of Landesman-Dwyer and Sackett (1978) provides evidence that even with individuals who are the most profoundly disabled, merely providing access to objects and peers results in behavioral changes. At the most basic level, providing the opportunity for behavior engagement can result in engagement as an outcome. McWilliam et al. (1985) concluded from their review of the research that engagement is a necessary, though probably not sufficient, condition for developmental change to occur.

Behavior engagement is a useful outcome measure at a number of developmental levels since the operational definition is in terms of time spent interacting. Thus, an individual may possess many skills, or only a very few; however, behavior engagement is concerned only with the actual time spent exhibiting those skills (McWilliam et al., 1985). Such engagement, while being a meaningful outcome in itself, does not necessarily provide a measure of the modifiability of an individual's responses (i.e., how sensitive he or she is to changes in the reinforcement contingencies). For such a measure, the operant conditioning literature, and the responses that are emitted during situations that have high levels of behavior engagement and provide appropriate consequences, must be reviewed to make those responses functional, not merely reactive.

Movements of the eyes, head, and limbs toward an object can be paired both with access to that object and to other stimuli that have reinforcing value for that individual. Indeed, the problem at this level may well be the determination of which sensory events serve a reinforcing function. However, it is possible to identify these stimuli using simple operant procedures (Dewson & Whiteley, 1987). The important outcome at this level is that an operant response be established. A behavior such as a head turn that activates a radio or a slide projector is an effective behavior because the individual is producing an effect upon the environment and, in turn, is being modified (i.e., learning) as well. If the critical effect of such a response is to "have fun," then this response may even meet that additional requirement. Haskett and Hollar (1978) report increased rates of vocalizing and smiling by the children with profound disabilities in their study. These responses were collateral to the response-dependent stimulation. Such behavior certainly gives the appearance of fun and enjoyment and of taking pleasure in one's mastery of an event. These behaviors can become functional if they draw others to the individual to share in the fun (cf. Meyer et al., 1983) and can potentially lead to further social interactions and other forms of behavior engagement.

Dunst, Cushing, and Vance (1985) have applied a social systems perspective to demonstrate how such simple beginnings can lead to more complex behaviors and social interactions. These authors suggest that "the impact of response-contingent learning extends beyond the immediate changes in behavior which are exhibited by the [individual]" (p. 43). There are effects that have a direct and indirect impact upon the individual and the behavior of the significant others in their lives (cf. Cochran & Brassard, 1979). The initial learning of a contingency is a first-order effect upon the individual himself or herself. Second-order effects upon the caregivers and significant others are those responses resulting from the acquisition of response-contingent behavior, such as amazement and enjoyment that learning has occurred, and the subsequent increase in attentiveness and responsiveness to the individual. Higher-order effects upon the individual and other persons occur as other operant responses are added to the repertoire, setting the occasion for facilitation and generalization of other responses. The caregivers then, in turn, "become more ingenious in devising strategies to evoke and sustain operant behavior from [the individual]" (Dunst et al., 1985, p. 45). Clearly, it is at this point that caregivers can assign certain functions to a response, such that a push of a buzzer no longer just turns on a light display; instead, it cues the caregiver to immediately interact with the individual for some period of time. A simple operant response then becomes an effective behavior that has the critical effect of initiating a social interaction. As Dunst et al. (1985) noted:

> Social systems theory, with its focus on the different order effects behavior has on intra- and inter-individual functioning, appears to provide the type of conceptual framework for broadening the perspective from which the benefits of even the simplest forms of learning can be viewed. (p. 45)

Quality of life, as defined by the meaningful outcome of effective behavior, thus becomes a reality for the individual with profound mental retardation.

Quality of life can be enhanced further through the provision of choice. At its most basic level, the process of choice or deciding is responding to one of two available stimuli (Skinner, 1950, 1953). Alternatively, choice may be regarded as response variability, such that one of two (or more) responses is made to a single stimulus. It is likely with persons who have profound disabilities that choices will have to be set up for them, in the sense that their mere expression of a preference (e.g., smiling, frowning) does not in itself lead to obtaining the preferred selection. The environment, in this case the social environment, must respond to the indication of preference in order for that behavior to be considered "effective." However, this does not diminish the effectiveness and function of their behavior once those choices (e.g., multiple stimuli, multiple responses) are available to them. Once again, the ingenuity of caregivers may be the limiting factor.

ALTERNATIVE OUTCOME MEASURES

The previous section discussed a number of novel approaches to the measurement of outcomes, as well as the criteria that can be used for evaluating the significance of a given outcome. In all cases, the outcomes were defined in terms of the client and his or her accomplishments or attributes. These outcomes were judged as allowing a more favorable or desirable relationship between the individual and his or her social and physical environment. In this section, outcomes that can be validated in terms of their effect on other persons, rather than just on the client, are addressed. These outcomes are still reflected in behavioral changes, but the importance of the outcome can be represented only by considering its significance for others.

Effect on Caregivers

As was noted in the discussion of the social systems perspective (Dunst et al., 1985), the caregiver who observes response-contingent behavior in a person under his or her care assumes and develops an interest in that individual that was not present when that person was viewed as unresponsive and incapable of learning. This interest leads to greater challenges for the person who is disabled, and, subsequently, to the aforementioned higher-order affects. The person with the profound disability who is capable of initiating a routine by signaling to the caregiver that it is time to perform that routine can come to be seen as in control and actively making decisions. The caregiver, no longer viewed as simply providing care, can be transformed further into the role of "care assistant." The caregiver becomes the individual who provides assistance to the person with profound disabilities at his or her initiation and request. This has the potential of transforming the person with disabilities from the passive role of patient (i.e., literally waiting for care) into the active role of consumer and director of his or her own care.

The effects on the caregiver can be equally noteworthy. Rather than following a set scheduled routine, such as "wake up 6:00 A.M., feed at 7:00 A.M., check hourly for incontinence," the care assistant can allow the individual who is disabled to help define the routine by his or her requests. Some limits would likely be necessary in order to ensure that adequate care was being provided. Even when such ability of the person is small and circumscribed (such as only indicating when he or she has been incontinent, or better, when he or she needs to be helped to a toilet to avoid incontinence), the effect can be a decrease in the performance of a redundant, high-frequency, and, perhaps, unpleasant task, such as hourly "diaper checks." Ideally, the effects would be to establish a positive attitude about the person's potential, spend more time in social interaction with him or her, and take advantage of these initiated routines as occasions for positive interactions. By not allowing the person with the profound disability to behave and attempt to initiate some routines, he or she will never do so, nor will caregivers ever know if the individual was capable of doing so. Furthermore, as Dunst et al. (1985) have suggested, parents of individuals with profound disabilities may become more willing to allow them to remain alone for periods of time, confident that they can entertain themselves or signal if they have any difficulties. This has the desirable effect of decreasing time demands that are placed on parents and allowing them to address other responsibilities and interests. The performance or outcome measurement in this area might involve monitoring the emergence of skills such as initiating, and then assessing, as a consequence, the collateral benefits on the social interactions between caregivers (e.g., family members, direct care staff) and clients. Measures such as the amount of time spent interacting during periods other than those set aside for direct care, the ratings of caregivers' attitudes toward clients and their own job satisfaction, and the amount of "free time" available to family members, may provide some initial outcome data reflecting the effect on caregivers.

The authors have already suggested that there are aspects of a person's skills that might alter the relationship between the client and the professional caregiver in a positive direction. The focus yet to be discussed is the relationship between the client and nonprofessional caregivers such as parents and family members. It is a well-established fact that the presence of a family member who is profoundly disabled poses an enormous burden of responsibility for day-to-day physical care, particularly on mothers (Wilkins, 1981). The amount of time spent in physical care is, understandably, directly proportional to the severity of the family member's disability (Ruhe, 1984). While many factors determine the actual difficulties experienced by families and their decision to eventually seek out-of-home placement (Cole & Meyer, 1985), the amount of time and effort spent in direct physical care is a very important factor mediating stress (Ruhe, 1984). Thus, any behavioral outcomes that are specifically able to ease the burden of direct care must be considered to be of great importance for persons whose handicaps require consistent and concentrated assistance.

As already explained, the steps involved in initiating a routine allow the person with the profound disability to maintain some degree of control over, and thus, ownership of, daily routines. However, from the caregiver's point of view, initiating by indicating needs or desires can be of great importance in, for example, reducing toileting accidents, or preventing outbursts of anger. Because people with profound handicaps often have a large number of associated medical problems, when the individual is able to monitor his or her own internal state, it can be very helpful (e.g., allowing a caregiver to administer medicine at the most appropriate time; recognizing the onset of a seizure by signaling the caregiver in warning, and moving to a location or position where the seizure would be least harmful).

Another way in which the client can be of assistance to those providing the care is through postural adjustments that make it easier to physically direct him or her. For example, in dressing, a person who learns to hold his or her body in a certain position to facilitate dressing can save the caregiver time that might more appropriately be spent in additional social interactions with the client. Lifting or positioning the client is another activity that can be difficult for family members, particularly mothers. Wilkins (1981) reported that this was one of the few activities in which mothers received assistance from fathers or older siblings. Again, there are positions and movements that make it easier to lift someone, and these would, therefore, be very desirable behaviors for the client to learn. Following the same logic, it is obvious that mobility skills become very significant in persons with profound handicaps. Walking or being able to locate one's way around a house makes a considerable difference to the assistance that must otherwise be provided.

Participation in Everyday Activities

One of the most interesting concepts that has recently emerged in evaluating programs for persons with severe and profound handicaps is that of *partial participation* (Brown et al., 1979). According to this perspective, an individual who may not be able to perform some activity independently should, nevertheless, not be denied the opportunity to participate in that activity. If the person can perform some small part of the activity, then he or she would be able to be included and integrated with others in this situation. F. Brown and her colleagues (Brown et al., 1987) suggested some additional criteria that would make partial participation meaningful. These authors argued that merely performing some fraction of an overall event would not guarantee that the participation was meaningful to that person or to others. In fact, it could be claimed that partially participating in some activities might be even more frustrating than not taking part at all. An analogy of such a situation might be to allow a younger sibling in a family to participate in a game, such as softball, but having him or her spend all the time in the outfield in a nonmajor role. For the younger sibling, this could be more frustrating than enjoyable.

Brown et al. (1987) have suggested some criteria for deciding what type of partial participation might or might not be meaningful. For example, the person's affect might be used to judge participation: does the affect seem to be appropriate to the task, or does the individual with the profound handicap have to be coaxed and encouraged to participate? External social criteria can also be used (e.g., would an independent judge view the participation as meaningful?). For instance, having your wheelchair placed so that you can hit the ball in a family volleyball game is probably more meaningful participation than being allowed to sit at the table when the family is playing Scrabble.

Acceptance

It has long been recognized that behavioral outcomes that make a person more acceptable to society are of great importance. However, it is sometimes possible to change societal attitudes and values, rather than trying to make individuals meet certain predetermined requirements. Professionals talk a great deal about how certain habits render a person less appealing to his or her peers and family (e.g., if a child were to drool less, then peers and teachers would increase their interactions with the child). There may be some truth to this; however, it has serious limitations when carefully examined. Those who are hypercritical or who are easily put off relating to someone because of that person's physical characteristics may not be greatly influenced by only minor changes in a child's behavior. Standards of this kind have a way of being constantly raised so that the person who is deviant will never quite be close enough to the criterion to be accepted.

Changing social attitudes is one major strategy that the authors feel must be employed; however, this chapter deals only with client outcomes and which ones are the most meaningful. (See Chapter 3, this volume, for more details on the issue of changing social attitudes.) Thus, the authors see some value in a limited or compromise position. One rule might be that if a primary and important caregiver has a particular personal concern, such as self-stimulatory behavior in public, then improving that particular behavior in that context could have some priority as an outcome. A second rule is that if the undesirable behavior would attract a great deal of negative public attention and avoidance, then again it might be a priority behavior for change. As an example, a person with a severe or profound handicap might have a threatening appearance to an uninformed person because of the way he or she stands or moves when around others. In this case, it can be predicted that a sufficient number of people will misinterpret the person's intent and, thus, the behavior becomes a priority for intervention. A third consideration is related to the presence of a few other behaviors that make people likeable, despite other specific negative habits. Some persons with profound handicaps are much more likely to attract the attention, interest, and liking of caregivers than others. Usually, the crucial difference is some relatively simple social behavior such as a smile, a relaxed disposition, or a comic style. Social behaviors such as smiling and greeting are most likely to be teachable and to have a very significant effect on acceptability, regardless of other characteristics.

Educational Validity

When conducting program evaluations based upon the various individual outcomes mentioned or when evaluating a particular client for the purpose of setting some future directions, it is necessary to take a somewhat broader perspective than measuring individual responses. According to the criteria for "educational validity" proposed by Voeltz and Evans (1983), it should be determined not only if a given measured outcome can be judged to be meaningful, but also if it has meaningful implications for that person's life situation. It can be argued that there are two dimensions to consider when evaluating specific behavioral outcomes more broadly. One of these is a lateral dimension and essentially poses the question of what percentage of a person's day is spent in meaningful activities. This could be assessed by real-time continuous observation of ongoing activities or by a number of random momentary samples throughout a day. It is no longer a sufficient outcome to report the change or progress of one behavior, unless the distribution of meaningful behaviors throughout the day is also enhanced.

The second dimension might be considered hierarchical and refers to the implications of the behavior change for the person's future. It is now rather clear that the goals of any treatment, whether clinical or educational, are never simply ends in themselves. Part of their value is contained in the implications that these changes have on future behavior and their role as the means to other desirable ends (Evans & Meyer, 1985). As has been pointed out, most of the outcomes described have implications for later developments. These implications could be: 1) direct, such as acquiring a behavior that is a prerequisite for another more complex skill; 2) indirect, such as creating opportunities for caregivers to spend more time in social interaction; or 3) causative, such as certain social behaviors that elicit further social interaction from someone else. In each case, these desirable ends are not inevitable and cannot be taken for granted. Thus, it is necessary to initiate a monitoring procedure to ensure that the targeted behavior change is indeed leading to the next desired outcome.

SUMMARY: A PERSPECTIVE ON EXPECTATIONS

The expectations of others are especially important when considering the evaluation of program outcomes for persons with profound disabilities for two predominant reasons. The first of these is that expectations about available outcomes tend to influence the kinds of programs that are implemented. Professionals who are involved in programming for persons who are profoundly handicapped frequently comment that their students will never be able to learn useful skills, work, or participate in the community. In fact, quite often when such outcomes are discussed, these professionals, with their focus on negative expectations, will continuously remind people of the sort of individuals that they are working with—the "really profoundly disabled." Work, in the sense that these professionals refer to it, is a particular activity (e.g., sorting mail, washing dishes), not a class of behavior. Functionally, work is a category of those behaviors that are performed because they are desired (or result in a product that is desired) by someone else. Obviously, it is a complex social process to find or create actual jobs (i.e., employment, supported employment) for clients who are profoundly disabled, but everyone is capable of functionally defined work. In fact, it is interesting to note that if the subjects of the studies reported in this chapter had been paid for their participation, then they all would have had employment for at least a period of time.

It is arguable that work behaviors do not have to be performed by everyone in society, a society that can clearly afford to exempt those with the most profound disabilities. However, it is also arguable that work, such as recreational and self-help behavior as functional classes, should occupy at least a percentage of one's day, and that work also affords other opportunities (e.g., pay, whether it be goods, monetary, or direct exchange of services, provides additional opportunities for the individual). Only if caregivers' expectations are oriented toward a functional definition of work would there be any chance for opportunities to be created that would allow persons with profound handicaps to perform these work behaviors. Similarly, if very positive expectations for persons with profound handicaps were linked to preconceived forms of behavior (e.g., "one day my child will be able to get a job as a janitor"; "this student might be able to sort transistors in a factory"), then instructional programs might be established to focus on outcomes that are, at present, unattainable to these individuals. Consequently, this could lead to undesirable social pressures on persons who are disabled, and produce diminished opportunity for reward.

Expectations determine the social and environmental conditions that are established for an individual who is profoundly disabled. This is probably true of all members of society. Despite some limitations in methodology, the famous Pygmalion experiments highlighted the point that expectations determine opportunities, to an extent (Rosenthal & Jacobson, 1968). The difference is that those opportunities are regulated by others according to an individual's degree of disability. Nonhandicapped students have many opportunities to create their own learning environments, and indeed do so. What prohibits persons with profound disabilities from creating such learning environments is that their chances of doing this are negligible, especially in structured care situations. The reason that institutional settings are disfavored as compared to the structure of the family-sized home is not because of normalization, expense, or other equally good reasons; it is because the social structure of these smaller settings enables the creation of desirable expectations. In a family-sized home, the expectation that the people living there should all take part in daily duties for the general good is much stronger than in a residential facility where the expectation is that the professional people should provide care, as in a hospital setting. Similarly, if a small group home has a structure that is oriented toward total care, so that the residents are expected to be like perpetual newborn infants in a typical family home, its "normalized" appearance will not matter since it will not afford opportunities for positive outcomes.

In this chapter, the authors have tried to influence expectations, not by being positive (i.e., look what persons with disabilities can do) or negative (i.e., look what persons with disabilities cannot do), but by focusing on dimensions of behavior that should be considered when thinking of outcomes. In the more elaborate behaviors of everyday life, function can often be inferred correctly by studying its form. For example, if we say that someone has learned to drive a car, this usually means that he or she can get to a destination without having to be driven there by someone else, and not that he or she has mastered the mechanical operations sufficiently enough for the vehicle to move forward in a straight line. However, with the simpler everyday behaviors form does not always reveal function. Expectations about daily activities are often tied to the amount of help typically needed for most activities. With persons who are profoundly disabled, social, self-help, recreational, and work functions can still be achieved, but often with very specialized (e.g., the use of technology to transform a simple manipulation into a complex communication) or minimal (e.g., body posture facilitating dressing) forms of behavior.

In addition to creating the conditions in which learning opportunities are embedded, outcome expectations also determine the satisfaction or happiness that a person feels toward whatever outcomes are achieved. Thus, these expectations ultimately determine the value that a person places upon the outcomes and the programs that produced them or failed to produce them (Evans, 1985b). If expectations are too low or are not keyed to meaningful dimensions, then there is a tendency to be satisfied with doubtful competencies and poor programs. On the contrary, if expectations are unrealistically overstated by present fascination with functional skills and the normalized forms of routines, it creates conditions of chronic disappointment and frustration, especially for families. Therefore, the key to successful program evaluation would seem to go beyond defining the meaningfulness of outcomes to the specification of behavioral characteristics that reflect intrinsically usable outcomes. In this way, criteria will emerge that designate the best outcomes achieved in some programs as the standard for other programs, and designate the best possible outcome as the goal for all.

REFERENCES

Brown, F., Evans, I.M., Weed, K.A., & Owen, V. (1987). Delineating functional competencies: A component model. *Journal of The Association for Persons with Severe Handicaps, 12*, 117–124.

Brown, L., Branston-McLean, M.B., Baumgart, D., Vincent, L., Falvey, M., & Schroeder, J. (1979). Using the characteristics of current and subsequent least restrictive environments as factors in the development of curricular content for severely handicapped students. *AAESPH Review, 14*, 407–424.

Burch, M.R., Clegg, J.C., & Bailey, J.S. (1987). Automated contingent reinforcement of correct posture. *Research in Developmental Disabilities, 8*, 15–20.

Cochran, M., & Brassard, J. (1979). Child development and personal social networks. *Child Development, 50*, 601–616.

Cole, D.A., & Meyer, L.H. (1985, August). *Impact of family needs and resources on the decision to seek out-of-home placement.* Paper presented at the annual convention of the American Psychological Association, Los Angeles.

Deiker, T., & Bruno, R.D. (1976). Sensory reinforcement of eyeblink rate in a decorticate human. *American Journal of Mental Deficiency, 80*, 665–667.

Dewson, M.R.J., & Whiteley, J.H. (1987). Sensory reinforcement of head turning with nonambulatory, profoundly mentally retarded persons. *Research in Developmental Disabilities, 8*, 413–426.

Dunst, C.J., Cushing, P.J., & Vance, S.D. (1985). Response-contingent learning in profoundly handicapped infants: A social system perspective. *Analysis and Intervention in Developmental Disabilities, 5*, 33–47.

Durand, V.M. (1982). Analysis and intervention of self-injurious behavior. *Journal of The Association for the Severely Handicapped, 7*, 44–53.

Evans, I.M. (1985a). Building systems models as a strategy for target behavior selection in clinical assessment. *Behavioral Assessment, 7*, 21–32.

Evans, I.M. (1985b). *Individual expectations and outcome evaluations: A strategy for judging the benefits of special education* (Tech. Report No. 9). Binghamton: State University of New York, Project SPAN.

Evans, I.M., & Brown, F. (1986). Outcome assessment of student competence: Issues and implications. *Special Services in the Schools, 2*, 41–62.

Evans, I.M., Brown, F.A., Weed, K.A., Spry, K.M., & Owen, V. (1987). The assessment of functional competencies: A behavioral approach to the evaluation of programs for children with disabilities. In R.J. Prinz (Ed.), *Advances in behavioral assessment of children and families* (Vol. 3, pp. 93–121). Greenwich, CT: JAI Press.

Evans, I.M., & Meyer, L.H. (1985). *An educative approach to behavior problems: A practical decision model for interventions with severely handicapped learners.* Baltimore: Paul H. Brookes Publishing Co.

Evans, I.M., Weed, K.A., Brown, F.A., & Weld, E.M. (in press). Differential generalization of component behaviors within routines: An experimental analysis of functional competence. *Child and Family Behavior Therapy.*

Favell, J.E., & Risley, T.R. (1984, November). *Organizing living environments for developmentally disabled persons.* Workshop presented at the convention of the Association for the Advancement of Behavior Therapy, Philadelphia.

Fuller, P.R. (1949). Operant conditioning of a vegetative human organism. *American Journal of Psychology, 62*, 587–599.

Green, C.W., Canipe, V.S., Way, P.J., & Reid, D.H. (1986). Improving the functional utility and effectiveness of classroom services for students with profound multiple handicaps. *Journal of The Association for Persons with Severe Handicaps, 11*, 162–170.

Haskett, J., & Hollar, W.D. (1978). Sensory reinforcement and contingency awareness of profoundly retarded children. *American Journal of Mental Deficiency, 83*, 60–68.

Kuhlenbeck, H., Szekely, E.G., & Spuler, H. (1964). Observations on the EEG of a hydranencephalic "decorticate" child in the resting condition and upon stimulation. In W. Bargmann & J.P. Schade (Eds.), *Progress in brain research: Topics in basic neurology* (Vol. 6, pp. 198–206). New York: Elsevier/North Holland.

LaMendola, W.F., Zaharia, E.S., & O'Brien, K.F. (1987). Foundation care: A treatment model for nonambulatory profoundly mentally retarded persons. *American Journal of Mental Deficiency, 91*, 341–347.

Landesman-Dwyer, S., & Sackett, G.P. (1978). Behavioral changes in nonambulatory, profoundly mentally retarded individuals. In C.E. Meyers (Ed.), *Quality of life in severely and profoundly mentally retarded people: Research foundations for improvement* (pp. 55–144). Washington, DC: American Association on Mental Deficiency.

McWilliam, R.A., Trivette, C.M., & Dunst, C.J. (1985). Behavior engagement as a measure of the efficacy of early intervention. *Analysis and Intervention in Developmental Disabilities, 5,* 59–71.

Meyer, L.H., Reichle, J., McQuarter, R.J., Evans, I.M., Neel, R.S., & Kishi, G.S. (1983). *The Assessment of Social Competence (ASC): A scale of social competence functions.* Minneapolis: University of Minnesota Consortium Institute for the Education of Severely Handicapped Learners.

Murphy, R.J., & Doughty, N.R. (1977). Establishment of controlled arm movements in profoundly retarded students using response contingent vibratory stimulation. *American Journal of Mental Deficiency, 82,* 212–216.

Parris Stephens, M.A., Norris-Baker, C., & Willems, E.P. (1984). Data quality in self-observation and report of behavior. *Behavioral Assessment, 6,* 237–252.

Piper, R.J., & McKinnon, R.C. (1969). Operant conditioning of a profoundly retarded individual reinforced via a stomach fistula. *American Journal of Mental Deficiency, 73,* 627–630.

Pollard, J. (Ed.). (1984). *Diagnosis and instructional programming: Student handbook.* Chelmsford, MA: Merrimack Special Education Collaborative.

Reid, D.H., Parsons, M.B., McCarn, J.E., Green, C.W., Philips, J.F., & Schepis, M.M. (1985). Providing a more appropriate education for severely handicapped persons: Increasing and validating functional classroom tasks. *Journal of Applied Behavior Analysis, 18,* 289–301.

Rice, H.K. (1968). Operant behavior in vegetative patients, III: Methodological considerations. *Psychological Record, 18,* 297–302.

Rice, H.K., & McDaniel, M.W. (1966). Operant behavior in vegetative patients. *Psychological Record, 16,* 279–281.

Rice, H.K., McDaniel, M.W., Stallings, V.D., & Gatz, M.J. (1967). Operant behavior in vegetative patients, II. *Psychological Record, 17,* 449–460.

Rosenthal, R., & Jacobson, L. (1968). *Pygmalion in the classroom: Teacher expectation and pupils' intellectual development.* New York: Holt, Rinehart & Winston.

Ruhe, L.A. (1984). *The impact of handicapped children on family time-budgeting, caretaking responsibilities, and the quality of life.* Unpublished master's thesis, State University of New York at Binghamton.

Skinner, B.F. (1950). Are theories of learning necessary? *Psychological Review, 57,* 193–216.

Skinner, B.F. (1953). *Science and human behavior.* New York: Free Press.

Stella, M.E., & Etzel, B.C. (1986). Stimulus control of eye orientations: Shaping S + only versus shaping S − only. *Analysis and Intervention in Developmental Disabilities, 6,* 137–153.

Voeltz, L.M., & Evans, I.M. (1983). Educational validity: Procedures to evaluate outcomes in programs for severely handicapped learners. *Journal of The Association for the Severely Handicapped, 8,* 3–15.

Weber, D.B., & Thaeler, D. (1987, May). *Daily exercise: Is it possible for profoundly mentally retarded individuals?* Paper presented at the annual convention of the Association for Behavior Analysis, Nashville.

White, O.R. (1980). Adaptive performance objectives: Form versus function. In W. Sailor, B. Wilcox, & L. Brown (Eds.), *Methods of instruction for severely handicapped students* (pp. 47–69). Baltimore: Paul H. Brookes Publishing Co.

Wilkins, D. (1981). A task-oriented approach to the assessment of the distribution of the burden of care, levels of support, and felt needs in the family. In B. Cooper (Ed.), *Assessing the handicaps and needs of mentally retarded children* (pp. 185–196). New York: Academic Press.

Wolf, M.M. (1978). Social validity: The case for subjective measurement, or how applied behavior analysis is finding its heart. *Journal of Applied Behavior Analysis, 11*, 203–214.

INTEGRATION FOR STUDENTS WITH PROFOUND DISABILITIES

5

Martha E. Snell
and Stanley J. Eichner

Although federal law has required for more than 12 years that all students with special needs be integrated to the maximum extent appropriate, the disappointing fact is that a significant percentage of those students still remain relegated to "handicapped-only" or segregated programs. Even in those educational systems where greater success toward integration has been achieved, there has been a continuing failure to integrate those students with the more severe and profound disabilities. (For clarification as to nomenclature, "children with disabilities," "children with special needs," and "children with handicaps" are intended to be understood as being synonymous. However, despite the use of the term "handicapped children" or "children with handicaps" in the major federal statute, the authors will use the term "disability" since that is the phrase of choice that is used by the disability community itself.) This disappointing record persists, many years after the passage of PL 94-142, the Education for All Handicapped Children Act of 1975, and after a significant number of educational systems have effectively transitioned to integrated programs and demonstrated the efficacy of educational integration. This chapter explores the legal and educational bases for integrating students with profound disabilities, and describes some of the factors that have impeded the attainment of integrated programming. Finally, it suggests some possible educational and legal strategies for enabling students with severe and profound disabilities to have functional and chronologically age-appropriate programs with their nonhandicapped peers.

Educationally, there is no program component or educational strategy that is provided in a segregated setting that cannot be implemented at least as effectively within a local public school. In addition, there are certain necessary elements to an appropriate education that cannot be provided in a "handi-capped-only" setting (e.g., socialization). Both federal law and compelling educational principles require that these students with special needs must receive their services within the local public school.

WHAT IS INTEGRATION?

Various terms such as *mainstreaming* and *integration* are sometimes used interchangeably, and frequently with quite different meanings intended. Prior to discussion of how and why to integrate students with special needs, it is important to clarify how these terms are used in this chapter.

Typically, the term mainstreaming refers to educationally placing students with mild disabilities in regular educational classes. Historically, integration has referred to the provision of special educational services to students with severe or profound disabilities within a local public school building. More recently, a growing number of authors have begun to argue in favor of placing students with severe disabilities in regular educational classrooms (e.g. Biklen, 1985; Stainback & Stainback, 1987). This chapter primarily addresses the integration of students with profound disabilities within the public schools.

Preliminarily, it should be noted that the principles of integration are defined or articulated within two separate but interconnected realms—legal and educational. The legal context is defined by the least restrictive environment (LRE) requirement found within PL 94-142. This statute requires that:

> To the maximum extent appropriate, handicapped children, including children in public or private institutions or other care facilities, are educated with children who are not handicapped, and that special classes, separate schooling, or other removal of handicapped children from regular educational environment occurs only when the nature or severity of the handicap is such that education in regular classes with the use of supplementary aids and services cannot be achieved satisfactorily. (20 U.S.C. §1415 [5][B])

Stated most simply, the law requires that all students with disabilities be educated alongside their nondisabled peers to the greatest extent possible, and that any move away from the regular educational setting occur only when it is not possible for that student's program, as supplemented with aids and services, to provide him or her with an appropriate education.

The educational description of integrated programming is different. The minimal essential components of an appropriate education for students with profound disabilities requires that: 1) the program be located on the same campus where the student's nonhandicapped peers attend school, and 2) there be ongoing and meaningful opportunities for both programmed and casual interaction between the students with special needs and their nondisabled peers (Brown et al., 1979). In addition to those two requisite characteristics, an appropriate educational program for these students should also: 1) employ functional skill targets, 2) establish chronologically age-appropriate skills, and 3) teach such skills in the community to facilitate generalization. As noted earlier, these components should not only be available within a local public school, but must be taught there since they cannot be provided within a segregated setting (Brown et al., 1979).

Historical Perspective on the Integration Imperative

To understand the legal mandate for integration, it is first important to review the historical context. Until the 1980s, the general pattern of treatment of students with disabilities was one of either de facto (i.e., from the practice) or *de jure* (i.e., legally mandated) exclusion. For example, in 1971, Pennsylvania's school code established, as a minimum entrance requirement to public school, that a student attain a mental age of five years (*Pennsylvania Association of Retarded Children (PARC) v. Commonwealth of Pennsylvania*, 1971). Similarly, in 1972 the District of Columbia's compulsory attendance law specifically allowed a child to be "excused" from attending school if the child was "found to be unable mentally or physically to profit from attendance at school" (*Mills v. Board of Education of the District of Columbia*, 1972). In each of these cases, existing laws barred students with severe and profound disabilities from attending public school.

These two landmark cases, *PARC (1971)* and *Mills (1972)*, successfully challenged the statutory exclusion and established most of the fundamental principles that were later incorporated into PL 94-142. One of these fundamental principles was zero-exclusion from an entitlement to a publicly supported education. Also included was the establishment of the central principle that stated that placement decisions must be made:

> Within the context of a presumption that, among the alternative programs of education and training required by statute to be available, placement in a regular public school class is preferable to placement in a special public school class and placement in a special public school class is preferable to placement in any other type of program of education or training. (*PARC* [1971], at §1260)

After the decision in the *PARC (1971)* and *Mills (1972)* cases, Congress held extensive hearings in preparation for its statutory response to the educational needs of these students. As a result, Congress made a fundamental educational decision that stated that children with handicaps need and benefit from placement in the regular educational environment with their nonhandicapped peers. The LRE requirement that expresses this congressional decision was first applied to special education in the Education of the Handicapped Act Amendments of 1974 (PL 93-380). The sponsor of the amendment, Senator Charles M. Mathias, Jr. (R–MD) made clear that the rights guaranteed by this change were intended to reflect and codify the findings of special education experts that children with handicaps require an integrated educational environment. Senator

Mathias (1974) stated, "My amendment supports the developing trend toward normalization, and mainstreaming, and will underscore the interlocking nature of special education with regular education." In the testimony heard from school staff, parents, advocates, and service providers, congressional committees were told repeatedly of three critical needs in the educational services of students with severe disabilities. These critical needs include: 1) need for normalized environments, 2) the need to move into the mainstream of education, and 3) society's need to use community schools as the country's "melting pot."[1] The committees considering Senate Bill 6 and the House of Representatives Bill 70 had learned that integration affected the quality of the special educational programs provided to children with disabilities. Dr. Ewald Nyquist (1974), Commissioner, New York State Department of Education, stated that, "The quality of many publicly operated or supported educational programs is related to the degree to which children with handicapping conditions are grouped or otherwise combined effectively with other children in the mainstream of our school and society" (*1974 House Hearings,* at §61).

It was just as important to understand that interlocking special education with regular education was critical for the full integration of students with disabilities into the postschool world, as it is, according to Senator Robert T. Stafford (R–VT) (1974), to show that:

> [w]e are concerned that children with handicapping conditions be educated in the most normal possible and least restrictive setting, for how else will they adapt to the world beyond the educational environment, and how else will the non-handicapped adapt to them.

Rehabilitation psychologist Dr. Fred Fay (1974) also expressed his concerns on this topic in his testimony to the Senate committee. He stressed his concern:

> About the effects of some special schools on children where they do not get a chance to develop normally in more than just school work, [to develop] their social skills with other able-bodied children . . . [T]o the extent possible, the students [should] be integrated with other able-bodied students so they get the maximum benefit of their education.

The integration imperative was not intended to benefit only high-functioning children with disabilities. As early as 1974, Congress had learned that children with severe disabilities could and, in fact, were benefiting from educational programs located in regular public schools. On the basis of 25 years of

---

[1]Such testimony can be found throughout the hearings held on the Senate and House bills that formed the basis of PL 94-142. See *Financial Assistance for Improved Educational Services for Handicapped Children Hearings on House of Representatives Bill 70 Before the Select Subcommittee on Education of the Handicapped of the House Committee on Education and Labor,* 93rd Congress, 2nd Session *passim* (1974) (hereinafter, *1974 House Hearings*); *Education for All Handicapped Children, 1973–74: Hearings on Senate Bill 6 Before the Subcommittee on the Handicapped of the Senate Committee on Labor and Public Welfare,* 94th Congress, 1st Session, 282 *passim* (1975) (hereinafter, *1974 Senate Hearings*).

experience in providing educational services, the United Cerebral Palsy Association, Inc. concluded that "[i]ntegration with non-handicapped children, wherever possible, is essential to the normalization process for severely and multiply handicapped children" (*1974 House Hearings,* at §369). Dr. Gunnar Dybwad (1974) from Brandeis University praised Senate Bill 6 for including institutionalized children within the scope of its integration imperative, stating:

> I welcome the emphasis placed on integration, to the maximum extent appropriate, of institutionalized children at regular schools.
>
> . . . [W]e must make sure that as many of these children as possible, even though they may have to reside in the institution for a certain time, get their schooling as close . . . to that of other children.
>
> And I am happy to report that at least it is being demonstrated in several parts of the country that it is feasible for children to reside in the State institution, for instance, for the mentally retarded and still go to school in the community. (*1974 Senate Hearings,* at §§371, 378–9)

The mandate for placement in the regular public school setting was intended by Congress to include children and youth with severe disabilities. The report of the House Committee of Education and Labor (1975) indicated that when students with severe handicaps could not receive a satisfactory education in the regular classroom, "the 'regular education setting' goal" could still be met "by having a separate class or separate wing in a regular school building." Even for students with severe disabilities then, the integration imperative mandates placement in the next least restrictive setting—when they cannot be mainstreamed into a regular class. The LRE requirement as stated by Senator Harrison Arlington Williams (D–NJ) (1974) thus "protects the rights of handicapped children to be educated together with their peers, and not to be educated in a separate educational system."

Legal Mandate for Integration of Students with Profound Disabilities

As the above review of the legislative history makes clear, Congress was mindful of the critical need for integrated educational programs for students with profound disabilities, and in PL 94-142, Congress issued a statutory mandate for regular school placement for such students. Simply stated, the congressional statutory mandate provides that if students with handicaps can be educated in the regular public school setting, then that is where they must be educated. The statute guarantees students with disabilities the substantive right to an education in the least restrictive environment. According to PL 94-142, the LRE principle requires that:

> To the maximum extent appropriate, handicapped children, including children in public or private institutions or other care facilities, are educated with children who are not handicapped, and that special classes, separate schooling, or other removal of handicapped children from regular educational environment occurs

only when the nature or severity of the handicap is such that education in regular classes with the use of supplementary aids and services cannot be achieved satisfactorily. [20 U.S.C. §1415(5)(B)]

The LRE requirement that is delineated in the federal statute is recapitulated in the federal regulations in two distinct parts [34 C.F.R. §300.550(b)]. The first part sets out the integration imperative—the mandate for placement in the regular public schools—that dominates the rest of the statute and its implementing regulations: "that, to the maximum extent appropriate, handicapped children should be educated with children who are not handicapped" [20 U.S.C. §1412(5)(B); 34 C.F.R. §300.550(b)(1)]. The second part establishes a presumption of regular class placement for children with disabilities and prescribes the limits on any removal from placement in such a class ("only when the nature and severity of the handicap is such that education in regular classes with the use of supplementary aids and services cannot be achieved satisfactorily" [20 U.S.C. §1412(5)(B); 34 C.F.R. §300.550(b)(2)]).

The strength of the congressional integration imperative is evident from the way in which it is woven throughout the rest of the statute and regulations. For example, the statute requires that the Individualized Education Program (IEP) that is prepared annually for each student with disabilities states "the extent to which such a child will be able to participate in regular educational programs" (20 U.S.C. §1401[19][C]). In the regulations, the mandate for integration is not limited to the physical location of the special educational program or to the traditional academic portion of the school day. Even in nonacademic services such as lunch, recess, and extracurricular activities, students with disabilities must be integrated "to the maximum extent appropriate" (34 C.F.R. §300.553). The regulations also include a specific section applying the integration mandate to those students who reside in institutions or who are so severely disabled as to require institutional care (34 C.F.R. §300.554). The comments to that section explain that "[r]egardless of other reasons for institutional placement, no child in an institution who is capable of education in a regular public school setting may be denied access to an education in that setting" (34 C.F.R. §300.554).

To reach its goal of regular public school setting and its presumption of regular class placement, Congress placed upon educational officials the burden of proving why a student with disabilities cannot be educated in the regular public school. Section 1412(5)(B) of the statute (PL 94-142) provides that students with disabilities, including those who have their residence in institutions, can be removed from the regular educational environment only when the use of supplementary aids and services in the regular environment will not provide them with a satisfactory education.

As a number of United States Courts of Appeals have recognized, the mandate of integration is so strong that it requires placement in the regular public school even though a superior program may be available in a segregated setting. If the student can receive educational benefit in the regular public school with the use of supplementary aids and services, the placement in the segregated facility violates PL 94-142. The clearest explanation of the requirements of the act occurred in the case of *Roncker v. Walter* (1983). This case concerned a 9-year-old student classified as trainable mentally retarded who had been assigned to Ohio's "county schools," attended exclusively by children with handicaps. In this case, the court framed the issue as "whether a proposed placement is appropriate under the act. In some cases, a placement that may be considered better for academic reasons may not be appropriate because of the failure to provide for mainstreaming . . . " (*Roncker*, 1983). The court in *Roncker* (1983) even questioned the validity of opinions that found segregated settings superior to integrated ones. "The perception that a segregated institution is academically superior for a handicapped child may reflect no more than a basic disagreement with the mainstreaming concept" (*Roncker*, 1983). Given the clear expression of congressional intent, "[s]uch a disagreement is not, of course, any basis for not following the Act's mandate" (*Roncker*, 1983).

To reinforce the general integration imperative for placement in the regular public school setting, the LRE requirement, in its second section, establishes a presumption of regular class placement for all students with disabilities. According to PL 94-142, if regular class placement with the use of supplementary aids and services will not result in a satisfactory educational program, then, and only then, can the child be removed from the regular class (20 U.S.C. §1412[5][B]). When such removal proves necessary, the general integration imperative still stands, requiring placement in the next least restrictive environment within the regular public school setting (20 U.S.C. §1412[5][B]).

Consistent with that goal, the pivotal placement criterion in the LRE requirement of PL 94-142 is whether the application of special educational services and technology—"the use of supplementary aids and services"—will result in a satisfactory education in the regular classroom or, if not there, then in the next most integrated setting (20 U.S.C. §1412[5][B]). In the *Roncker* (1983) case, the court saw in the LRE requirement precisely this relationship between educational feasibility and the integration imperative. Even:

> [i]n a case where the segregated facility is considered superior, the court should determine whether the services which make that placement superior could be feasibly provided in a non-segregated setting. If they can, the placement in the segregated school would be inappropriate under the Act. (*Roncker*, 1983, at §1063)

This critical relationship between feasibility and integration is precisely why the ongoing existence and viability of integrated educational programs for students with severe and profound disabilities is so fundamentally important, not just from an educational standpoint but from a legal one as well. By establishing a fluid standard in PL 94-142 that is tied to the current best practice, Congress articulated the requirement that if integration is feasible, then it must be implemented. When the viability of such integrated programs has long passed the point of being model programs or demonstration projects, those programs then become established standards against which all other less integrated programs must be educationally and legally judged.

RATIONALE FOR INTEGRATION

The literature on integration indicates that all people benefit from the integration of persons with disabilities into the mainstream of school, work, and community (e.g., Biklen, 1985; Brinker, 1985). In particular, the beneficiaries are those persons with disabilities; their families; their peers who do not have disabilities (and, indirectly, the families of those peers); and the caregivers employed to teach, administer, or otherwise work in integrated settings. Support for the existence of these benefits ranges from experimental research to logical common sense. In this section of the chapter, the rationale for integration is discussed in terms of integration's benefits for persons with severe and profound disabilities and their families, for students without disabilities, and for professional staff.

Benefits for Students with Profound Disabilities

Influence of Learning Characteristics   The need for integrated school settings has clear support from the knowledge about learning in students with profound disabilities. Three undisputed learning characteristics of these students are their slow rates of learning; loss of skills resulting from disuse; and difficulty in generalization or transfer of a learned skill to other settings, materials, and people. These characteristics influence how all skills are learned, including social skills. In order to counter these deficiencies, educational programs must exhibit two basic features. First, because these students acquire skills slowly, only the skills that are actually needed by a particular student to function as independently as possible, now and in the future, should be targeted for instruction. There is little time to teach skills that will not be used or will be outgrown once mastered. Second, educational programs must teach students to generalize the skills so that changes in the surroundings will not result in forgotten or dysfunctional skills. For the person with profound disabilities, only integrated settings offer the medium in which social skills can be practiced meaningfully and learned as generalized behaviors (Brinker, 1985; Voeltz, 1984).

Social skills are learned through daily interactions, both planned and spontaneous, between people with disabilities and their nondisabled peers. Research has shown that there appears to be little substitute. The presence of nonhandicapped peers creates more social opportunities for students with handicaps than segregated environments offer. Brinker's (1985) work and that of others (Gaylord-Ross & Peck, 1985; Strain & Kerr, 1981; Youniss, 1980) offer strong support for the position that interaction with nonhandicapped peers leads to more generalized use of social skills by students with severe disabilities. Social skills also cannot be learned when interaction is infrequent. For example, monthly or even weekly trips to the world outside the segregated school or work setting are too episodic to provide enough practice for mastery. Furthermore, these skills cannot be learned in "handicapped-only" settings where nondisabled peer interaction does not exist and social interaction is restricted to adult staff. The stimuli in "handicapped-only" settings are very different from those in the integrated world. Recall what the halls of a junior high are like between classes, the bus loading area at 3 P.M., or the cafeteria at lunchtime: groups of adolescents talking and laughing; their dress, conversation, and social exchanges are characteristic of their age, the location, and that year's style. Similarly, integrated work and leisure settings stand in stark contrast to sheltered workshops and special recreation groups in terms of the narrow range of social experiences that enable social competence and the development of meaningful social relationships (Voeltz, 1984).

Individual Variations of Social Skills All students need to learn social skills. Students with profound disabilities are no exception to this rule. Depending on the particular person (i.e., age, presence or absence of additional physical handicaps, mode and extent of communication), these social behaviors and forms of interpersonal interaction that are targeted will vary, and must be individually defined (Certo & Kohl, 1984; Gaylord-Ross & Pitts-Conway, 1984). The social skills targeted for a student might be as basic as refraining from stigmatizing behavior in public (i.e., talking aloud to oneself or rocking), raising a hand in greeting; or more sophisticated skills such as wearing age-appropriate clothes, learning when to speak to strangers and when to remain silent, and knowing how to communicate with nonhandicapped peers who speak faster, use slang, and expect different reactions than professionals do of persons with disabilities.

The benefits of having social skills are at least twofold. They contribute directly to one's enjoyment of others through friendship and they enable a person with profound disabilities to reduce or even overcome the "stigma" that many associate with being different. Perhaps, more importantly, the absence of appropriate social behavior reduces the opportunities that one has to enjoy life (e.g., to be able to eat in a public restaurant, to use a grocery store or a library, to enjoy a movie, to hold a job, to remain in one's natural home or in a small community-based residence). The more socially deviant a person appears to be in public, despite the presence of a multitude of academic, daily living, or vocational skills, the more probable it is that he or she will be barred from the use of community resources and employment. Social skills are central to community survival.

Other Benefits Many other benefits exist when students with profound handicaps attend school, play, and work in integrated settings (Halvorsen, 1983). These benefits include:

1. Students have age-appropriate, nondisabled peers as role models.
2. Positive behavior changes occur as a result of contact with and imitation of nonhandicapped peers.
3. Students are often more motivated in learning activities when working alongside of a nondisabled peer.
4. Students can partake in a variety of school activities suited to their chronological age (e.g., recess, lunch, assemblies, music, art, dances, clubs).
5. New mutual friendships are developed between students and their nondisabled peers that may extend beyond the day.
6. Students encounter and learn to deal with the expectations for performance and diversity present in schools and society.
7. Students' parents, caregivers, and teachers are also integrated in the regular school and thus experience new relationships, less isolation, and new ideas to benefit their interactions with students having disabilities.
8. Students have more opportunity to learn in natural contexts, including the presence of cues, corrections, and reinforcement that are typically available to nonhandicapped peers.

Benefits for Students without Disabilities and Professional Staff

How do segregated settings affect the nondisabled peers and coworkers of students with handicaps, and the professional and nonprofessional staff in schools and work settings? Many report that nondisabled peers' expectations for the performance of students or clients with disabilities are depressed in nonintegrated school and work sites. Others have found that when nondisabled children and adults see themselves as similar to peers with profound disabilities (e.g., appropriate in dress, activity, interests), they evaluate these peers more positively (Bak & Siperstein, 1987; Bates, Morrow, Pancsofar, & Sedlak, 1984). Staff in segregated settings operate without any proper age-norms for judging what is age-appropriate for their students. The absence of nonhandicapped peers may lead teachers to use an interaction style of teaching, to target skills, and to select materials and classroom decorations suited to much younger children. By contrast, when school, community, and work settings allow for interactions to occur between people with disabilities and people without disabilities, many benefits can exist. The following are examples of existing benefits:

1. Attitudes toward persons with disabilities improve.
2. Expectations of persons with disabilities increase and become more realistic.
3. Students experience appreciation and increasing acceptance of individual differences (Halvorsen, 1983).

4. Meaningful friendships between people can grow without regard to the presence or absence of disability.
5. The future parents of children with disabilities can confront their situation with more knowledge and optimism and with less prejudice.
6. The majority of future taxpayers can approach legislation that is influencing persons with disabilities in a more sensible manner.
7. Students who have a relative with a disability may establish a greater understanding of these family members.

PARTICULAR CONSIDERATIONS FOR STUDENTS WITH THE MOST SERIOUS DISABILITIES

Extraordinary Medical and Behavioral Problems

It is debatable which disabilities constitute the "most serious." Many disabilities are in this category due to their association with medically fragile conditions. For example, children and adolescents who are in need of regular "medical" attention during the school day in order to remain physically healthy are in this group. The physical and psychological conditions that are actually responsible for making some disabilities the most serious is less clear. Also, whether the mere presence of these conditions constitutes an adequate reason for exclusion from the public school is often the center of the controversy. Consider the following situations:

1. In Montgomery County, Maryland, the schools have hired an aide to walk a girl with "brittle bone" disease to and from classes to make sure that others do not bump into her (Viadero, 1987).
2. In numerous school districts, children are fed by their teachers or aides through a tube, often during instruction.
3. In some school buildings, students who require a respirator to breathe acquire watchful assistance from their schoolmates.
4. In a public school classroom in Albuquerque, New Mexico, a child receives regular suctioning of a tracheostomy tube from an attendant in order to maintain a clear breathing passage, while another child with heart problems is monitored by an aide at recess (Viadero, 1987).

In all instances, the students attend a regular school because the school system was able to introduce into that school the services needed for each person's medical condition. The medically disabling conditions that lead to education in separate facilities vary for different school districts. The determining factors appear not to be the medical condition as much as the current attitudes of the school administrators, the school's past history with other students having medical problems, the persistence of the parents of the student with disabilities, recent litigation, and the perceived or actual cost.

The same phenomenon seems to operate with students who have disruptive behavior as a result of their disability. If the school system has staff trained to design and implement skill training and behavior management programs, the problem is reduced or disappears. A history of success with students who are disruptive leads to a more positive outlook on their placement in regular schools with special services and staff. When the competence to deal with serious behavior problems is missing, the problem is exacerbated, sometimes to the point where exclusion of the student appears to be the only choice.

Are there any medical, behavioral, or cognitive conditions or problems that generally require exclusion from an integrated school setting? The answer to this question should not vary with the changing competence of the receiving school, but must pertain directly to the disability itself. Students cannot be held responsible for the inadequacies of different school systems. Schools must identify and supply the resources and training needs to serve students with extensive disabilities, rather than use the absence of these resources as the reason for exclusion or include students in their programs without being able to care properly for their special needs.

To answer the question posed in the previous paragraph, there are very few individuals with disabilities for whom an integrated program is not appropriate. The reason for these few students' segregation is not educational. For example, it is recognized that there is a very small population of students for whom integration would pose a risk, either to themselves or to others. By way of illustration, those school-age people who might possibly pose a risk to other students, disabled and nondisabled would fit in this small category. The risks to others might be due to the presence of seriously assaultive behavior despite the efforts of appropriately trained staff; or the risks might pertain to a highly contagious disease that a student may carry such as chicken pox or impetigo. Furthermore, children who are temporarily sick, who require extended bed rest, who are too medically fragile to be moved to the public school, who are too dependent upon constant medical attention to leave the hospital, or who are attached to nonportable life support equipment generally are best served in hospitals or their own home, not in schools. This group of people is very small. Their separation from the regular school environment is due to reasons that are not educational, and, in many cases, their separation should be temporary.

Ability to Learn

There are some school-age persons whose ability to learn has been questioned (Ellis, 1981; Kauffman & Krouse, 1981). Schools have either excluded or argued against accepting such persons based upon the rationale that people who belong in school must be able to learn. It is interesting to note that, like those who have been medically excluded in the past, the composition of this group has also changed over time. In the 1950s, there were many people who felt that children with moderate mental retardation as well as Down syndrome did not have the proper entry skills or simply did not learn adequately enough to qualify for attendance in regular public schools. Today, in the United States, these students are not in the group that is labeled "uneducable," simply because they can learn valuable skills when taught appropriately.

There has been little research on persons with profound mental retardation who have minimal levels of awareness and responsiveness and still reside in state institutions. Since many of these people are older than age 21, have had little or no educational or therapeutic intervention, are often nonambulatory, and have been institutionalized for most of their lives, legitimate questions can always be raised about what their repertoires would have been had they received appropriate, long-term programming in community settings. The existing research acknowledges that a complex array of variables also influences the state of being of these people, including nutrition, physical activity, position, presence of peers, activity in the surrounding environment, room temperature, comfort, and drug dosage (Guess, 1987; Landesman-Dwyer & Sackett, 1978). Because these people are dependent upon others for all their care and generally are given little or no control over their physical state, the importance of careful and intelligent arrangement of environmental variables must be recognized and the role of choice and control by the individual warrants investigation. Guess (1987) has stated that the knowledge about these people is still too primitive to conclude how much they can learn or how to design the best conditions under which they might learn. However, researchers are generally optimistic about the potential that such individuals may have for learning and the importance of their quality of life. Their presence in integrated school settings should be an issue of their chronological age and physical health, not location or incomplete knowledge of appropriate educational approaches.

Another group of people identified as having minimal levels of awareness include those who are unconscious or in severe comatose states due to traumatic head injuries. By comparison to the former group of people, researchers are still uncertain as to how much these individuals perceive while in this state, whether they can learn given their minimal responsivity, and what intervention beyond medical care is appropriate (Begali, 1987). By contrast, individuals with flat electroencephalograms (EEG) are not regarded as being in a comatose state. The term *brain-dead* is defined as the absence of brain activity including brain stem reflexes. This state is evidenced by a flat electroencephalogram (EEG) and no breathing reflex over a 3-minute period once a respirator has been turned off. Coma patients do not usually have flat EEGs, and most will recover; however, the degree of recovery depends upon many variables. People in comas rarely remain in that state for long; typically, they either die or recover. The small number of people who remain comatose for long periods of time require total care and close medical supervision to live. Despite the uncertainty about whether people in an unconscious or comatose state have meaningful awareness and potential for learning, professionals generally argue that these individuals are best served in hospital settings with medical intervention or at home with medical supervision, not in schools. However, these conclusions must be viewed as tentative due to the lack of knowledge of awareness and learning in this small group of people, in contrast to medical capacity to save lives.

Thus, any response to the question of whom, if anyone, should be excluded from regular school settings should be time-defined and regularly revised, since these answers must be tied to educational and medical technology, rather than to the characteristics of the student. Some students might require exclusion until the means are discovered to include them. For example, the realization that clean intermittent catheterization (CIC) did not require sterile conditions, as determined in the Supreme Court decision of *Tatro v. Texas* (1983), enabled that process to be carried out in schools by nonmedical staff with a minimum of in-service training and expense. Medical research made it feasible for students with myelomeningocele who had received only homebound education to attend schools. However, in most of these cases, the students did not attend school until the courts and/or parents forced schools to reverse their exclusionary practices and prepare their staff to provide the CIC.

Current educational practices (i.e., appropriate practices) must be recognized as direct products of: 1) the current level of knowledge and technology, 2) universities' and schools' capacities to transmit that knowledge and technology to school personnel and students, 3) the laws and regulations at the state and federal levels and their enforcement, and 4) the attitudes and values about education. Each factor has an influence on integration, whether prevailing conditions favor and facilitate integration or not. While each of these factors can vary over time, they all must change in a complimentary direction before educational practices in any given school system can improve. Any single factor or combination of factors can impede integration.

BARRIERS TO IMPLEMENTATION
OF THE INTEGRATION IMPERATIVE

Although in many respects people are justifiably proud of the results that have been achieved since the passage of PL 94-142, the implementation of the LRE requirements has been comparatively disappointing. Given the clarity of the requirements in the law, why has it been so difficult to see widespread acceptance and implementation of the act's integration requirements? The primary reason that implementation has lagged behind other provisions of the law is because those people who are charged with effecting the federal requirements on a statewide and local level have at best passively resisted, and at worst, actively fought implementation of it. This resistance on the part of the intended implementors has two major underpinnings: philosophical inertia and nonacceptance and territorial self-interest.

Philosophical Inertia and Nonacceptance

On a local level, for the vast majority of special educational administrators as well as the staff people under them, there simply has not been heartfelt acceptance of the principle that maximum integration of students with special needs is something that is worth working toward. Far beyond the acceptance of the principle, integration typically requires a substantial initial investment of time, effort, energy, and political capital. In places where there is a history of separate, "handicapped-only" programs, there is the strong and persistent view that "this is how we have always done it." This, in turn, provides the basis for the growth and nourishment of the principles and rationalizations for segregated schooling for students with disabilities.

For the most part, these educators have simply not seen successfully integrated programs. Without ever having had that exposure, educators and administrators will not take the first step of making the significant effort and commitment that is needed in order to effectively integrate programs for all students with disabilities. Only in places where there has been a history of meaningful integration do the administrators and students have a real basis for being emotionally attached to the value, excitement, and ideology of integration. When this positive exposure is absent, the important task of attaining compliance with the integration imperative of PL 94-142 has been and will continue to be significantly more difficult. The changing of these attitudes is compounded by past history, when most separate schools were programmatically superior to the programs in the regular schools that were literally hidden away in the basements and closets of the public schools.

These same attitudes appear at the state level as well. Most state departments of education in the United States fail in their statutory leadership role. PL 94-142 very clearly places upon state departments of education the responsibility: 1) to monitor and enforce compliance with the requirements of the law (20 U.S.C. §1412[6]), and 2) to assume a leadership role in the areas of personnel training, development, encouragement, and promotion of demonstration projects (20 U.S.C. §1413[a][3]). For the most part, the state departments of education have not upheld these responsibilities. While many states might give lip service to the principle of LRE, they have been unwilling or unable to provide the necessary leadership for public school programs. Their role in terms of monitoring and compliance issues has also not been particularly positive.

This issue is perhaps best illustrated by a recent case study that was conducted in Massachusetts (Landau, 1987). This extensive study analyzed why the percentage of students in segregated schools had increased over an 11-year period. Landau found that the State Department of Education's failure to monitor and enforce the LRE requirements was one of the key bases for the increase in segregated programming. Moreover, the study found that, to a large extent, the necessary data needed to monitor compliance with LRE requirements was not even being kept by the State Department of Education (Landau, 1987).

Territorial Self-Interest

In addition to the resistance based upon a philosophical rejection of the integration principle, a second factor contributes to the segregation of students with disabilities. Nonintegrated, parallel, separate schools have a built-in constituency for their continued existence and growth. Educators, administrators, and other staff who work in those facilities are understandably slow to work toward the gradual shrinking or dissolution of those facilities. They are not anxious to dissolve the very facilities that currently provide them with positions of employment and influence. It is worth pointing out that sometimes these facilities are publicly administered, such as in Missouri, where more than 3,000 students are educated in segregated programs. Other programs are in private schools, such as in Massachusetts, where a significant number of students are in "handicapped-only" settings. This understandable self-interest, coupled with an honest belief that an integrated program is, at best, no better than the separate program, and, more probably, academically inferior to the separate school, combine to form a significant roadblock to a thorough implementation of the LRE requirements of PL 94-142.

STRATEGIES FOR OBTAINING INTEGRATED PROGRAMS

Legal and Political Strategies

There is no single approach for attaining integration for students with profound disabilities. Because states, regions, communities, and even individual school buildings differ in the variables that are pertinent to successful geographical and social integration in the public schools, methods chosen for accomplishing integration must be matched to these individual differences (Biklen, 1985; Piuma, Halvorsen, Murray, Beckstead, & Sailor, 1983; Taylor, 1982). While there is no single strategy that will be uniformly effective, there is an underlying principle that is relevant to any such analysis: the move to an integrated service delivery model should be understood as being nothing less than effecting social change. Thus, the process and context of the debate is essentially a political one. The extent to which advocates for integration are successful will depend upon whether those persons can effectively marshall the political forces within that community. Stated in its simplest terms, the measure of success will be whether the decisionmakers find the appropriate steps to integration easy enough to follow.

As Figure 5.1 illustrates, there are an array of forces that can be brought to bear upon the school system. However, prior to a review of the outside forces, it is important to realize that there are multiple layers of decisionmakers within the local school district. Superseding the special education director is the superintendent of schools, with the superior authority of the system being the local

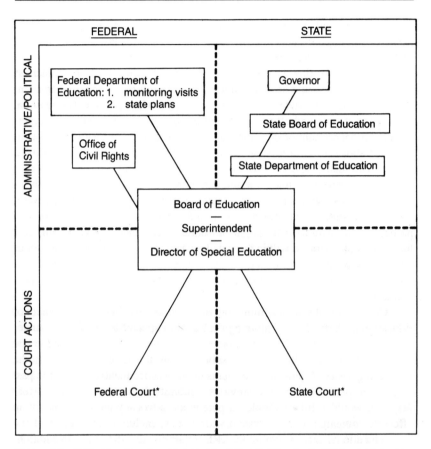

Figure 5.1. Political forces pertinent to integration in local public schools. (*State and federal law requires that, absent special circumstances, the party exhaust his or her administrative remedies prior to filing an action in court.)

board of education (typically an elected body). Each of these "layers" should be examined to identify individuals who are supportive of integration. For example, school board members, as elected officials, are subject to all of the traditional political forces, including: moral/ethical principles, legal compulsion, fiscal concerns, and enlightened self-interest. A political campaign promoting integration could consist of demonstrating that integration is: 1) the ethically and educationally correct approach, 2) the approach that is required by the law, and 3) ultimately the more cost-effective approach for a district. These arguments could be made to a school board; however, if that attempt fails, an alternate approach would be to obtain the election of prointegration candidates for the school board.

dimensional influences across the three key elements in the change process (i.e., values, operations, systems) as shown in Figure 5.2, and through horizontal exchanges between peers as shown in Figure 5.3. Thus, if any of the key administrators are opposed to integration, peer influence can be an effective force to change attitudes. For example, principals who are resistant to the inclusion of students with severe and profound handicaps in their building are most likely to listen to other principals who have already integrated a school, especially when the school is of similar size and has the same age range. Observing successfully integrated schools can motivate administrators who are fearful of the needed changes or who have little experience with special populations. Beyond attitude change in the central administration and at the principal level, the work of developing an integration plan must be completed.

Developing an Appropriate Service Delivery Model Assessing the quality of the educational program prior to integration can provide pertinent data to teachers, upcoming parents, and administrators as to whether change is warranted and what changes are needed. For example, the special education teachers in Indianapolis became convinced of the need for making major program improvements once they studied the activities of former students who had graduated from their segregated school programs (Johnson, 1987). The most restrictive educational placements were not preparing students for the least restrictive "placements" in adult life. The results indicated that a "postsecondary nothing" phenomenon was commonplace among graduates.

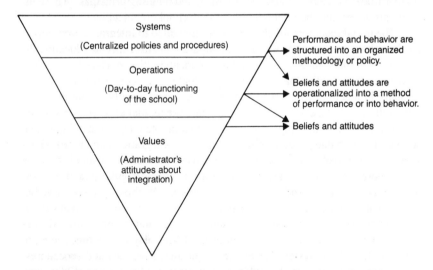

Figure 5.2. Key characteristics in the process of changing a school or an entire system from being segregated to being integrated. Multidimensional influences working from the bottom up and the top down. (Source: Piuma, C., Halvorsen, A., Murray, C., Beckstead, S., & Sailor, W. [1983]. *Project REACH administrator's manual.* San Francisco: San Francisco State University and San Francisco Unified School District, Project REACH.)

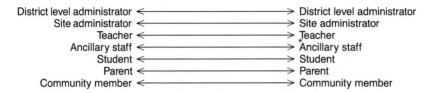

Figure 5.3. Key characteristics in the process of changing a school or an entire system from being segregated to being integrated. Horizontal exchanges (i.e., interactions between peers at the same level of decisionmaking) that also affect values, operations, and systems. (Source: Piuma, C., Halvorsen, A., Murray, C., Beckstead, S., & Sailor, W. [1983]. *Project REACH administrator's manual.* San Francisco: San Francisco State University and San Francisco Unified School District, Project REACH.)

Besides convincing special education staff of the need to revamp their program, these data on graduates' employment, daytime activity, current residence, and amount of government assistance served two additional purposes: 1) its analysis dictated necessary program changes—functional age-appropriate curricula in life skill domains, community-based instruction, and regular interaction with nonhandicapped peers; 2) its publication in the local media provided an alarm to the public and brought the issue before the school agenda.

The first step in planning for integration includes developing a "contact protocol" (Piuma et al., 1983, p. 18) that specifies the lines of authority in a school system. The second step is to assess the needs and strengths of the school system in terms of: 1) the number and types of students with severe disabilities and their ages; 2) their current locations; 3) the equipment and program needs of the students and classes to be integrated; 4) the location of available classrooms as possible integration sites (close to the students' homes and that allow community programming), the respective building modifications needed, and the receptivity of the building principals; 5) teachers', ancilliary staffs', and parents' attitudes toward change; and 6) potential problems anticipated by teachers, parents, and others familiar with the students. The third step is to create an integration planning committee (Piuma et al., 1983) or task force (Taylor, 1982) to use this information to develop a long-term plan for integration. Members include "downtown" administrators, integration site administrators, regular and special education teachers, ancillary staff, parents, and possibly nonhandicapped student representatives; in short, everyone who will be affected by the changes. Piuma et al. (1983) found that significant adaptations were needed in the following school policies or procedures in San Francisco's school system: transportation, accounting, attendance, budget and finance, personnel, student assignment, curriculum, custodial services, personnel evaluation, facilities planning, food services, and staff development. The integration plan should address or assign to others those aspects of the school program that will be affected by the change.

When classes of students with disabilities are moved from a segregated school with its own administrative staff into a regular school, a plan for ongoing management responsibility must be developed. Piuma et al. (1983) used two different plans to handle changes in administration: 1) the site principals have total responsibility, and 2) the special education administrator is responsible for several integrated facilities, and discussed in detail their pros and cons. In both cases, the building principal must be in favor of the change and have accurate information on the rationale for integration as well as input on the integration process.

Other concerns that must be addressed in the plan include who will be integrated first, where integration will occur, which staff will be involved (e.g., administrative, teacher, ancillary, paraprofessional), and what will be the program criteria.

Selecting Initial Sites and Staff for Integration   Stetson (1984) found in a study of integrated systems that "freeing up" the staff who provide administrative assistance and instructional leadership to make them more available during the implementation phase enhanced the success of integration efforts. When there is a choice of which members of the teaching staff from whom to elicit assistance in the initial sites chosen for integration, Piuma et al. (1983) suggest that well-trained teachers be recruited who have a history of success and good peer interaction skills. Furthermore, these staff (e.g., principals, regular and special education teachers), as well as the schools selected for integration, need to be the recipients of incentives such as strong administrative support and curricular assistance. For example, having the school board and the superintendent speak favorably of the planned changes and hold open forums to give information and answer questions would provide important early administrative support. Curricular support could include eliciting the assistance of a speech therapist to devise more effective communication systems for integrated students. In larger systems, hiring a person to help develop special friends (Voeltz, 1984) and peer tutoring programs (Certo & Kohl, 1984) would enable teachers to obtain social integration more quickly following geographical integration. In smaller systems, and those already partially integrated, there would be less of a choice of which staff or students to include in the initial integration plan. If attitudes toward the planned changes are poor, then more effort is needed to inform these staff and/or parents who are involved of the benefits that will result from the integration and the steps necessary to achieve a successful bridge. Also, by including these people in the planning process, the result could possibly be a more positive involvement for these individuals (Biklen, 1985; Piuma et al., 1983).

Implementing a Responsive Staff Development Program
While this element may be the most crucial for successful integration, staff development or in-service will need to be ongoing from the initial decision to integrate through the late phases of implementation when different problems and needs arise. The content of in-service will vary over time but must be responsive to the changing staff concerns and needs. Initially, all staff will need

information on the benefits of integration; later, they will require advice on the facilitation of social integration. Most staff will need to know some basics about students with profound disabilities with an emphasis placed on students' skills and potential, rather than their deficits. Introducing individual students who will be integrated to staff and students in the receiving school is another important step. While it is true that students with profound disabilities who engage in age-appropriate social behavior may be better accepted when moved to the regular school (Hamre-Nietupski, Nietupski, Stainback, & Stainback, 1984), appropriate social skills are not a prerequisite to integration. In fact, social skills taught in segregated settings are less likely to generalize to the conditions that integrated schools present for interaction. Piuma et al. (1983) suggest that students with high-frequency, extremely aberrant behavior not be included in the first group that is integrated into the regular school; however, some socially responsive students who clearly have disabilities should be included in this first group.

Later, but still prior to implementation, different groups of staff will require in-service to highlight the specific ways in which integration will affect their duties. As the number of students with the more severe disabilities increases, the amount of focused in-service will also increase. For example, kitchen staff will need advice on necessary changes in meal preparation, while bus drivers will need information on behavior management, interaction with nonvocal students, and seizures. Regular classroom teachers and special activity teachers (e.g., music, art, and gym teachers) will benefit from some instruction on interaction with students who have different means of communication. An adequate number of school staff should have current cardiopulmonary resuscitation (CPR) certification. Administrators will also need training in order to provide teachers and ancillary staff with meaningful supervision, to understand the functional curriculum used, to promote school-wide social integration, and to effectively participate in IEP meetings.

Important focal points of in-service training for special education teachers and all ancillary staff before implementation should highlight integrated therapy, social skills, community-based instruction, functional life curriculum, and systematic instruction. The use of needs assessment instruments, observation, and interview of staff before planning the in-service content will enable relevant topics to be chosen and deficient staff skills to be remediated (Stetson, 1984). Follow-up observation in the classrooms of participating staff will further the effects of in-service training by individualizing the application of that program's content.

Fostering a Positive Attitude toward the LRE Concept in the School It has been widely documented that the successful inclusion of students with severe and profound disabilities in the regular school environment is dependent upon the combined attitudes of staff and students in the receiving school (cf. Condon, York, Heal, & Fortschneider, 1986; Stainback & Stainback, 1981). Positive attitude changes are dependent primarily upon having one's concerns about integration addressed and having adequate information concerning students with severe and profound disabilities.

Initial in-service on integration benefits and methods may be best accomplished by dynamic consultants who have assisted with successful integration programs in other school systems. These individuals along with supportive and high-ranking school administrators need to allow repeated opportunity for questions to be answered and staff fears and concerns to be aired.

Nondisabled students should have their own instruction, one that is geared to their level of understanding and interests. Stetson (1984) reported the use of instructional modules prepared by parents of students with disabilities together with parents of nondisabled children. The primary message is the understanding and acceptance of the wide range of differences and similarities that exists in any group of peers. Whenever possible, a suitable staff member should be designated to assist teachers and students in establishing special friends and peer tutoring programs so that social interactions are facilitated and integration is implemented (Kohl, Moses, & Stettner-Eaton, 1984; Voeltz, 1984). Piuma et al. (1983) used grant funds to hire a team to work with students and school staff in this manner.

Promoting Community Acceptance of the LRE Concept Schools are intertwined with communities. School systems generally operate under the guidance of a school board that is made up of active community members. Most people in a community have some connection with schools at some point in their lives. Despite this blending of community and schools, the public generally is unfamiliar with people who have profound disabilities. In most cases, the public has no direct contact with this group and, thus, has an inaccurate picture of their potential. When schools undertake a plan to integrate students with disabilities, the community deserves accurate and positive forewarning of these plans, along with the rationale. Sharing outcome data on graduates' accomplishments, in contrast to what is possible with "best practices," can be convincing if the plans for change are portrayed as being cost-effective. Furthermore, generous information on integration must be provided to the school board long before the integration plan is developed. The community serves as the logical extension of classroom instruction for students with severe disabilities, since the student will be spending an increasing amount of time there as he or she prepares for adult life. Community members need to be shown how they can contribute positively toward enhancing the integration efforts initiated by the schools.

Parental Acceptance of the LRE Concept Many have identified parental fears as the strongest barrier to integration (viz., H. D. B. Fredericks, personal communication, February 18, 1986; L. Meyer, personal communication, February 3, 1986; Stetson, 1984). Parents of the older students with severe and profound disabilities have often fought hard for the segregated school since its presence in many LEAs was preceded by no services or inferior services. By comparison, parents of younger students may be more receptive to integration (Johnson, 1987). Stetson (1984) identified three typical integration worries of these parents, including:

> a) concern that their child would be ridiculed, b) concern that they would be harmed, and c) concern that the instructional and related services to be provided in the integrated setting would not be as comprehensive or as available as they had been in the segregated setting. (p. 75)

These fears appear uninfluenced by the severity of the disability. While these worries are legitimate, careful planning can prevent their realization. Ironically, parents of nondisabled children have similar fears, including: 1) that the curriculum will be weakened with the influx of students with handicaps due to the anticipated costs of these changes, and 2) that their children will be harmed or have unpleasant experiences through these new contacts.

When the parents of both groups of children are involved in planning integration, they can serve as the representatives for other parents. The parents who have invested in planning and whose concerns are addressed become more committed to the plan. If these parents participate in parent-to-parent discussions, the resulting communication is often more convincing to the inactive parents than the presentations and official memoranda from school administrators (see Figure 5.2). Besides including parents in the planning phases, open forums should be held by school officials early on to hear and address parental concerns. Stetson (1984) reported that parents in the LEAs that she studied frequently complained that the schools had inadequately explained the legal and educational bases for the LRE concept. Question and answer sessions, chaired by parents from other LEAs with successful integration, may provide more credible information to parents than school staff or even local parents. Other sessions can focus on specific topics of concern (e.g., reduction in therapy) in which the LEA plans are presented and discussed. In any case, successful integration is possible only when parents are supportive; furthermore, schools must be sensitive to parents' concerns as well.

Particular Considerations for Students with the Most Serious Disabilities

Students with special health care needs and those with high-frequency disruptive or dangerous behavior present particular challenges to their teachers as well as to the regular school system. Past history is a reminder of the changing nature of what constitutes the "most serious" handicaps. Examples of creative solutions by school systems for including students with special health needs or disruptive behavior in the regular school include: 1) training a classroom aide to perform a CIC for a child with myelomeningocele; 2) having an aide walk beside a student with "brittle bone" disease to prevent accidental bumps in the halls between classes; 3) working with parents to decide the best way to transport an 8-year-old with brain injury that was sustained from nearly drowning and who is now paralyzed and unable to breath without regular cleaning of his tracheostomy tube, and to determine what the school's liability would be for any medical complications and who would pay for a medical attendant; and 4) having both special education and regular school staff with training in nonviolent means for stopping and handling seriously aggressive behavior in the school and at community sites.

When school systems practice and support integration of students with severe and profound disabilities and when parents come to expect it, the barriers to moving children with special health needs from hospital or home-bound settings are mainly ones concerning cost and liability. Three solutions to cost are currently employed by most schools. First, the Education of the Handicapped Amendments Act of 1986 (PL 99-457) includes a mandate to serve all children ages 2–5 and financial incentives to serve children from birth to 2 years. Many special education teachers predict that this law will push the issue of serving medically fragile and seriously aggressive children in the public school to the forefront, which in turn will stimulate the sharing of creative solutions among school systems (Viadero, 1987). Second, some school systems in Illinois and Pennsylvania are filing claims for educational services (e.g., occupational therapy, physical therapy, audiology) with the insurance company of the student's parents, with the company paying 80% of these claims and the school, not the parent, paying the remainder. Third, other schools make use of Medicaid, the federal health insurance program for low income patients, to pay for some of these services (Viadero, 1987).

Students with high-frequency aggressive behavior pose different, but equally difficult, challenges to the LRE doctrine. Frequently, state formulae for giving aid to schools act as disincentives to the integration of these children, even when the school is equipped with staff to teach such students effectively. For example, under the Massachusetts reimbursement formula, the state pays for more than half of the cost of a residential program; however, in a less restrictive program, the cost of the program and the cost of transportation is not paid for by the state. The result of this type of funding formula is that the LEA has little or no incentive to provide the necessary supplementary aids and services that are required in order to provide educational services within the local public school (Landau, 1987). When regulations exist that make integration more costly than segregation, then these regulations need to be targeted for legislative change by exposing their disincentive effects.

Piuma et al. (1983) suggest that students with the most aggressive behavior be moved out of segregated schools last, after the students in the regular schools have come to accept the more socially appropriate students with severe disabilities. In the meantime, a team of competent educators could be hired as consultants in order to assist teachers to educate those students who still remain in the segregated schools to develop socially appropriate behaviors. Durand and Kishi (1987) reported a technical assistance model using this approach. One clear problem that requires solution with such a plan is the absence of peers who can model appropriate social behavior. Scheduling community-based instruction first on a weekly basis, and then daily, along with gradually increasing the students' time in the regular school, are ways in which educational professionals avoid the impossible dilemma of "getting students ready for" integration by keeping them segregated with other students who have seriously aberrant behaviors.

SUMMARY

Integration is required by federal law, as well as by most state education statutes. However, practice does not reflect these laws; as many as three-quarters of the states fail to place school-age children, adolescents, and young adults with disabilities into the regular schools with their nonhandicapped peers. Segregated schooling means that students with profound disabilities, in particular, are unable to learn social skills since they have little opportunity to interact with their nonhandicapped peers. They are limited in their school associations to the adults who teach them and to their fellow students with disabilities who also have limited interaction skills. There are many reasons for this discrepancy between what was intentionally written into the laws—a mandate for the least restrictive environment—and current practices in most local school districts. The primary theme of these reasons or barriers to integration is fear: fear of the unknown (i.e., people with severe and profound disabilities) and fear of change (i.e., movement from segregated to integrated schooling).

Because breaking these barriers requires social change, the process and context is a political one and necessitates the cooperation of various political bodies at the local community level (e.g., school board, parents, school administrators, staff); at times, state, federal, and judicial bodies may be involved as well. Methods that are successfully used to facilitate the closing of segregated school facilities have widely varied. While there is no formula for a successful educational strategy, there does appear to be some essential elements involved in such a program, including: 1) attaining organizational support for the LRE concept, 2) developing an appropriate service delivery model that incorporates integration, 3) selecting initial sites and staff for integration, 4) implementing a responsive staff development program, 5) fostering a positive attitude toward the LRE concept in the school, and 6) promoting community and parental acceptance of the LRE concept. While students with the most profound disabilities may pose particular integration challenges for the schools and parents, their inclusion is not less possible nor less important than that of students with milder disabilities being placed into regular public school.

REFERENCES

Bak, J.J., & Siperstein, G.N. (1987). Similarity as a factor effecting change in children's attitudes toward mentally retarded peers. *American Journal of Mental Deficiency, 91*, 524–531.

Bates, P., Morrow, S.A., Pancsofar, E., & Sedlak, R. (1984). The effect of functional vs. nonfunctional activities on attitudes/expectations of non-handicapped college students: What they see is what we get. *Journal of The Association for the Severely Handicapped, 9*, 73–78.

Begali, V. (1987). *Head injury in children and adolescents*. Brandon, VT: Clinical Psychology Publishing Co.

Biklen, D. (1985). *Achieving the complete school: Strategies for effective mainstreaming*. New York: Teacher's College Press.

Brinker, R.D. (1985). Interactions between severely mentally retarded students and other students in integrated and segregated public school settings. *American Journal of Mental Deficiency, 89*, 587–594.

Brown, L., Branston, M.B., Hamre-Nietupski, S., Pumpian, I., Certo, N., & Gruenewald, L.A. (1979). A strategy for developing chronological–age appropriate and functional curricular content for severely handicapped adolescents and young adults. *Journal of Special Education, 13*, 81–90.

Certo, N., & Kohl, F.L. (1984). A strategy for developing interpersonal interaction instructional content for severely handicapped students. In N. Certo, N. Haring, & R. York (Eds.), *Public school integration of severely handicapped students: Rational issues and progressive alternatives* (pp. 221–244). Baltimore: Paul H. Brookes Publishing Co.

Condon, M.E., York, R., Heal, L.W., & Fortschneider, J. (1986). Acceptance of severely handicapped students by nonhandicapped peers. *Journal of The Association for Persons with Severe Handicaps, 11*, 216–219.

Durand, V.M., & Kishi, G. (1987). Reducing severe behavior problems among persons with dual sensory impairments: An evaluation of a technical assistance model. *Journal of The Association for Persons with Severe Handicaps, 12*, 2–10.

Dybwad, G. (1974). Education for All Handicapped Children, 1973–1974: Hearings on Senate Bill 6 before the Subcommittee on the Handicapped of the Senate Committee on Labor and Public Welfare, 94th Congress, 1st Session, 282 Passim (1975). *Congressional Record, 120*(15), 269.

Ellis N.R. (1981). On training the mentally retarded. *Analysis and Intervention in Developmental Disabilities, 1*, 99–108.

Fay, F. (1974). Education for All Handicapped Children, 1973–1974: Hearings on Senate Bill 6 before the Subcommittee on the Handicapped of the Senate Committee on Labor and Public Welfare, 94th Congress, 1st Session, 282 Passim (1975). *Congressional Record, 120*(15), 269.

Gaylord-Ross, R., & Peck, C.A. (1985). Integration efforts for students with severe mental retardation. In D. Bricker & J. Filler (Eds.), *Severe mental retardation: From theory to practice* (pp. 185–207). Reston, VA: Division on Mental Retardation of the Council for Exceptional Children.

Gaylord-Ross, R.J., & Pitts-Conway, V. (1984). Social behavior development in integrated secondary autistic programs. In N. Certo, N. Haring, & R. York (Eds.), *Public school integration of severely handicapped students: Rational issues and progressive alternatives* (pp. 197–219). Baltimore: Paul H. Brookes Publishing Co.

Guess, D. (1987, March). *Implications of biobehavioral states for the education and treatment of persons with profound and multiple handicaps*. Paper presented at the meeting of the Profoundly Mentally Handicapped Symposium, "New Directions," South Carolina Department of Education, Columbia, SC.

Halvorsen, A.T. (1983). *Parents and community together.* San Francisco: San Francisco State University and San Francisco Unified School District, Project REACH.

Hamre-Nietupski, S., Nietupski, J., Stainback, W., & Stainback, S. (1984). Preparing school systems for longitudinal integration efforts. In N. Certo, N. Haring, & R. York (Eds.), *Public school integration of severely handicapped students: Rational issues and progressive alternatives* (pp. 107–141). Baltimore: Paul H. Brookes Publishing Co.

House Committee on Education and Labor. (1975). *H.R. Report No. 332,* 94th Congress, 1st Session 9.

Johnson, V. (1987, October). *Fallacies, barriers, and possibilities: An administrator's perspective on social integration.* Presentation at the meeting of the Middle Tennessee Association for Persons with Severe Handicaps, Nashville, TN.

Kauffman, J.M., & Krouse, J. (1981). The cult of educability: Searching for the substance of things hoped for; the evidence of things not seen. *Analysis and Intervention in Developmental Disabilities, 1,* 53–60.

Kohl, F.L., Moses, L.G., & Stettner-Eaton, B.A. (1984). A systematic training program for teaching nonhandicapped students to be instructional trainers of severely handicapped schoolmates. In N. Certo, N. Haring, R. York (Eds.), *Public school integration of severely handicapped students: Rational issues and progressive alternatives* (pp. 185–195). Baltimore: Paul H. Brookes Publishing Co.

Landau, J. (1987, May). *Out of the mainstream: Education of disabled youth in Massachusetts.* Boston: Massachusetts Advocacy Center.

Landesman-Dwyer, S., & Sackett, G.P. (1978). Behavioral changes in nonambulatory, profoundly mentally retarded individuals. In C.E. Meyers (Ed.), *Quality of life in severely and profoundly mentally retarded people: Research foundations for improvement* (pp. 55–144). Washington, DC: American Association on Mental Deficiency.

Mathias, C.M., Jr. (1974). Education for All Handicapped Children, 1973–1974: Hearings on Senate Bill 6 before the Subcommittee on the Handicapped of the Senate Committee on Labor and Public Welfare, 94th Congress, 1st Session, 282 Passim (1975). *Congressional Record, 120*(15), 269.

Meyer, L.H., & Kishi, G.S. (1985). School integration strategies. In K.C. Lakin & R.H. Bruininks (Eds.), *Strategies for achieving community integration of developmentally disabled citizens* (pp. 231–252). Baltimore: Paul H. Brookes Publishing Co.

Mills v. Board of Education of the District of Columbia, 348 F. Supp. 866 (D.D.C. 1972).

Nyquist, E. (1974). Financial assistance for improved educational services for handicapped children: Hearing on House of Representatives Bill 70 before the Select Subcommittee on Education of the Handicapped of the House Committee on Education and Labor, 93rd Congress, 2cd Session passim (1974). *Congressional Record, 120*(15), 271.

Pennsylvania Association for Retarded Children v. Commonwealth of Pennsylvania, 334 F. Supp. 1257 (E.D. Pa. 1971).

Pennsylvania Association for Retarded Children v. Commonwealth of Pennsylvania, 343 F. Supp. 279 (E.D. Pa. 1972).

Piuma, C., Halvorsen, A., Murray, C., Beckstead, S., & Sailor, W. (1983). *Project REACH administrator's manual.* San Francisco: San Francisco State University and San Francisco Unified School District, Project REACH.

Public Law 94-142, *Education for All Handicapped Children Act of 1975,* 20 U.S.C. §§1412-1415 (5)(B), 1975.

Public Law 93-380, *Education of the Handicapped Act Amendments of 1974*, 20 U.S.C. §§1401-1461, Supp. 1975.

Public Law 99-457, *Education of the Handicapped Amendments Act of 1986*, 1986.

Roncker v. Walter, 700 F.2d 1058-1063 (6th Cir. 1983).

Stafford, R.T. (1974). Education for All Handicapped Children, 1973–1974: Hearings on Senate Bill 6 before the Subcommittee on the Handicapped of the Senate Committee on Labor and Public Welfare, 94th Congress, 1st Session, 282 Passim (1975). *Congressional Record, 120*(15), 272.

Stainback, W., & Stainback, S. (1981). A review of research of interactions between severely handicapped and nonhandicapped students. *Journal of The Association for the Severely Handicapped, 6*(3), 23–29.

Stainback, W., & Stainback, S. (1987, April). Educating all students in regular education. *TASH Newsletter, 13*(4), pp. 1,7.

Stetson, F. (1984). Critical factors that facilitate integration: A theory of administrative responsibility. In N. Certo, N. Haring, & R. York (Eds.), *Public school integration of severely handicapped students: Rational issues and progressive alternatives* (pp. 65–81). Baltimore: Paul H. Brookes Publishing Co.

Strain, P.S., & Kerr, M.M. (1981). *Mainstreaming of children in schools: Research and programming issues*. New York: Academic Press.

Tatro v. Texas, 625 F.2d 557 (5th Cir. 1980).

Tatro v. Texas, 703 F.2d 823 (5th Cir. 1983).

Taylor, S.J. (1982). From segregation to integration: Strategies for integrating severely handicapped students in normal school and community settings. *Journal of The Association for the Severely Handicapped, 8*(3), 42–49.

Viadero, D. (1987, March 11). "Medically fragile" students pose dilemma for school officials." *Education Week, 6*(24), 1, 14.

Voeltz, L.M. (1984). Program and curriculum innovations to prepare children for integration. In N. Certo, N. Haring, & R. York (Eds.), *Public School integration of severely handicapped students: Rational issues and progressive alternatives* (pp. 155–183). Baltimore: Paul H. Brookes Publishing Co.

Williams, H.A. (1974). Financial assistance for improved educational services for handicapped children: Hearing on House of Representatives Bill 70 before the Select Subcommittee on Education of the Handicapped of the House Committee on Education and Labor, 93rd Congress, 2nd Session, Passim (1974). *Congressional Record, 120*(15), 271.

Youniss, J. (1980). *Parents and peers in social development: A Sullivan-Piaget perspective*. Chicago: University of Chicago Press.

Issues in The Education of Students with Complex Health Care Needs

6

Donna H. Lehr
and Mary Jo Noonan

One of the requirements of PL 94-142 (Education for All Handicapped Children Act of 1975) states that a student be provided with free appropriate public education in the least restrictive environment. Since this law's enactment, school districts have been increasingly challenged to incorporate its requirements as they relate to children with severe and profound handicaps. The latest challenge is that of serving students with complex health care needs (Viadero, 1987). Districts have been providing educational services to some students with chronic health care problems for years, with the assistance of a small body of literature regarding educational service delivery to this population of students (Kleinberg, 1982). However, as Hobbs, Perrin, and Ireys (1985) have stated, relative to the general population of students with handicaps, little attention has been focused on children with chronic illnesses. Additionally, a review of the literature reveals that when the needs of children with chronic illnesses are addressed, the emphasis is on those children with health problems such as diabetes, asthma, spina bifida, cleft lip, renal diseases, sickle cell anemia, hemophilia, cystic fibrosis, and muscular dystrophy (cf. Hobbs et al., 1985; Kleinberg, 1982). According to Kleinberg (1982), little attention has been given to the 20% of children who are described as having chronic illnesses with other handicapping conditions such as mental retardation. Likewise, little emphasis has been placed on the delivery of services to those students whose special health care needs are complex or who require medical technology for breathing, suctioning, ventilation, or feeding. The reasons for this omission of information on such complex health care needs are understandable: until recently, these students were not a concern of the public school system, but the responsibility of their parents or institutions (Shayne, Walter, Perrin, & Moynihan, 1987; Viadero, 1987).

EMERGENCE OF A NEW POPULATION

The presence of this "new" population of students, those children with chronic illnesses, in the public school can be attributed to a number of factors. These factors include: improved technology, principle of normalization, and early childhood programs.

Improved Technology

In the past, students with such complex health care needs, either due to congenital birth defects or acquired problems through accident or injury, did not survive the neonatal period or the period immediately following the traumatic event (Khan & Battle, 1987; Perrin, 1986; Viadero, 1987). Improved technology has greatly increased survival rates of such individuals to the point that they are now living long enough to attend school. Improved technology has also enabled family members and teachers to conduct various medical procedures in less controlled settings (Ekstrand, 1982), resulting in the transfer of the sophisticated care that was traditionally provided by physicians and nurses to families (Stein, 1986). Consequently, children with very complex medical needs no longer have to reside exclusively in hospitals or residential facilities that are specially equipped to meet their needs. Instead, they are able to live in their own homes or in community-based settings and to have portable equipment, such as apnea monitors, portable suctioning machines, and portable ventilators. Since these children reside in their home school districts with school-provided transportation, attendance inevitably becomes an issue.

Principle of Normalization

Since the late 1960s, service provision for individuals with serious handicaps has led to increased participation in the normal activities of life. The principle of normalization (Wolfensberger, 1972) is the guiding philosophy that has resulted in the movement of many individuals with handicaps from very restrictive large institutions into less restrictive settings, including convalescent hospitals, group homes, and family homes. For individuals with special health care needs, this principle has been further assisted by the Katie Beckett Program (TEFRA, 1982) that has permitted the provision of Medicaid and Supplemental Security Income (SSI) to individuals who are residing in environments other than hospitals or institutions, regardless of family income. Prior to this, the lesser restrictive environments, including family and group homes, were not an option for such individuals; residence in such a setting would mean the loss of essential funds to pay for the care.

The least restrictive environment (LRE) requirement of PL 94-142 stems from the principle of normalization and has halted the automatic placement of students with special health care needs in home- or hospital-bound instruction. The LRE requirements state that students should be educated in an environment that is as close as possible to the "regular" school environment; the most desirable environment is the regular class with other nonhandicapped children, and the most restrictive environment is an institutional setting. Increasingly, decisions are being made to educate students with significant handicaps in the more normalized settings of regular classes and schools (Certo, Haring, & York, 1984). The consequence of implementing the LRE requirements with students who have special health care needs is that local educational agencies (LEAs) must assume responsibility for such students in their schools, not just in the institutional settings that may be situated within their district boundaries.

Early Childhood Programs

PL 94-142 mandated the provision of educational programs to children beginning at age 5 with incentives to serve children at 3 years of age. The later amendments to that law, PL 99-457 (Education of the Handicapped Amendments of 1986), have indicated an even stronger commitment to this young population by mandating that services be provided to children beginning at age 3, with further incentives offered for those agencies that provide services to children from birth to 3 years of age. The consequence of these amendments is that more young children are attending school at an earlier age, and it is these younger children who have benefited the most from the technological advances and improved survival rates beyond the neonatal period. In this group is found the greatest number of students with special health care needs. As LEAs assume responsibility for serving young children, they also assume responsibility for assisting and educating students with complex health care needs.

DEFINING STUDENTS WITH
COMPLEX HEALTH CARE NEEDS

Who are these students with complex health care needs? In this chapter the authors focus on those students who, in addition to having mental retardation and/or significant neuromotor disabilities, have such needs as catheterization, tracheostomy suctioning, or respiratory ventilation. The prevalence of complex health care needs is higher among students with profound handicaps than among those who are nonhandicapped or have less severe handicapping conditions (Abromowicz & Richardson, 1975; Hotte, Monroe, Philbrook, & Scarlata, 1984). This higher prevalence of complex health care needs is due to the extensiveness of the physiological and/or neurological conditions that characterize most students with profound handicaps.

Students with complex health care needs are generally not ill, but require some health services in order to participate in special education. Students with profound handicaps who are ill are not included in this definition of students with complex health care needs. Infectious diseases, feeding tubes, respiratory conditions, and catheterization are categories of special health care needs.

Infectious Diseases

Infectious diseases are illnesses that can be transmitted from one person to another, typically through saliva, blood, or other bodily secretions. The most serious infectious diseases that are of concern in the schools are hepatitis B, herpes, acquired immune deficiency syndrome (AIDS), and cytomegalovirus (CMV). The major concern in serving students with infectious diseases in the schools is the risk of transmitting that disease to other students, teachers, or school personnel. Teachers of students with profound handicaps must be scrupulous in their hygiene habits because necessary daily care and interaction with these students frequently involves extensive physical contact, including positioning, feeding, diaper changing, and other care routines.

Hepatitis B Hepatitis B is a disease characterized by infection and inflammation of the liver. Secondary symptoms may include fever, headache, abdominal pain, mild upper respiratory infection, headache, dark urine, sluggishness, fatigue, anorexia (i.e., lack of appetite), nausea, and vomiting. As the disease progresses, jaundice occurs (American Academy of Pediatrics, 1982). There is no cure for hepatitis B. Persons with hepatitis B who are asymptomatic (i.e., no longer evidencing symptoms) continue to be carriers of the disease and may still be contagious. Hepatitis B is transmitted through close personal contact, specifically through blood, saliva, and semen; environmental surfaces (e.g., floor mats, teaching materials) contaminated with hepatitis B can also transmit the disease for up to 1 week (Bauer & Shea, 1986).

Hepatitis B is considered to be a major public health problem. Each year approximately 200,000 Americans contract this disease, and several thousands die from disorders or complications associated with it (Immunization Practices Advisory Committee, 1985). Hepatitis B is of particular concern in special education because of its prevalence among residents and staff of institutions for persons with mental retardation, and because many of these students who have been deinstitutionalized are now being served in the public schools (Bauer & Shea, 1986).

Herpes A number of skin conditions are referred to as herpes; the diseases that are of most concern to special educators are the herpes simplex virus (HSV), oral or Type 1 (HSV-1), and genital or Type 2 (HSV-2). HSV-1 and HSV-2 are typically differentiated by the location of the symptoms on the body (although they are not always separated by placement): HSV-1 is usually above the waist in the oropharynx (i.e., the portion of the throat continuous with the mouth), eye, brain, and skin; and HSV-2 is usually below the waist in the genitalia (Guess et al., 1984). Illnesses symptomatic of herpes may include gingivostomatitis (fever and bleeding ulcers in the mouth and pharynx), "cold sores" (lesions on the lips or nose), keratoconjunctivitis (red eye with a discharge that may lead to corneal scarring), and genital herpes (i.e., symptoms such as ulcers on the genitalia, pain or tenderness in the genital tract, swollen glands in the groin, rectal pain or burning, increased urination, fever, and/or headache) (American Academy of Pediatrics, 1982). Although there is no cure for herpes, there are treatments to aid the healing of the symptoms.

HSV-1 is most commonly transmitted by saliva or respiratory droplets. HSV-2 is transmitted through skin contact with the infected area (American Academy of Pediatrics, 1982; Bettoli, 1982). Unlike hepatitis B, the herpes virus does not survive on inanimate objects (Bureau of Epidemiology, 1983). Outbreak following exposure and transmission averages 6 days and may vary from 2–20 days (Alford & Pass, 1981).

Acquired Immune Deficiency Syndrome   Acquired Immune Deficiency Syndrome (AIDS) is caused by a virus called human immunodeficiency virus (HIV) and is also referred to as human T-lymphotropic virus type III-lymphadenopathy-associated virus (HTLV III/LAV) (Centers for Disease Control, 1985a, 1985b). In addition to causing AIDS, this virus may be asymptomatic or may cause symptoms that are not typical of AIDS. This is known as the AIDS Related Complex (ARC) (Centers for Disease Control, 1985a, 1985b). AIDS is characterized by a defect in the human immune system's ability to ward off disease. Because the body's natural immunity to disease is defective, individuals with AIDS are vulnerable to many serious diseases and infections. From 1981 to 1986, more than 20,000 cases of AIDS were reported in the United States; approximately 54% of the cases resulted in death (U.S. Department of Health and Human Services, 1986).

The diagnosis of AIDS is usually made following the development of the secondary "opportunistic" diseases and infections that indicate the loss of immunity. Antibodies present in the blood can also be used for the diagnosis of AIDS. Early symptoms associated with AIDS include tiredness; fever; loss of appetite and weight; diarrhea; night sweats; and swollen glands (lymph nodes), usually in the neck, armpits, or groin (U.S. Department of Health and Human Services, 1986). AIDS is transmitted through sexual contact (i.e., homosexual, heterosexual) or through the introduction of the virus into the bloodstream by contaminated hypodermic needles, transfusions of infected blood, or transfusions of components/products of infected blood. Transmission of AIDS to children usually occurs through their mother during the perinatal period (i.e., before, during, or after birth) or through blood transfusions, as in the case with some children with hemophilia (Centers for Disease Control, 1985a, 1985b).

Cytomegalovirus   Cytomegalovirus (CMV) is a prevalent infection among young children. It is usually asymptomatic, and when symptoms do occur, they are usually so mild that the infection goes unnoticed (Pass & Kinney, 1985). Children with CMV shed the virus intermittently in saliva and urine. The virus may be shed for a few months or for several years. Transmission of the virus occurs through direct, prolonged, or repeated contact with the virus (Pass & Kinney, 1985). For example, CMV can be transmitted through coughing and sneezing.

Studies of daycare and infant development centers indicate that the virus is usually present in 20% of the children in these programs; about 10% of children in the United States acquire CMV during their first year of life, and 10%–20% more children acquire the infection by age 6. In a study of daycare workers, antibodies to CMV were present in 50%–100% of the staff indicating past infection. CMV is so prevalent, and often undetected, that it is virtually impossible for childcare workers to avoid coming into contact with it.

CMV is of most concern to pregnant women because infection during the first trimester can have devastating effects on the development of the infant, including spontaneous abortion, central nervous system damage, hearing loss, and mental retardation (Pass & Kinney, 1985). Pregnant child care workers obviously should be concerned about the hazard of CMV. This virus is also a hazard for pregnant women whose children attend daycare because the children may carry the infection home to their mothers. Although a large percentage of pregnant women have antibodies for CMV, they are still at-risk for infection by a different strain of CMV. Special education teachers serving infants, toddlers, or preschoolers with profound handicaps are likely to come into contact with children who have congenital CMV. Good hygiene habits, such as careful handwashing after diaper changing, wiping a child's nose, and sanitizing toys, can substantially reduce the chances of acquiring CMV.

Feeding Tubes

Feeding tubes (i.e., "gavage" feedings) provide an alternative means for feeding individuals who are unable to eat normally. Medication can also be administered through a feeding tube. Conditions that may lead to the use of feeding tubes include disorders such as cerebral palsy accompanied by severe oral motor difficulties; chronic gagging or vomiting; hypersensitivity in the mouth, tongue, and throat; muscle or nerve disorders in the face or cranium; or refusal to eat (i.e., a behavioral problem) (Pathfinder & School Nurse Organization of Minnesota, 1986). Because some students with profound handicaps have very severe feeding problems due to central nervous system damage, feeding tubes may be used to ensure that the student is receiving adequate nutrition. In most cases, it is advisable to continue efforts to improve mouth feeding (i.e., "sham feeding").

School health concerns related to tube feeding include infection or aspiration (i.e., when food or fluid gets into the lungs through the oral or nasal tube that is used for feeding) (Pathfinder & School Nurse Organization of Minnesota, 1986). If oral or nasal tubes are inserted for each feeding (some nasal tubes are kept in place for extended periods of time), caution must be exercised to ensure that the tube is inserted correctly (the tube must not be inserted into the trachea or "wind pipe").

Gastrostomy   A gastrostomy is a small incision or *stoma* made in the wall of the abdomen (Pathfinder & School Nurse Organization of Minnesota, 1986). A rubber tube is inserted through the stoma so that it opens into the stomach; the other end can be attached to a feeding device and is closed with a clamp and taped to the stomach when not in use (Pathfinder & School Nurse Organization of Minnesota, 1986). Food is administered through one of two methods: the gravity method or a pump method (i.e., kangaroo bag). In the *gravity method,* food or "feeding fluid" is placed in a large syringe. The syringe is attached to the gastrostomy tube and together they are elevated about 4–5 inches above the individual's abdomen. The food or fluid passes slowly through the gastrostomy tube into the stomach. Feeding takes about 20–45 minutes. Water is usually administered through the tube after feeding. The *pump method* is similar; however, a pump is used to move the food from the kangaroo or feeding bag, through the gastrostomy tube, and into the stomach.

Nasogastric and Oralgastric Tubes   When a feeding tube is inserted through the nose or mouth, it is referred to as a nasogastric (i.e., Levin tube) or oralgastric tube, respectively. The tube is made of plastic or rubber (Pathfinder & School Nurse Organization of Minnesota, 1986). Insertion of the nasogastric and oralgastric tubes requires special training, and in most cases, schools will require that a licensed physician or school nurse insert the tube (California State Department of Education, 1980; Pathfinder & School Nurse Organization of Minnesota, 1986). When the tube is in place, food is administered through a gravity method as in gastrostomy feeding. Nasogastric tubes are taped in place when feeding is completed; however, oralgastric tubes are almost always removed following feeding.

Respiratory Conditions

Children who have difficulty breathing may need aids to assist with respiration. Respiratory conditions may be temporary due to an illness (e.g., child may have a tracheostomy following surgery); acute due to a periodic condition (e.g., allergy, asthma); or chronic due to disease (e.g., cystic fibrosis may require frequent suctioning). Because breathing problems may be life threatening and require emergency procedures, children with respiratory problems are of special concern for school personnel. Students with respiratory conditions must be monitored on a regular basis throughout the school day for signs of breathing difficulties (e.g., irregular or stressful respiration, blue or dark lip and/or nail color) and thick, yellow or green colored mucous or fever that indicates infection (Pathfinder & School Nurse Organization of Minnesota, 1986). When oxygen is required to provide respiratory assistance, it may be administered via an oxygen tent or headset, a nasal or oral tube, a mask, or a tracheostomy tube (Waechter, Phillips, & Holaday, 1985). Care must be taken to ensure that children with respiratory conditions are adequately hydrated and nourished; water is lost when children breathe primarily through their mouths, and children who have difficulty breathing typically do not eat well because it is difficult to swallow and breathe at the same time.

A tracheostomy is an incision through the neck into the trachea (i.e., *windpipe*) that enables an individual to breathe. A tracheostomy tube is inserted into the stoma (i.e., the hole in the trachea). The tube or *cannula* may be metal or plastic. A metal tracheostomy tube usually involves two cannulas. One cannula is inserted inside a larger one; the smaller cannula can be removed for cleaning while the larger one holds the airway open (Pathfinder & School Nurse Organization of Minnesota, 1986). If the tube is plastic, only one is generally used. The tracheostomy tube is secured in place with a tie around the person's neck. Care of the tracheostomy tube requires suctioning to keep the airway clear of mucous. A special tracheostomy suctioning machine and a small catheter (i.e., a plastic tube) is usually used. Suctioning is required daily, and in some cases, it may be needed frequently throughout the day. Caution must be exercised in inserting the catheter to avoid tissue damage. Because the tracheostomy is essentially an open passage to the lungs, the risk of infection is of serious concern. Clean or sterile suctioning techniques are necessary to prevent infection.

Other respiratory conditions may require suctioning, ventilators, or apnea monitors. A ventilator is a mechanical aid that supplies oxygen through the nose, mouth, or tracheostomy tube (Scipien, Barnard, Chard, Howe, & Phillips, 1986). The ventilator may be attached to an endotracheal (ET) tube that is inserted to support the airway. In some situations an ET tube is used in conjunction with a tracheostomy (usually when long-term ventilator assistance is needed). ET tubes may be inserted through the oral or nasal cavities. Generally, nasotracheal tubes are preferred over oraltracheal tubes; oraltracheal tubes are less stable than nasotracheal tubes and are associated with a buildup of secretions, greater risk of infections, and a possibility of causing damage to the trachea (Scipien et al., 1986).

Frequent suctioning is required when a ventilator is used in conjunction with the ET tube (approximately once an hour). Children who receive mechanical ventilation must be monitored frequently for color and even, unlabored diaphragm movements (Scipien et al., 1986). It is also important to be certain that the ET tube is firmly secured to the cheek with tape so that it does not accidentally get displaced or removed (i.e., extubation). The ventilator itself must also be checked regularly to ensure that the respiratory settings are correct, that there is no tension on the tracheostomy or ET tubes, that the ventilator tubes are free of kinks and water, and that the "alarms" are set (Waechter et al., 1985).

Children with ET tubes cannot be fed orally and must receive hydration and nourishment intravenously or through stomach tubes (i.e., gastrostomy). The child must be gradually weaned from dependence on the ventilator when mechanical respiratory assistance is to be terminated. It is frequently difficult to terminate mechanical ventilation when the ventilator has been used for an extended length of time. Intermittent mandatory ventilation (IMV) is the procedure typically used to wean a child from a ventilator (Waechter et al., 1985).

Apnea is a condition in which breathing temporarily ceases (Thomas, 1985). This condition is obviously quite serious and may be seen in conjunction with meningitis, coma, heart disease, kidney disease, or a cerebral concussion. Infants or children who are prone to this condition are typically checked with an apnea monitor.

Catheterization

Catheterization is a procedure for emptying an individual's bladder. Students with profound handicaps who are paralyzed below the waist due to spina bifida or some other disability may be unable to void and empty their bladders without assistance. Catheterization is accomplished by inserting a small tube or "catheter" into the urethra. When the catheter is inserted far enough, urine will begin to flow (Pathfinder & School Nurse Organization of Minnesota, 1986). In some instances, pressure to the lower abdomen may be needed to express residual urine from the bladder (i.e., *Crede's Method*).

Catheterization is usually done *intermittently* (i.e., the catheter is inserted each time the student needs to void and is removed immediately afterwards). Intermittent catheterization is generally preferable to an indwelling catheter that provides continuous catheterization because there is less risk of kidney or bladder infection (Pathfinder & School Nurse Organization of Minnesota, 1986). In many cases, it is not necessary to use sterile procedures for inserting the catheter; however, clean intermittent catheterization (CIC) procedures are frequently recommended by the student's physician (i.e., soap, rubber gloves, and other good hygiene practices are followed, but strict sterile procedures are not practiced). Catheters must be washed after each use to reduce the chances of infection. School concerns related to catheterization are proper insertion of the catheter and prevention of infection.

ISSUES

Students with complex medical conditions are coming to schools that have a "new set of unclearly defined responsibilities for school administrators" (Viadero, 1987, p. 1) since they are surviving long enough to live in nonhospital settings and attending regular schools in the community. For these reasons, the number of programs for these young children is increasing. Never before have educators dealt with questions like, Should children on ventilators with oxygen come to school? or Who will administer prescribed medical treatments? Currently, few states or districts have policies that serve to guide the provision of educational services to students with complex medical conditions (Palfrey, DiPrete, Walker, Shannon, & Maroney, 1987; United States Congress, 1987;

Wood, Walker, & Gardner, 1986). As has been previously noted, educators' experiences in this area are limited.

Currently, very difficult case-by-case decisions are being made each time a new student enters the educational system (Palfrey et al., 1987). The decisions seem to revolve around two central issues: the provision of related services and the restrictiveness of the placements.

Provision of Related Services

The requirements in PL 94-142 that state that related services must be provided to persons with handicaps to enable them to benefit from special educational programs has generated much disagreement when determining which services must be provided for students with severe and profound handicaps (Lehr & Haubrich, 1986). The disagreement has centered on the issue of the school district's responsibility as it relates to transportation and health/medical services that need to be provided for these new students (United States Congress, 1987).

The questions are simple regarding transportation for students with complex medical problems: How will they get to school? And, can they be transported on regular school buses, specially equipped vans, or ambulances? All of the aforementioned options are being used with various children, but while it is not known whether there have been any due process hearings regarding who pays for the costly ambulance service, it is hard to imagine that such services have been provided without debate within school district administration. While transportation is clearly specified as a related service in PL 94-142, is ambulance service at $600 per day what the lawmakers had in mind?

A number of issues exist regarding the provision of related medical and school nursing services. Students are coming to school with health care needs beyond those that were traditionally addressed by school nurses. PL 94-142 specifies that school districts must provide only those medical services that are required for the purposes of diagnostic evaluation. The issues involve questions of which procedures are medical services and which are health-related services and, consequently, the responsibility of the schools. That is, if suctioning and tube feeding are medical services, not diagnostic in nature, it would appear that under PL 94-142, these procedures would not have to be provided by school district personnel. But, what if they are health-related procedures necessary to enable a student to benefit from special educational services? The question then is what procedures should and should not be implemented at school and by school personnel (United States Congress, 1987). Several court cases have clarified the parameters of school-related services. In *Irving Independent School District v. Tatro* (1984), the Supreme Court established that CIC was a health-related procedure and that it must be provided by the school district. CIC was considered to be a related service rather than a medical service because it could be performed by a nurse or other qualified persons (i.e., as stated in

PL 94-142). Relying on *Irving Independent School District* (1984) and the PL 94-142 distinction between health-related services and medical services, the *Department of Education, State of Hawaii v. Dorr* (1982) established that reinsertion of a tracheostomy tube was within the parameters of a school health service and was thus to be provided under the health-related services provision of PL 94-142.

Two other cases, *Detsel by Detsel v. Board of Education of Auburn* (1986) and *Bevin H. by Michael H. v. Wright* (1986), had different outcomes. In these cases, it was decided that the school districts should not be responsible for administering the health-related services. In both cases, it was stated that these procedures were much more complex and time consuming than that of CIC, as in *Irving Independent School District* (1984), which was not considered to be a health-related service.

Melissa Detsel was a 7-year-old student attending a special education class. Melissa had severe physical disabilities and required constant respiratory assistance with a continuous supply of 40% oxygen. Prior to entering school, Melissa was provided with 16 hours per day of nursing services in her home that were funded by the county department of social services. Upon entrance into school, the county refused to continue to pay for nursing services during school hours. The school district agreed to pay, but only until the parents determined whether other sources of payment were available. The parents requested an impartial hearing, resulting in the hearing office determining that the school district was, in fact, responsible for paying for the nursing services. An appeal by the school district to the state Commissioner of Education resulted in reversal of the impartial hearing decision. The Commissioner found that the health care services were beyond the requirements of PL 94-142. This decision was based upon the determination that the services required by Melissa, including checking her vital signs, administrating medication through a tube to the jejunum (i.e., a portion of the small intestines), assuring the ingestion of saline solution into the lungs, and suctioning of mucous from the lungs, were beyond those typically required of a school nurse. These services were not health-related but medical services that, according to PL 94-142, were not the responsibility of the school district.

Bevin (Bevin, 1986) was a 6-year-old student with profound mental retardation and multiple handicaps. She required tracheostomy suctioning, gastrostomy tube feeding, administration of medication through the gastrostomy tube, chest physical therapy (that took approximately 35 minutes), and emergency respiratory aid within 30 seconds of distress. The parents had been paying for nursing services for their child while she attended a special education school with partial reimbursement from Major Medical coverage. Projecting future costs and anticipating depletion of resources, the parents requested an impartial hearing to appeal the school district's decision to not cover the costs. As in

Detsel (1986), the impartial hearing officer recommended that the school district assume this responsibility. However, as in *Detsel* (1986), after an appeal by the school district, the State's Secretary of Education reversed the decision, again stating that "the level of skill, complexity, and frequency of nursing services and excessive costs of providing such services fall beyond the scope typically required of public schools."

When it is determined that the health-related procedure is, in fact, the responsibility of the school district, the question becomes one of who will perform the service. Questions asked include:

Whose job is it anyway?
What is the role of the teacher?
Shouldn't a teacher just teach?
Since tube feeding is done solely for the purpose of providing nourishment, is
    that what a teacher should be doing?
What is the role of the school nurse?

Mulligan Ault, Guess, Struth, and Thomas (1988) asked teachers of students with severe multiple handicaps in Kansas which procedures they considered their responsibility and which should be those of paraprofessionals or school nurses. Their responses can be seen in Table 6.1. It should be noted that there were differences between descriptions of what procedures the teachers thought were the responsibility of others and those that they did, in fact, implement. In other words, while they often assumed responsibility for implementing procedures, they perceived it as someone else's job.

Many states have Nurse Practice Acts that specifically state which procedures can and cannot be provided by school nurses. In some programs in various states, this act seems to dictate who will provide what services to the students with disabilities. In other states, the act seems to have little effect on who performs the services, in some cases due to limited knowledge of its existence. Similary, Mulligan Ault et al. (1988) found that teachers of students with complex health care needs often were not aware of whether or not there were district policies.

In some programs, the "If a parent can do it . . . " policy (a criterion set as a precedent in the *Irving Independent School District* [1984] case) seems to be in effect. Parents of children with complex health care needs are routinely taught to implement the necessary health-related procedures to care for their children at home. Many programs are simply saying if the parents can learn to perform the procedures, school district personnel should be able to implement the procedures also.

Union contracts in school districts also effect decisions regarding who implements what health-related procedures. Some contracts specifically state what an employee can and cannot do. For example, in *Department of Education*

Table 6.1. A comparison of the assignment of responsibility for health-related procedures

Health-related procedure	Teacher should be responsible		Paraprofessional should be responsible		Nurse should be responsible	
	Teacher using procedure (%)	Teacher not using procedure (%)	Paraprofessional using procedure (%)	Paraprofessional not using procedure (%)	Nurse using procedure (%)	Nurse not using procedure (%)
75%–100% of classes						
Seizure monitoring	96	100	63	70	56	40
Teeth and gum care	*85*[a]	*36*	*70*	*27*	38	64
Medication administration	48	54	14	31	*85*	*54*
Emergency seizure procedure	88	86	68	57	79	67
50%–75% of classes						
Prevention of skin breakdown	*86*	*61*	*63*	*39*	61	68
Establishing bowel habits	*87*	*50*	*60*	*27*	40	53
25%–50% of classes						
Treatment of skin breakdown	*70*	*44*	48	33	78	84
Diet monitoring/ supplementation	63	59	43	27	*86*	*61*
Postural drainage	*84*	*56*	62	42	48	69
Handling and positioning	88	77	65	53	44	51
CPR	82	85	82	71	86	81
Shunt care	*65*	*19*	*38*	*6*	92	91
Percussion	*86*	*43*	59	43	*45*	*75*

(*continued*)

Table 6.1. (continued)

Health-related procedure	Teacher should be responsible		Paraprofessional should be responsible		Nurse should be responsible	
	Teacher using procedure (%)	Teacher not using procedure (%)	Paraprofessional using procedure (%)	Paraprofessional not using procedure (%)	Nurse using procedure (%)	Nurse not using procedure (%)
0%–25% of classes						
Gastrostomy feeding	73	52	55	33	55	68
Prosthesis care	***89***	***61***	67	44	56	58
Cast care	53	46	37	32	63	63
Monitoring glucose levels	12	16	12	6	88	87
Colostomy/ ileostomy	57	32	36	18	79	78
NG tube feeding	38	44	13	19	50	79
Catheterization	17	16	0	8	83	95
Machine suctioning	40	13	***40***	***7***	80	93
Nasal cannula	67	28	0	18	67	94
Oxygen supplementation— humidifed air	100	36	50	25	50	82
—bulb syringe	67	29	33	13	67	84
—oxygen mask	100	38	0	23	100	86
—mechanical ventilation	—	—	—	—	—	—
Changing trach tubes	0	6	0	3	100	97
Changing trach ties	0	16	0	9	100	91
Administering enema	0	9	0	4	78	84
Delee suctioning	—	—	—	—	—	—

From Mulligan Ault, M., Guess, D., Struth, L., and Thompson, B. (1988). Implementation of health-related procedures in classrooms for students with severe multiple impairments. *Journal of The Association for Persons with Severe Handicaps*; reprinted by permission.

[a]Bold/italic numbers indicate significant differences at the .05 level, using a Chi square analysis.

State of Hawaii (1983), grievance petitions were filed by three unions that were representing teachers and principals a few days after a physician began training school personnel in tracheostomy care and emergency procedures. The parents of Katherine D. (*Department of Education, State of Hawaii*, 1983) refused the public school placement offered by the Department of Education because of the staff's reluctance to cooperate in learning the special health care procedures that Katherine might have needed. The United States district court judge in this case noted that, "the attitude of the school's personnel toward the plan made it completely unworkable and ineffectual" (*Department of Education, State of Hawaii*, 1983). The union grievances represent more than just a conflict between personnel contracts and the federal mandate of PL 94-142; the professionals represented by these grievance petitions were understandably frightened by the potential responsibility for providing emergency lifesaving interventions. Do educational personnel have a right to refuse students if they are fearful of performing health-related procedures that might be needed? Unfortunately, this issue has yet to be resolved. If school districts decide that only select personnel (e.g., registered nurses) are permitted to administer certain health-related procedures, then it is likely that the range of placement options for a student with complex health needs will be limited to the locations where those personnel are based. Such policies may lead to another issue in providing education for students with complex health needs—the issue of limited and restrictive placement alternatives.

Restrictiveness of Placement

A unnamed federal special education official was quoted in a recent article as saying, "When the handicapped-education laws were written 10 years ago, I don't think anybody imagined that we'd have kids with this kind of machinery showing up at the school door" (Viadero, 1987, p. 1). The fact of the matter is that these students are attending school, and the question is now which ones should they attend: schools exclusively for children with handicaps or those for the nonhandicapped. Or, perhaps, do these students continue to stay at home and be taught by homebound teachers? As has been previously discussed, the LRE requirements in PL 94-142 are being taken into consideration as placement decisions are being made.

Only one court case was located in the records that addressed the issue of the least restrictive placement of children with complex health care needs. Katherine D. (*Department of Education, State of Hawaii*, 1983) was a student with cystic fibrosis and tracheomalacia who required tracheostomy tube suctioning, reinsertion, and periodic medication. The school district offered an educational program for her that consisted of speech therapy and parent counseling that were to be provided at home. The parents rejected this placement offer and Katherine continued to attend a private daycare center. Upon appeal of the district's decision, the impartial hearing officer determined that the placement offer being made did not, in fact, represent a least restrictive alternative. The decision was affirmed by the district court.

The complexity of the problems presented by students with special health care needs makes the decisionmaking and delivery of special education and related services in the least restrictive environment difficult (Great Lakes Area Regional Resources Center, 1986). The Great Lakes Area Regional Resources Center (1986), in a policy research paper entitled "Medically Fragile Handicapped Children." It describes four questions asked by educators regarding least restrictive placement decisions:

1. Does the risk to the child's health justify placement in the least restrictive environment?
2. Does the benefit that the child receives justify the cost of service delivery and placement in the least restrictive environment?
3. Do the rights of other individuals whose health might be adversely affected prevail over the rights of the child to be placed in the least restrictive environment?
4. Is the child necessarily better served and educated in the least restrictive environment. (Great Lakes Area Regional Resources Center, 1986, p. 13)

To a large degree, these questions reflect administrative concerns about the intent of the least restrictive placement mandate. For example, asking if the benefit justifies the cost of services implies that students with complex health needs are only entitled to less restrictive placements if it can be demonstrated that educational progress greater than that expected in a more restrictive placement is likely. This reasoning leads to the premise that if the placement is more restrictive (and a more administratively convenient placement) it would be considered to be acceptable and appropriate. This strategy for judging the appropriateness of placement is contrary to the LRE requirements that begin with the assumption that a regular class placement or minimally restrictive placement is most appropriate, unless the student is unable to benefit from education "with the use of supplemental services." Some students may be too dependent upon continuous medical attention or may require medical equipment that is not portable, making hospital or home care more appropriate (United States Congress, 1987; see also Chapter 5, this volume). However, Snell (Chapter 5, this volume) emphasizes that, in all cases, that very restrictive placements should be considered temporary and frequent review of the placement decision should occur.

PROBLEMS INVOLVED WITH PROVIDING SERVICES

Because the delivery of educational services to students with complex health care needs depends on many issues and state policies and lacks historical precedents, the services are often variable and inconsistent (Hobbs et al., 1985; Palfrey et al., 1987). A survey conducted by the departments of education and public health in all states indicates that services to this population of children are being addressed at the local and not the state level (United States Congress, 1987). Currently, different answers are being generated in different school districts within the same state in regards to the provision of services to students with complex health care needs. For example, one school district has developed a policy that nurses will be the only school professionals authorized to provide tube feedings. In other districts in the same state, classroom teachers and even paraprofessional aides implement such procedures. A survey of 150 teachers of students with severe and multiple disabilities in the State of Kansas revealed several interesting findings including the following:

1. Teachers lacked an awareness of school district policy regarding the provision of health-related services.
2. Teachers assumed more responsibility than school nurses for the provision of health-related services.
3. Teachers did not utilize the school nurse as a source of information regarding the provision of health-related services. (Mulligan Ault et al., 1988)

The inconsistency in the provision of services does not seem to be based upon the individual needs of students. Instead, it is based upon lack of precedents, guidelines, and experience; concern for liability; and availability of services.

Additional concerns of these authors (Mulligan Ault et al., 1988) relate to the day-to-day delivery of appropriate educational programs for students. Since experience in serving students with complex health care needs is limited and concerns are high, two prevalent areas of concern have been noted. One concern that has been observed is that these individuals are being treated as patients rather than as students. That is, observation of such students has revealed that the entire focus of the program has been on meeting the health care needs of the students and little on what would be indentified as addressing their educational needs. For some students, the distinction may not be readily apparent; however, this is clearly an area that must be addressed.

A second concern is the nature of the relationship between the classroom teacher and other persons (e.g., nurses) who are responsible for providing health care services to students with complex medical needs. Unfortunately, teachers and nurses do not have a history of working closely together; too often cooperation across disciplines has focused on creating clear delineation of roles. The transdisciplinary model (Hutchinson, 1978) calls for the coordination of services among occupational, physical, and speech therapists with special educators, but fails to emphasize the involvement of nurses. The new population of students with their present health-related problems necessitates the extensive involvement of nursing staff with special educators (Hertel et al., 1984). An even more complex situation is created when students come to school with their own nurse, not the school district's nurse. In such a case, the child may be attended to by the school nurse, private care nurse, teacher, and paraprofessional aide, who are all trying to communicate and coordinate his or her education and health-related efforts.

CURRENT EFFORTS

A number of groups and individuals have focused their attention on the needs of this new population of students. The Office of Special Education and Rehabilitative Services (OSERS) and the office of Maternal and Child Health and Crippled Children's Services (MCH/CCS) are providing federal leadership by funding programs that are focusing on this population. The United States Congress's Office of Technology Assessment in Special Education (OTA-SE) conducted a study on the technology dependent child (United States Congress, 1987). Both the Council for Exceptional Children (CEC) and The Association for Persons with Severe Handicaps (TASH) have established committees to study the needs of students with special health care needs. In 1987, the Council for Administrators in Special Education (CASE) sponsored a series of institutes on the topic of the education of students considered to be medically fragile (Council for Administrators in Special Education, 1987).

Several programs have developed manuals to assist personnel in administration of health-related procedures. The California State Department of Education (1980) published the first of such guidelines that specifically describes how to implement 16 specific procedures such as catheterization, tube feeding, and providing tracheostomy care; similarly, manuals were produced by Campbell, Cohen, and Rich (1987); Graff, Ault, Taylor, and Guess (in press); and the Western Hills Area Education Agency (1987). While these manuals are an important first step in meeting specialized health care needs, they are only a beginning. Every school district in the nation needs clearly delineated procedures for implementing specific health-related procedures to ensure that students receive adequate and appropriate care. Such guidelines are also essential for addressing liability concerns. However, procedures manuals do not address the more difficult policy issues such as agency responsibility, personnel roles, or placement guidelines.

RESEARCH AND PROGRAM DEVELOPMENT

The information and materials for providing educational services to students with complex health care needs are slowly becoming available; however, those who are faced with implementing these services still have no guidelines. To better enable the public schools to assume their new set of responsibilities, much additional research and program development must be undertaken. Answers must be sought in areas that effect educational service delivery for children with complex medical needs. The following are several priority areas that need to be addressed: an estimate of children with complex health care needs, descriptions of appropriate programs, information regarding pertinent policies, current "best practices," and dissemination of educational program information.

First, researchers need to estimate the number of children with complex medical needs and the nature of those needs. Currently, no such data base exists (Viadero, 1987).

Second, descriptions are needed of the characteristics of programs for students with complex health needs. While there is great variability regarding the models and methods of service delivery, there are no clear accounts of those various models and methods in the literature. Sharing information regarding the characteristics of current educational programs has the potential of assisting districts in identifying methods of providing services that might have otherwise gone unrecognized. Such information might include descriptions of:

1. Educational settings
2. Transportation alternatives
3. Health care needs that should be addressed in school
4. Implementation guidelines for specific health-related procedures
5. Linkages between school and other health care providers or agencies

Third, information is needed regarding what policies have been developed in various districts and states. Furthermore, those policies need to be analyzed to determine the effect that they have on delivering educational programs to these targeted children.

Fourth, "best practices" resulting in effective service delivery to this population of students must be identified. And last, dissemination of this information is essential to increase the knowledge of those persons working with these students with complex health care needs.

SUMMARY

The purpose of this chapter is to present information regarding a relatively new population of students who are receiving educational services—those with complex health care needs. These students, due primarily to improved medical care, are surviving long enough to attend school and are bringing with them many challenges for school personnel relative to methods for appropriately meeting their complex health care and educational needs.

REFERENCES

Abromowicz, H.K., & Richardson, S.A. (1975). Epidemiology of severe mental retardation in children: Community studies. *American Journal of Mental Deficiency, 80,* 18–39.
Alford, C., & Pass, R. (1981). Epidemiology of chronic congenital and perinatal infections of man. *Clinics in Perinatology, 8,* 397–414.

American Academy of Pediatrics. (1982). *Report on the committee on infectious diseases.* Elk Grove Village, IL: American Academy of Pediatrics.

Bauer, A.M, & Shea, T.M. (1986). Hepatitis B: An occupational hazard for special educators. *Journal of The Association for Persons with Severe Handicaps, 11,* 171–175.

Bettoli, E. (1982). Herpes: Facts and fallacies. *American Journal of Nursing,* 924–929.

Bevin, H. by Michael H.v. Wright, 666 F. Supp. 71 (W.D. Penn. 1987).

Bureau of Epidemiology. (1983). *Recommendations: Management of herpes infections in educational and residential institutions.* Topeka: Kansas Department of Health and Environment.

California State Department of Education. (1980). *Guidelines and procedures for meeting the specialized physical health care needs of students.* Sacramento: California State Department of Education.

Campbell, M.S., Cohen, S.L., & Rich, M. (1987). *Guidelines for the management of health impaired students.* Portland: Providence Child Center.

Centers for Disease Control. (1985a). Education and foster care of children infected with Human T-Lymphotropic Virus Type III-Lymphadenopathy-Associated Virus. *Morbidity and Mortality Weekly Report, 34,* 517–524.

Centers for Disease Control. (1985b). Summary and recommendations for preventing transmission of infection with HTLV-III/LAV in the workplace. *Morbidity and Mortality Weekly Report, 34,* 681–695.

Certo, N., Haring, N., & York, R. (Eds.). (1984). *Public school integration of severely handicapped students: Rational issues and progressive alternatives.* Baltimore: Paul H. Brookes Publishing Co.

Council for Administrators of Special Education (CASE). (1987). Proceedings of the 1987 CASE Institutes: Medically related special education and related services. Indianapolis, IN: Author.

Department of Education, State of Hawaii v. Dorr. U.S. District Court, 727 F. 2d 809 (D.H. Cir. 1983).

Detsel by Detsel v. Board of Education of Auburn, 637 F. Supp. 1022 (N.D.N.Y. 1986).

Ekstrand, R.E. (1982). Doctor, do you make (school) house calls? *Children Today, 11*(3), 2–5.

Graff, C., Ault, M.M., Taylor, M., & Guess, D. (in press). *Health related procedures information manual for the classroom teacher.* Unpublished manuscript, University of Kansas, Lawrence.

Great Lakes Area Regional Resource Center. (1986). *"Medically fragile" handicapped children: A policy research paper.* Columbus: Ohio State University.

Guess, D., Bronicki, M.A., Firmender, K.H., Mann, J.M., Merrill, M.A., Olin-Zimmerman, S.J., Wanat, P.E., Zamarripa, E.J., & Turnbull, H.R. (1984). Legal and moral considerations in educating children with herpes in public school settings. *Mental Retardation, 22,* 257–263.

Hertel, V., Brainerd, E., Desrostus, C., Hatfield, M.E., Lewis, P., Markendord, J., & Quinne, H.N. (1984). National association of state school nurse consultants define role of school nurse in: "PL 94-141—Education for All Handicapped Children Act of 1975." *The Journal of School Health, 54,* 475–478.

Hobbs, N., Perrin, J.M., & Ireys, H.T. (1985). *Chronically ill children and their families.* San Francisco: Jossey-Bass.

Hotte, E.A., Monroe, H.S., Philbrook, D.L., & Scarlata, R.W. (1984). Programming for persons with profound mental retardation: A three year retrospective study. *Mental Retardation, 22*(2), 75–78.

Hutchinson, D.J. (1978). The transdisciplinary approach. In J.B. Curry & K.K. Pepper

(Eds), *Mental retardation: Nursing approaches to care* (pp. 65–74). St. Louis: C.V. Mosby.

Immunization Practices Advisory Committee. (1985). Recommendations for protection against viral hepatitis. *Morbidity and Mortality Weekly Report, 34,* 313–334.

Irving Independent School District v. Tatro, 468 U.S. 883, 82 L. Ed. 2d 664, 104 S. Ct. 3371 (1984).

Khan, N.A., & Battle, C.U. (1987). Chronic illness: Implications for development and education. *Topics in Early Childhood Special Education, 6*(4), 25–32.

Kleinberg, S.B. (1982). *Educating the chronically ill child.* Rockville, MD: Aspen Publishers Inc.

Lehr, D.H., & Haubrich, P. (1986). Legal precedents for students with severe handicaps. *Exceptional Children, 52*(4), 358—365.

Mulligan Ault, M., Guess, D., Struth, L., & Thomas, B. (1988). Implementation of health-related procedures in classrooms for students with severe multiple impairments. *Journal of The Association for Persons with Severe Handicaps, 13*(2), 100–109.

Palfrey, J., DiPrete, L., Walker, D., Shannon, K., & Maroney, E. (1987). *School children dependent on medical technology.* Washington, DC: ATA Institute.

Pass, R.F., & Kinney, J.S. (1985). Child care workers and children with congenital cytomegalovirus infection. *Pediatrics, 75* (5), 971–973.

Pathfinder & School Nurse Organization of Minnesota. (1986). *Managing the student with a chronic health condition: A practical guide for school personnel.* St. Paul, MN: Medical Education and Research Association of Gillette Children's Hospital.

Perrin, J.M. (1986). Chronically ill children: An overview. *Topics in Early Childhood Special Education, 5*(4), 1–11.

Public Law 94-142, *Education for All Handicapped Children Act of 1975,* 20 U.S.C. §121,(1975).

Public Law 99-457, *Education of the Handicapped Amendments of 1986,* 20 U.S.C. §§619, 676, (1986).

Scipien, G.M., Bernard, M.U., Chard, M.A., Howe, J., & Phillips, P.J. (1986). *Comprehensive pediatric nursing.* New York: McGraw-Hill.

Shayne, M.W., Walker, D.K., Perrin, J.M., & Moynihan, L.C. (1987). Health impaired children deserve a break. *Principal, 66*(3), 36–39.

Stein, R. (1986). Promoting communication between health care providers and educators of chronically ill children. *Topics in Early Childhood Special Education, 5*(4), 70–81.

TEFRA. (1982). Katie Beckett Program, 42 U.S.C. § 1396(a)(c)3.

Thomas, C.L. (Ed.). (1985). *Taber's cyclopedic medical dictionary.* Philadelphia: F.A. Davis.

United States Congress. (1987). *Technology-dependent children: Hospital vs. home-care—A technical memorandum* (OTA Publication No. TM-H-38). Washington, DC: United States Government Printing Office.

U.S. Department of Health and Human Services. (1986). *Facts About AIDS.* Washington, DC: Author.

Viadero, D. (1987, March). 'Medically fragile' students pose dilemma for school officials. *Education Week, 1,* 14.

Waechter, E.H., Phillips, J., & Holaday, B. (1985). *Nursing care of children* (10th ed.). Philadelphia: J.B. Lippincott.

Walker, D.K. (1986). Chronically ill children in early childhood education programs. *Topics in Early Childhood Special Education, 5*(4), 12–22.

Western Hills Area Education Agency. (1987). *Procedures for management of children with special health needs in educational settings.* Sioux City, IA: Author.

Wolfensberger, W. (1972). *Normalization: The principal of normalization in human services*. Toronto, Canada: National Institute on Mental Retardation.

Wood, S.P., Walker, D., & Gardner, J. (1986). School health practices for children with complex medical needs. *Journal of School Health, 56*(6), 215–217.

II

PRACTICES

DYSFUNCTION IN POSTURE AND MOVEMENT IN INDIVIDUALS WITH PROFOUND DISABILITIES
Issues and Practices

Philippa H. Campbell

Many individuals with profound disabilities have disorders that result in limitations in posture and movement. Some of these limitations result from damage to the brain during or after birth. Some result from genetic or chromosomal abnormalities, multiple congenital anomalies or malformations, or other factors. These disorders in posture and movement can be so severe in some individuals that special health and medical care is required to ensure proper nutrition and growth, reasonable respiratory status, and freedom from secondary medical problems such as skin breakdown, infections, malnutrition, or dehydration.

Difficulty learning to move against gravity due to limitations in the sensory systems, dysfunctional muscle tone, or inadequate environmental stimuli is a common characteristic of an individual with a profound disability (e.g., Campbell, 1987b; Wilson, 1984). Programming designed to remediate disorders in posture and movement and to stimulate gross motor development is seldom effective. Many individuals with disabilities involving posture and movement may not learn to stand or even sit independently. Few will learn to walk without assistance. Many may remain dependent on others for self-care needs. Some may develop even greater limitations in posture and movement over time, resulting from secondary development of muscle tightness, structural limitations in the joints, and orthopedic deformities (Campbell, 1987c).

PROGRAM FOCUS

The majority of programming approaches used to enhance functioning in posture and movement are based upon a *remedial perspective* (Campbell, 1984; Hanson & Harris, 1986; Scherzer & Tscharnuter, 1982). An assessment of performance of gross motor skills results in identification of skills that cannot yet be performed. Physical and occupational therapists may supplement skill performance assessments with procedures to determine deviancies in muscle tone and strength, in range of motion at joints, and in other physical areas. This information becomes the basis for establishing goals and objectives that represent the areas of skill or overall functioning that are in need of remediation. Goals that include sitting independently, increasing range of motion at the elbow joint, toning up the abdominal muscles, or eating with one's mouth, result from a remedial approach toward assessment and programming.

Disorders in posture and movement abilities are frequently so severe in individuals with profound disabilities that remediation cannot be achieved through currently used treatment and intervention approaches. Remediation that is designed to enable an individual to achieve developmental milestone skills is particularly ineffective with teenage or adult individuals who may have acquired a number of disorders in posture and movement that are secondary to their original dysfunction in muscle tone or coordination of movement patterns (Campbell, 1987c; York & Rainforth, 1986). Secondary disorders that relate specifically to posture and movement include: 1) variations in muscles, 2) changes in joint structures, 3) orthopedic deformities, 4) decreased strength in muscles, and 5) diminished motor planning abilities. Other secondary disorders may also result indirectly from severe movement impairment, including limited motivation to interact with objects or people, diminished abilities to solve environmental problems, decreased communication, and limited acquisition of critical skills (Campbell, 1987b, 1987c).

Alternate Program Approaches

One alternate program approach to secondary disorders is to focus intervention in such a way as to prevent acquisition of these handicapping conditions. A *prevention-intervention approach* is most often used with infants who are known to be biologically or environmentally "at risk" for developing handicaps (Campbell, in press). Professionals implement intervention strategies early in the life of the infant for the purpose of preventing development of generalized secondary handicaps, such as mental retardation, language dysfunction, or social-emotional disorders. A prevention-intervention approach also has remarkable applicability with children and adults with profound disabilities when applied with a slightly different focus.

A known outcome as determined through various studies conducted with individuals with profound disabilities who have been institutionalized has been established (e.g., Landesman-Dwyer & Sackett, 1978). In general, when physical dysfunction accompanies other disabilities, individuals who have been institutionalized for long periods of time are known: to be dependent in all self-care skills; to demonstrate limited abilities to interact with objects and people in the environment; and to have numerous secondary physical disabilities, including contractures and deformities (Bricker & Campbell, 1980). Professionals in all disciplines have identified difficulties in locating motivators to use in programming these individuals (Bricker & Campbell, 1982), pinpointed problems with fabricating appropriate adaptive equipment (Staller, 1984), and expressed difficulties in designing unique training strategies that are effective in enabling individuals to perform essential skills (Campbell & Bricker, 1980; Campbell, Cooper, & McInerney, 1984). Programming designed to prevent development of each of these known disorders or to alleviate further disability can be more effective with these individuals than that designed to remediate dysfunction.

A second alternate approach to programming also has great applicability in addressing the needs of individuals with profound disabilities. A *compensatory approach* recognizes that not all disorders can be either remediated or prevented. Rather, some disorders are so restricting that strategies are required to compensate for their severity (York & Rainforth, 1987). Use of adaptive equipment to properly position an individual with contractures and deformities is one example of the application of a *compensatory* focus. Proper equipment allows supported performance of postural skills, such as sitting, that may be impossible for an individual with severe motor dysfunction and, when specifically designed, compensates for the atypical muscle tone and lack of postural alignment that may be preventing the performance of particular skills (Bergen & Colangelo, 1982; Trefler, Tooms, & Hobson, 1985). Switch interface devices have gained popularity in programming individuals with profound disabilities because various types of devices may enable these individuals to interact in his or her physical or social environment in the absence of coordinated manipulation skills (Esposito & Campbell, 1986; York, Nietupski, & Hamre-Nietupski, 1985).

Application of Program Approaches

Quality of previous programming; intensity and quality of current, available programming; extent of disability; and age are all factors to consider when selecting programming approaches to be used with a specific individual. A remedial approach is least likely to be effective with individuals with profound disabilities, even during infancy and early childhood. A compensatory approach, by itself or used as a method to prevent further disabilities, is most likely to benefit the majority of individuals with profound disabilities regardless of age, degree of disability, or other factors.

Realistically, the extent of disability demonstrated by an individual, irrespective of age, partly determines the degree to which programming is directed toward strategies that compensate for existing impairments. Some individuals with profound disabilities use vision and hearing appropriately and may have limited involvement in motoric abilities. Others, even in infancy, demonstrate disorders in vision, hearing, and movement. These children, in particular, are at great risk for developing secondary disorders in communication, cognition, and social interaction. Development of secondary disorders are more easily preventable in younger children with profound disabilities when programming uses compensatory approaches for prevention-intervention and integrates information from various disciplines (Campbell, in press).

The amount and type of programming that has been received in the past is a significant factor in determining the number and type of secondary handicaps. Children with profound disabilities who may have received early intervention services may not have received physical or occupational therapy or may have received only "consultative" or "maintenance" programming due to the severity of their disabilities. The longer an individual waits without proper and sufficient programming, the greater the probability that numerous secondary disorders will develop. The greater the number of secondary disorders that develop, the more intense, systematic, and compensatory the current programming must be if both original and secondary disabilities are to be addressed adequately.

Quality and intensity of available programming influences the extent to which children and adults will acquire functional skills. Disorders demonstrated by older individuals, in particular, can sometimes be altered only with intensive, systematic, and, often, one-on-one programming that integrates information from necessary professionals and caregivers (e.g., Campbell & Bricker, 1980; Durand & Kishi, 1987). Longitudinal, sequenced, and coordinated programming, provided by well-trained individuals of various disciplines, can be successful in teaching functional skills to individuals with profound disabilities of various ages (Bricker & Campbell, 1980; Campbell, 1987b).

Secondary disorders in cognition, communication, and social interaction, in themselves, cause individuals to acquire more numerous disabilities than those with which they were born. Older students or adults who have not received programming to prevent such secondary disabilities are likely to have more significant disabilities than their similarly involved younger counterparts. However, the effect of extensive secondary disorders on areas of functioning can be compensated for at any age, given sufficient means, including a functional programming curriculum (Sailor & Guess, 1983; Snell, 1987), adaptive and prosthetic devices, and personnel trained to use those devices appropriately in programming (e.g., Garner & Campbell, in press; York et al., 1985).

OVERALL PROGRAM EMPHASIS

Individuals with profound disabilities need to be able to perform as many age-appropriate activities in as many age-appropriate environments as possible. In this sense, the instructional needs of this group of individuals with the most severe disabilities are no different from those of their peers with less serious handicaps. The challenge to the various disciplines which are involved with these individuals lies in determining the unique combinations of instructional and therapeutic strategies that will enable as much independence as possible.

Posture and movement skills allow persons with profound disabilities to express their thoughts, feelings, and ideas. They are also an essential component in skill areas, such as self-care/personal management, mobility, recreation/leisure, and work. As such, posture and movement disabilities are not simply a problem area in themselves but modify an individual's ability to perform essential life skills, to communicate, or to solve environmental problems (e.g., use functional cognition or thinking). Overall programming focuses on preventing secondary disabilities and on ensuring that opportunities are available for use with whatever abilities are possible for the individual as a means to independence, however limited. Individuals with profound disabilities who develop additional (i.e., secondary) motor problems, for whatever reason, become even further restricted in expression of communication or cognition and even more limited in performance of basic skills. Those who are not encouraged to use their present abilities for independence may learn to be helpless instead of independent, a situation that can be extremely difficult to overcome through programming (e.g., Bricker & Campbell, 1980).

Preventing Secondary Physical Disabilities

Multiple disorders in posture and movement skills are common among individuals with the most challenging programming needs. These disorders originate in difficulties with muscle tone that may be of sufficient severity to prevent the individual's independent antigravity posture and coordinated movement abilities. Discrepancies in muscle tone may range from mild to severe and may vary from too low (i.e., hypotonic) to too high (i.e., hypertonic). Conditions of low or high tone prevent an individual from performing independent antigravity postures, such as sitting or standing. An individual may lack sufficient muscle power and control to achieve antigravity postures when muscle tone is low. Coordinated movements may be absent or extremely restricted when an individual is unable to control the head, limbs, or body against the influences of gravity. Contrarily, individuals with high muscle tone are typically stiff and, although their high tone keeps them up against gravity if supported, the tone is so high that malalignment of the body results and coordinated movements are either extremely limited or impossible to produce.

Extreme deviations in muscle tone hinder acquisition of antigravity postures and limit production of coordinated movement patterns, making those individuals with such muscle tone abnormalities dependent on caregivers to reposition their bodies or change their body position from one posture to another. Individuals who are not frequently realigned by a caregiver or whose positions are not changed frequently because they are unable to do it themselves are at-risk for developing permanent changes in muscle length, joint structures, and skeletal system. Thus, an individual who is positioned in an adaptive chair for most of the day will eventually develop hip and knee flexion contractures due to being restricted in the same position and being unable to readjust body position independently. Similarly, an individual who leans to the side when in an adaptive chair will eventually develop a permanent C-shaped curve or C-shaped scoliosis in the spine due to inability to sit with a normally aligned spine.

Positioning to Maintain Muscle Length   Preventing the almost inevitable development of changes in muscle length is a challenge when dealing with individuals who have significant discrepancies in muscle tone. However, certain areas of the body are at greater risk than others, depending on the number and variety of postures in which individuals are placed. Many nonambulatory individuals are positioned for most of the day in some form of sitting. This seems to be a typical practice for a number of reasons. First, most individuals function better in an upright position than when in stomach, back, or sidelying positions. Second, many individuals may own only one piece of adaptive equipment. An adaptive wheelchair is the equipment of choice when only one option is possible. Third, sitting is an age-appropriate position for persons who are more than 6 months of age and it is becoming the most normalized position since greater numbers of individuals with profound handicaps are being integrated into regular education and work settings.

Changes in muscle length will occur with high probability in the spine, pelvis or hips, knees, and feet when individuals are situated for long lengths of time in the sitting position. Changes in the length of spinal musculature will be dependent on the type of muscle tone that is present in the trunk. An asymmetrical distribution of muscle tone (e.g., higher on one body side than the other) may cause the spine to pull in on one side, tipping the individual to the same side on which the spinal musculature is shortened. Increased tone (i.e., high tone) throughout the trunk is unusual except with individuals with the most profoundly disabling conditions. The extensor muscles in the spine may become shortened, pulling the individual into a backward orientation. A variety of types of shortened muscles are possible when muscle tone is low in the spinal or trunk musculature. These individuals often "fall into" supports placed on adaptive chairs or into gravity itself, resulting in either shortening of either the lateral flexors (due to leaning to the side) or the muscles in the lower back area (from the trunk falling forward over the pelvis).

Muscle overlengthenings also occur in each position, including sitting, and result from immobility of the body. Overlengthenings can vary from person to person, dependent upon the particular distribution of high or low muscle tone. For example, an individual who has shortened lower back muscles is also likely to have overlengthened abdominal muscles. Shortened hip flexor muscles, in turn, overlengthen the hip extensors. Falling into and stabilizing the shoulders on shoulder straps or harnesses may result in shortening of the shoulder girdle flexors with corresponding overlengthening in the thoracic spine (i.e., upper back). Muscle shortenings are more obvious than muscle overlengthenings; however, the overlengthenings are often more debilitating since the muscles lose their ability to contract against gravity to bring the body into alignment or to produce coordinated movement patterns.

Restricting the amount of time that is spent in a sitting position, in itself, will not prevent the development of muscle shortenings and overlengthenings that result from immobile positions. Alternate positions must be selected systematically in order to place those muscle groups at greatest risk for developing shortenings and overlengthenings into the opposite length. Supported weight-bearing standing positions are appropriate opposite postures for individuals who spend a great deal of time sitting. The hip and knee muscles that are flexed in sitting are extended in standing. Alignment of the trunk can be achieved through supports used, for example, on supine standers, prone boards, or other types of supported standing devices. The amount of time spent in weight-bearing standing positions should be equal to that spent in sitting for the benefits and liabilities of each position to balance the other. Additional therapeutic activities may also need to be implemented to overcome the negative aspects of immobility in each position.

Many individuals, particularly those who have been immobile for many years, may have developed deformities and secondary physical changes that prevent him or her from being situated in weight-bearing standing positions. Particularly problematic are foot or ankle deformities that eliminate the feet as a weight-bearing surface or that induce painful dislocations or subluxations of the hip (Fraser, Hensinger, & Phelps, 1987). Supported standing using adaptive equipment can be achieved, when an individual has some limitations in full hip and knee extension, by using pads that support the knees in a flexed position while obtaining as much extension at the hips as possible. Alternative positions that maximize hip and knee extension with a normally aligned spine must be selected if further deformity is to be prevented. Sidelying and backlying positions provide alternatives that are appropriate from a physical management standpoint; however, this may not be age-appropriate. These positions should be used, where possible, outside functional classroom activities. For example, they should be used during a recreational activity, such as watching television, or during sleep.

Therapeutic Activities to Restore Muscle Length   Tightness and overlengthenings develop very quickly when infants and children are unable to move into different positions without assistance. While these changes in muscle length can technically be prevented through proper positioning and adequate therapeutic intervention, more often than not, therapeutic activities must be provided regularly in addition to proper positioning in order to maintain muscles at as close to normal length as possible. Shortenings that have already occurred can be reversed, where necessary, through use of active and passive range of motion and muscle stretching procedures or through surgical correction.

Deep pressure provided to a muscle group through positioning or by placing the hands over the muscle (or both) provides tactile and proprioceptive input that is necessary in order to lengthen muscle fibers (e.g., Campbell, 1987c). This procedure assists in lengthening fibers to their most physiologically possible extent; however, this will not stretch out contractures in muscle fibers. Deep pressure techniques can be used independently or in conjunction with range of motion and muscle stretching activities to stretch permanently shortened muscle fibers. The sensory stimuli provided by the deep pressure applied to the muscle causes it to relax to the fullest extent that is possible. Passive range of motion techniques can be implemented following deep pressure. The muscle can then be stretched passively and held at its maximal possible length to obtain further lengthening.

Both passive range of motion and stretching can be painful techniques that can result in further damage to the muscles if passive movement occurs too rapidly or if the muscle is stretched beyond the ideal length. The inherent risks in these procedures are greater when used with an individual who may not be able to speak or indicate pain. The procedures are best used when scheduled and regularly monitored by a physical or occupational therapist who has trained others to implement the procedures with a particular individual. Deep pressure is a less intrusive technique and can be used with relatively little risk.

Passive Deep Pressure through Dynamic and Static Positioning Muscles that are weight-bearing on a surface are receiving deep pressure through contact with that surface. The degree of pressure that is provided can be enhanced through additional input from the caregiver's hands or by readjusting the student's body alignment to maximize weight-bearing on a particular body surface. Deep pressure can be used in conjunction with both dynamic and static positioning. For example, if an individual is placed in a sidelying position with the underlying arm placed above the head, deep pressure is applied to the muscles that are on the side of the body. That is a positioning procedure that is used with an individual with shortening on one side or to lengthen shortened muscles under the arm.

Deep Pressure over a Muscle Group The caregiver's hands provide sensory input to muscles in specific therapeutic handling procedures as well as any time a student is moved or touched. Deep pressure techniques can be easily incorporated into positioning, repositioning, and all caregiving routines that are frequently necessary with individuals with severely dysfunctional posture and movement skills. They can also be effectively used with older individuals to help return body musculature to a more normal length (Smith, 1984). Figure 7.1 illustrates a sequence of deep pressure obtained through positioning and direct pressure over a group of muscles. Initially, the child was positioned

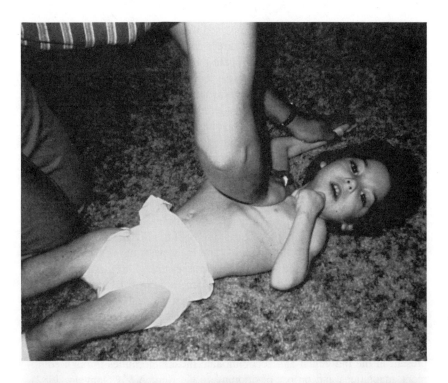

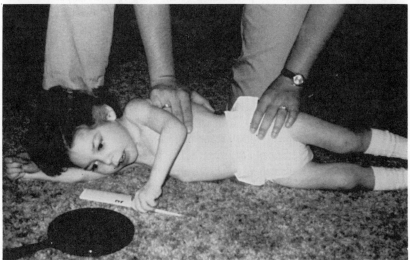

Figure 7.1. Top: Deep pressure over the shoulder muscles lengthens these muscles to facilitate range of motion of the right arm in preparation for moving a child into a sidelying position.
Bottom: The sidelying position provides pressure through weight-bearing on the right side to further facilitate muscle lengthening.

on her back with direct deep pressure used over the shoulder girdle flexors to obtain necessary lengthening. This direct deep pressure was combined with passive range of motion, used to prepare the arm for full extension in a side-lying position in order to obtain passive lengthening of the scapular-humeral muscle groups. Direct deep pressure was used in a sidelying position to reinforce the pressure provided through positioning to obtain spinal alignment during reaching. These procedures, used in one-on-one treatment, were also incorporated into dressing and playing routines.

Orthopedic Deformities Deformities of the skeletal system are a direct consequence of changes in muscle length and joint structures. Dislocated hips and variations in spinal alignment (e.g., scoliosis, kyphosis) are the most common deformities. Most individuals, even those with severe posture and movement disorders, are born without deformities. The types of deformities that are acquired are related to positioning of the individual, distribution of muscle tone, extent of tonal deviations, and the type of physical management that is provided for each individual (e.g., Fraser et al., 1987). All deformities cannot be corrected; however, those that can, are correctable only through orthopedic management and surgery. Even when surgical correction is possible, the respiratory status and other basic functions of some individuals may be too impaired to risk necessary surgery. Physical management procedures, such as positioning and handling, must take into account the deformities that are present in the individual and accommodate those deformities through equipment adaptations and proper positioning (e.g., Bergen & Colangelo, 1982). Implementing necessary management procedures to prevent the acquisition of orthopedic deformities is easier than designing equipment for these individuals in an effort to correct their secondary physical disabilities.

Preventing Learned Helplessness

The phenomena of learned helplessness among individuals with profound disabilities was originally described by Seligman (1975) and has since been expanded upon by educators who work with individuals with severe handicaps (e.g., Bricker & Campbell, 1980; Campbell, 1987c; Robinson & Robinson, 1987). This concept describes a depressive state where individuals learn how to function as if they were helpless instead of performing tasks independently. Many individuals who have been institutionalized for long periods of time appear to have learned to be helpless. However, the same phenomena can be observed even in younger children with severely restricted movement repertoires and/or multisensory impairments who reside at home (Campbell, 1987b, in press).

Fostering Independence Infants and young children typically are motivated to move and explore their environments. Children are the change agents who modify adult behavior in their drive for independence. For example, a young child may grab for food or the spoon long before his or her mother sets self-feeding objectives, or the child may insist on doing things for him- or herself, often at times when his or her parents would prefer the expediency of doing the task for their child. Infants and children with severe and profound disabilities seldom demonstrate this drive for independence; furthermore, if that drive is present, it is not easily identified by adults. Adults may continue to physically care for children as if they were infants, establishing a pattern where even the child's most basic needs are met by the caregiver. This would inadvertently eliminate or limit opportunities for the child to demonstrate his or her independent skills. Many service delivery approaches also reduce opportunities for individuals to demonstrate independence. For example, therapists may focus on the physical needs of an individual and select floorlying positions (e.g., supine, prone, sidelying) that may be helpful in establishing alignment but do so using methods that foster dependence. Also, therapists may overfocus on the qualitative aspects of movement, preventing a child from performing a skill that he or she can do independently because the pattern or coordination is qualitatively poor (Scherzer & Tscharnuter, 1982). An individual may be able to perform a skill independently, but only at a rate of movement that is so reduced that adults eventually do the skill for him or her. For example, many individuals in institutions and nursing homes are able to feed themselves; however, because feeding is so slow that food becomes cold or the meal is not finished before the dishes need to be returned to the kitchen, these individuals are usually fed by caregivers (Perske, Clifton, McLean, & Stein, 1986).

A first step in fostering independence is to allow an individual to perform whatever skills are possible without adult assistance. Vocal or motor responses that are performed independently by an individual can be incorporated into programming, even when those responses are believed to be "involuntary" or "reflexes" (e.g., Campbell, 1987b; Campbell et al., 1984; York & Rainforth, 1987). Adults must develop an expectation for performance from the individual, however limited it may be. Adults who have learned that an individual is unable to do much independently will operate on expectations that do not foster whatever independence is possible.

Using Compensatory Strategies Infants and young children with severe and profound disabilities are at great risk for learning to be helpless. Remedially based early intervention models, designed to identify developmental areas in need of remediation, penalize these young children by assuming that they are least likely to make progress in early developmental skills that are so heavily rooted in motoric competence (Campbell, in press). Approaches that recognize the significant disabilities of these young children and use methods that compensate for disabilities rather than remediating them are more likely to enable children to perform skills independently; however, they often use somewhat unconventional responses. For example, an infant can be taught to vocalize before being fed a mouthful of food or to move the hand and arm to a specific location on a wheelchair tray before being pushed. These responses are unconventional but allow use of whatever limited movement is possible to give individuals some degree of independence and control over their environments.

Adaptive equipment and devices enable an individual to gain independence that he or she may not be capable of without aids. Equipment is used to position an individual in whatever degree of postural alignment that he or she is capable of so that head or limb movements can be used. Existing responses expressed with the head, eyes, arms, hands, or legs can be used to determine partial or total independent responses. These responses may be made more functional through the use of switch interface devices or other forms of adaptive devices (e.g., York et al., 1985). The use of devices is a programming necessity for many individuals with profound disabilities. However, to be effective, devices must be selected on the basis of their activation rate and the individual's overall cognitive abilities (e.g., Esposito & Campbell, 1986; Campbell, 1985).

MOTOR EXPRESSION IN COGNITION

Many individuals with profound handicaps appear to have primitive, non-complex cognitive and communicative skills. Acquisition and use of cognitive and communication abilities are vulnerable when individuals have profound disabilities, due to both the extremely limited repertoire of posture and movement skills that may be available for use in such expressions, and the decreased number of opportunities that may be present in which expression is recognized and responded to by adults. Most individuals demonstrate at least basic sensorimotor cognitive competence. However, the motoric expression of these abilities may be so restricted and so unconventional that early attempts in these areas may go unrecognized by adults.

Secondary disabilities in cognition develop when: 1) programming does not match abilities, 2) opportunities are not provided for individuals to use whatever cognitive abilities are present and to build more sophisticated skills on this ability base, and 3) learned helplessness has developed. Programming for posture and movement is directed generally toward preventing secondary physical disabilities and, specifically, toward the use of posture and movement (however limited or abnormal) for functional purposes. Functional movement results when existing posture and movement patterns are used for intentional or self-directed purposes that solve environmental problems (e.g., Campbell, 1987b, 1987d).

Preventing Secondary Cognitive Handicaps

The extent of the individual's disability in cognition is, to a large extent, a function of the degree of brain damage that is present, the number of related biological impairments (e.g., vision, hearing), and the opportunities for learning that have been provided. Those cognitive impairments that are the result of specific brain damage cannot be prevented. However, the extent to which impairments limit an individual's ability to use cognition to direct functional use of movement can be influenced. Appropriate early intervention can have an effect on the extent to which an infant with severe and profound disabilities learns to become either helpless or competent. Programming that is sensitive to the state and neurobehavioral level of an infant, establishes joint reciprocity between an infant and his or her caregiver(s), and supports independence in basic skills through prevention-intervention and compensatory strategies is more likely to foster continued use of movement for functional purposes. In contrast, programming that is designed to remediate deficits and to teach an infant with severe and profound disabilities to perform behavior that is typical of nonhandicapped infants is likely to establish a base of incompetence and helplessness that will limit the use of functional movement (Campbell, in press).

Coping with Cognitive Handicaps

Infants and young children acquire cognitive competence through interaction with their physical and social worlds (e.g., Dunst, 1981; Piaget, 1952). Movement patterns that are in the repertoires of newborns are believed to be manifested through coordinated patterns available through genetic preadaptation (Bower, 1982; Kopp, 1979). Such general response patterns include sucking and grasping, and appear each time when specific stimuli are provided. These responses become adapted through the infant's experiences with objects and people. A child is able to use movement intentionally for functional use within the environment at the point at which cognitive abilities such as looking or means-ends concepts are paired with coordinated movement patterns for self-directed movement.

Individuals with profound disabilities may have both restricted movement repertoires and diminished cognitive competence (i.e., learned helplessness). More importantly, cognitive abilities may be difficult to determine due to these individuals' inability to use conventional motor response patterns (e.g., reaching, looking, grasping, smiling) or to communicate through vocal or nonvocal means. In addition, other factors such as concomitant sensory problems, medication for seizures, and other medical management procedures (e.g., ventilated breathing) may also complicate an individual's ability to respond to stimulation in conventional ways.

Matching Cognitive Stimuli to Behavior State

Recent research (e.g., Guess et al., 1987; Wilcox & Campbell, in press) indicates that some individuals with profound disabilities may have difficulties maintaining a sufficiently alert state long enough to be sensitive to stimulation in their environments. Wilcox and Campbell (1987), drawing largely from the work of Brazelton (1961), and Brazelton and Als (1979) with infants, developed a rating system by which a child's interaction with an adult could be analyzed. Results of a pilot study with four preschool children with severe and profound disabilities indicated that these children seldom interacted with objects or people. Furthermore, these stimuli were as likely to produce responses that resulted in "removing" a child from the situation (e.g., eye gaze aversion) as they were to encourage the child to engage in the interaction. Similar results have been reported by Guess et al. (in press) who used a live observation, time-sampling procedure to record state levels of students with severe disabilities who were attending school in regular classrooms. Many students never engaged in interactions with instructional stimuli while others appeared to be "overloaded" and responded by withdrawing from stimuli.

Individuals with profound disabilities may have fragile and primitive neurological organization, and/or poor neurobehavioral organization of their respiratory and other autonomic nervous system functions, motor system functions, and overall state. Levels of medication necessary for effective seizure control may also influence the individual's state levels. Instructional and therapeutic procedures that are sensitive to state level and neurobehavioral organization can be adapted from such procedures that are used with infants who are preterm or who are born with severe neurological dysfunction. They can be used in an effort to match stimuli to the individual's levels of behavioral organization. In general, these techniques include: 1) presenting single stimuli in a slow, graded manner (rather than presenting multimodal stimuli that may "bombard" the individual and result in aversion or withdrawal rather than attention or engagement, 2) analyzing stimuli to determine which are the most easily attended to by an individual, 3) waiting for sufficient lengths of time for a response to occur since latency between stimuli and response may be low, and 4) reading the behavioral cues of the individual in an effort to determine when to increase the complexity of stimuli presented when he or she is in an alert state and when to withdraw stimuli that may result in an overload.

The effectiveness of these methods with a specific individual is best determined through ongoing data collection and sensitive reading of neurobehavioral cues. Responses such as head/neck posturing away from an individual or stimuli, eye aversion, eye shutting, increased respiratory rate, difficulty breathing, grunting, and increased muscle tone are all indicators of nonengagement, diminished attention state levels, and poorly organized neurobehavioral functions. Head/neck orientation, eye gaze toward a person or object, and movement toward an object or person (i.e., reaching, vocalization, smiling) are all indicators of engagement and interest on the part of the individual. Programmers must first engage attention before expecting an individual to acquire information or actively participate in an activity. Instruction is wasted on an individual who may be seizuring, in respiratory distress, or in a state of nonengagement.

An engaged state is expanded upon once the type of stimuli that results in engagement are determined. For example, a programmer may find that an individual posturally orients and looks toward a specific object, such as a taperecorder that is playing music. The response requirements can be increased systematically within this particular activity by using the following sequence: 1) the individual orients his or her attention toward the taperecorder both posturally and with his or her eyes, after music is turned on; 2) when the music plays and then stops, the individual orients his or her attention toward the object again, both posturally and with his or her eyes to continue activity; 3) the individual again orients his or her attention toward the object, posturally and with his or her eyes, while vocalizing or reaching toward it to continue the activity, regardless of whether the music is on or off; and 4) the individual orients his or her attention toward the taperecorder and reaches and/or vocalizes to indicate initiation of the activity.

Determining an Appropriate Response Mode

Postural orientation responses are possible with all individuals with profound disabilities, even those with severe hypertonus or hypotonus or limited repertoires of postural and movement skills. However, these responses are often difficult to recognize as they may be performed in quite unconventional ways. Responses are likely to be qualitatively modified by abnormal muscle tone, secondary changes in muscle length, or orthopedic deformities. For example, an individual with asymmetrically distributed muscle tone may turn the head and trunk away from a stimuli, thereby activating an *asymmetrical tonic neck reflex* (ATNR). The orientation of this posture remains away from the stimuli even though the response may be achieved through asymmetrical distribution of hypertonus. In essence, the function of the response indicates nonengagement while the form is characterized by asymmetrical high tone. For example, an individual with a scoliosis to the left side may have postural orientation to the side (due to the scoliosis) but may rotate his or her head toward the object as an indicator of engagement.

Postural orientation cues may be difficult to recognize and read during programming. Cues such as eye movement, arm motions, and vocalization are more conventional cues and, therefore, more easily read by other individuals. Eye movement, arm motions toward or away, and vocalization are paired with the postural orientation cues to provide more salient cues concerning the individual's state of engagement and interest in an activity. These responses can, subsequently, be trained for functional use in relation to environmental events. Specific responses are selected in relation to each individual's pattern of disabilities. Obviously, eye movement is not possible for an individual who is blind; arm motioning toward or away from an object or person may not be feasible for an individual with severe contractures in his or her arms and hands; and vocalization may not be effective with an individual with hearing impairment or with severe hypotonus that limits the rate and intonation of vocalization patterns (e.g., Campbell, 1987b).

Selecting a particular response occurs on the basis of conventionality and rate. The response that is the most ideal is the one that can be identified most easily by the greatest number of caregivers and the one that can be produced at the highest rate within an individual's repertoire. However, selecting the response on these two criteria ignores the extent to which a response occurs with atypical muscle tone (e.g., produced with hypertonus) and with an abnormal pattern of coordination. The most conventional responses or those of the highest rate may also be classified as abnormal in tone or pattern (e.g., Campbell & Wilcox, 1987). An abnormal response that is practiced and functionally used will eventually result in development of additional secondary physical changes (e.g., muscle length, joint mobility). An abnormal response is selected for use when it is the response produced at the highest rate but is shaped into a more normally organized pattern once the pattern is functionally used in self-directed situations (e.g., Campbell, 1987b).

Training Cognitive Abilities—Use of Functional Movement

Movement patterns are combined with self-directed cognitive skills and used to solve environmental problems, such as bringing a spoon to the mouth, moving from one location to another to obtain a particular object or to participate in an activity, or performing work. Functional movement can be trained under the following conditions if: 1) a response that occurs at a reasonable rate can be identified; 2) objects, activities, or people that are potentially reinforcing can be located; and 3) state levels indicate engagement for some portion of time, during which instruction or therapeutic procedures can be implemented (e.g., Campbell, 1987b; Campbell & Bricker, 1980).

Initial programming efforts are designed to enable the individual to build sufficient abilities in each of these areas before combining them in an effort to train movement that could be functionally used. Later, programming is directed toward all areas, simultaneously, and within the context of age-appropriate routines. For example, emphasis can be directed toward increasing the level of state awareness (as described above) while simultaneously strengthening functional use of the selected response mode during alert or engaged states (Wilcox & Campbell, in press-b). The most critical factor in establishing functionally used movement patterns is identifying the potential reinforcing objects, activities, or people (Campbell, 1987d).

Procedures that are used for determining the individual's possible reinforcers range from observing his or her behavior during programming to using specifically designed procedures, such as two-choice discrimination protocols (Bricker & Campbell, 1982). Baumgart et al. (1982) have suggested "partial participation" as a means for incorporating students with profound handicaps into age-appropriate routines. These researchers usually have little regard for reinforcers or motivating situations and assume that what is age-appropriate for the individual will be reinforcing. Individuals with profound limitations in behavior, while not able to participate in each aspect of a task, learn functional use of movement through partial participation in one or more carefully selected steps of a particular task.

More specifically designed programming uses behavioral principles that are embedded in group instruction within age-appropriate (and functional) routines (e.g., Campbell et al., 1984; Cooper, 1985). These strategies that are used to develop functional use of movement while synthesizing cognitive and motor abilities have been described in detail by Campbell and Bricker (1980), and by Campbell (1983, 1987b, 1987d). These strategies are briefly summarized in Table 7.1.

MOTOR EXPRESSION IN COMMUNICATION

Most individuals with profound disabilities have some form of communication, however primitive or nonintentional. Parents or caregivers may be able to read communication cues more easily than other adults, especially if cues are nonconventional, as is likely to be the case (Wilcox & Campbell, in press-a; in press-b). Typically used cues include: postural adjustment; head/neck movement; upper extremity movement; eye movement (in individuals without severe visual impairment); and vocalization that may be pleasurable or distressful. These cues are often missed by caregivers and, if identified as communication cues, may be interpreted with different meanings and, therefore, responded to in different ways. For example, a vocalization made by an individual may be

Table 7.1. Strategies for developing functional uses of posture and movement skills

Level	Representation	Strategies
Basic movement pattern	S → R	Strengthen existing posture or movement pattern through consistent reinforcer
		Parameters: 1) Existing pattern at reasonable rate 2) Known reinforcer
Differentiated use	S → (M) → R	Strengthen use of two different patterns through differential use of reinforcement
Functional use	S → (M) → R → S → R	Chain two or more differentiated patterns to solve environmental problems

S = stimulus.
R = response.
M = medication.

interpreted by one caregiver as indicating "more" and by another as indicating the desire to stop an activity (Campbell & Wilcox, 1987).

Preventing Secondary Communication Handicaps

Severe communication disabilities are preventable through early and clear identification of communicatively used behavior, consistent response to that behavior, and systematic programming to increase the complexity of functionally used communication (Wilcox, in press). Effective programming depends upon the competence and consistency of the caregivers who interact with an individual. When caregivers recognize the communicative aspects of a behavior and then respond to that behavior as if it had the same meaning, it comes to communicate that meaning.

Identifying Communicative Behavior Most individuals with profound disabilities are not likely to demonstrate intentional and recognizable use of communication (e.g., speech or sign). Communication cues are likely to take the form of posture and movement since these skills are within the individual's repertoire. Posture and movement, used for communication, reflects atypical muscle tone, patterns of coordinated movement, and any secondary physical changes, as well as any concomitant disabilities (e.g., vision or hearing loss) that may also be present. Figure 7.2 illustrates two communication cues for a 4-year-old child with low muscle tone and severely uncoordinated patterns of movement. Both cues reflect the atypical muscle tone and severely uncoordinated patterns of movement that characterize this child's posture and movement abilities.

Identification of the communication cues of an individual with profound handicaps is a three phase process that is best accomplished with videotaped samples of that person's behavior (Campbell & Wilcox, 1987). Live observation of an individual can be conducted; however, the videotaped sample allows for observation of subtle and unconventional cues that are not as easily observed while they are occurring. Procedures include: 1) obtaining samples of behavior during a variety of activities; 2) synthesizing a 5-minute sample of tape that reflects episodes identified as "most communicative" by caregivers who are familiar with the individual; and 3) establishing an individual viewing of the 5-minute sample by each of the persons with whom the individual has regular contact, including teachers, therapists, parents, or other caregivers (e.g., Campbell & Wilcox, 1987; Wilcox, in press). Communicative analysis procedures are based upon the perceptions of the adults who view the videotape. Each caregiver identifies: 1) the point at which communication occurs, 2) the specific forms of behavior viewed as communicative (e.g., postural adjustment, eye movement), and 3) the meaning given to the behavior by the various adults (e.g., wants more, is unhappy). This information is synthesized with the assistance of the persons who are involved to identify areas of agreement on occurrence, behavior type, and meaning. Those areas in which agreement

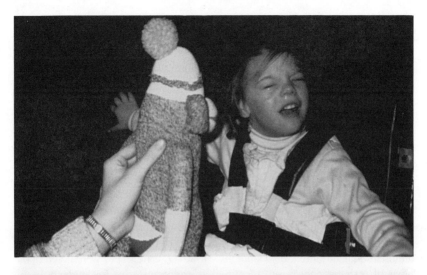

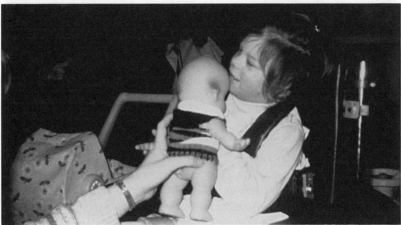

Figure 7.2. Top: A response of postural adjustment and head/arm orientation away from an object or person communicates displeasure, disinterest, and general lack of engagement in an activity, object, or person. Bottom: The opposite orientation toward an object or person communicates interest and availability for interaction.

occurs concerning behavior types and meaning become the focus of communication training for the child's caregivers. Similarly, where limited agreement occurs, the caregivers agree on particular behavior types/meanings and respond consistently to strengthen functional use of the identified behavior-meaning cues.

Obtaining caregiver agreement and consistency on communicative cues is frequently the most difficult aspect of this type of assessment programming. Campbell and Wilcox (1987) used the identification procedure described above to identify communication cues in a group of seven school-age students with profound multiple handicaps who ranged in age from 6 to 10 years of age. Teachers and therapists who worked with these students identified four students as being totally without understandable communication, and three as having some form of communication that was frequently not understandable by the caregivers. Few differences were noted in frequency of communication for students in each group. Analysis of the 5-minute composite videotape samples yielded an average of 39 communication acts for those students identified as preintentional and 41.33 communication acts for students who were intentional. More than 80% of the identified acts were classified as responses by the caregivers; however, independent ratings of student behavior indicated that some attempts to initiate communication were virtually missed by the majority of the observing caregivers. A higher percentage of communication acts were identified by caregivers for the students who were preintentional; the mother was found to be able to identify the highest number of communication acts for both preintentional and intentional students. However, differences were noted in the types of responses that were identified as communicative for students in the intentional and preintentional groups. Vocalization was the most common behavior identified as communicative for preintentional students; contradictorily, upper extremity and eye movements were the most frequently identified responses for students in the intentional group. Whereas the caregivers agreed that communication acts had occurred 77% of the time, they agreed only 67% of the time on the type of behavior demonstrated by a student. Agreements on the meaning of the communication occurred in only 52% of the episodes. Both the type of behavior and its meaning were similarly identified in only 46% of all communication acts.

Lack of agreement among caregivers on the amount of communication that occurred, the type of behavior that was demonstrated, and the meaning that was conveyed has significant implications for communicative competence of individuals with profound disabilities. Communication cues that go unrecognized or, more importantly, that are inconsistently identified by different caregivers will not be acknowledged systematically enough for the behavior to be strengthened. However, inconsistent recognition, when accompanied by differing interpretations of the meaning being conveyed, is likely to become even more confusing for the child. Such interactions are likely to result in weakening of the behavior as well as potential extinction of communication attempts.

Establishing Essential Communication   Even communication that is nonvocal and nonintentional can convey specific, essential meanings such as engagement, pleasure, displeasure, or discomfort. State levels of individuals interact with initial communication in many ways. For example, an individual who is nonengaged or not in a maximal state of alertness is displaying communication cues of nonavailability for interaction (or instruction). Other general meanings, such as requesting, may also be conveyed by individuals whose communication remains nonintentional and nonsymbolic. The communicative meaning of a particular behavior form must be responded to systematically in order for the individual to realize that his or her responses communicate messages to other individuals. Effective training strategies are those that are focused on the caregivers who interact with the individuals with disabilities. These strategies direct the caregivers' attention to the occurrence of a particular type of behavior, and train them to respond to these occurrences consistently in terms of meaning (Wilcox, in press). Training strategies also encourage the caregivers to recognize a type of behavior and its meaning in self-initiated and response situations; thus, these strategies provide individuals with increased opportunities for strengthening the communicative function of various behavior types.

Various behavior types are less well-used in some environments than in others. For example, a behavior of upper extremity movement in an upward direction (e.g., hand raising) can be used to attract adult attention by a student in a classroom or work setting. However, this same behavior type might not be effective at home where the same student might not be in visual range of his or her caregiver. A compromise of pairing vocalization with upper extremity movement provides a consistent response that will work equally well in both classroom and home situations. Behavior types and their meaning, used for communication, are selected by parents or team members, as a whole, on the basis of the videotaped samples of current communicative competences. Existing types of behavior that are not functional in a variety of situations can be strengthened through systematic reinforcement and paired with other forms of behavior to increase usefulness. Thus, if the student described above were only able to vocalize to attract attention, parents and all team members would respond to the communicative meaning (i.e., need attention) of the vocalization while training the student to simultaneously use upper extremity movement.

Potentially abnormal characteristics of a communicative behavior type are considered when developing the use of functional communication. Responses that are characterized by abnormal muscle tone, patterns, or coordination and are reinforced through systematic responses from the caregivers will be strengthened. This would create a situation where individuals may simultaneously acquire functional communication skills and secondary physical deformities. The often severely restricted posture and movement repertoire in individuals with profound disabilities may necessitate use of abnormal responses for communicative purposes, requiring similar strategies to counteract development of secondary physical disabilities, as were earlier described in terms of programming for functionally used movement.

Establishing Symbolic Communication Individuals with the most profound handicaps may never acquire fully symbolic communication. A great deal of nonverbal and communicative meaning is conveyed without use of symbols, although they allow greater expression of thoughts, ideas, and feelings. Words are the primary symbols used for communication by most individuals. Pictures or objects, symbol systems such as Bliss or Pictographs, gesture systems, and sign language are alternate means for symbolic expression. The use of one or more of these alternatives to speech is selected on the basis of competence in posture and movement abilities in combination with consideration of the individual's other disabilities that may be present. An individual with severely limited posture and movement abilities, in combination with visual impairment, would be an unlikely candidate for sign language or visual symbol systems; however, an individual with reasonable manipulation abilities and well-coordinated movement of the upper extremities might be taught simple signs.

Symbolic expression is based upon the extent to which an individual is alert and "available for interaction" as well as whether he or she has developed an understanding of the communicative process as a way for interacting with others. Programming for individuals with profound handicaps has often been initiated with symbolic expression of very complex ideas (e.g., yes and no). Expression of these ideas may meet immediate demands of parents and other caregivers but may not match the current competency levels of an individual with profound disabilities. As a result, the individual may ignore existing nonsymbolic communication. Those nonsymbolic (and potentially, nonintentional) behavior-meaning types, that are consistently used by an individual in ways that appear to be intentionally self-directed, can be represented by symbols that are paired with existing behavior. The posture and movement cues subsequently can be faded, leaving the symbolic expression of a meaning already in the individual's repertoire (e.g., Reichle & Keogh, 1986).

ARRANGING AND ORGANIZING
SERVICES FOR EFFECTIVE PROGRAMMING

Above all, programming for individuals with profound disabilities must integrate the expertise of a wide variety of professionals in an effort to prevent the development of secondary handicaps through compensation for disorders in posture and movement and in other biological systems, such as vision and hearing. The various medical, educational, therapeutic, social, and vocational services that may be required to meet the needs of individuals with profound disabilities must be organized and coordinated using programming that focuses on the underlying commonality among services. For example, discontinued and poorly organized services for an individual may result when physical and occupational therapists approach programming from a remedial perspective and educators focus on enabling that person to gain the independence needed through the use of compensatory approaches (Wetherbee, Campbell, & Garner, 1987).

Coordinated services are more difficult to arrange for individuals with profound disabilities than for those with less complicated needs. The team of professionals involved in providing services are not likely to be employed by the same agency or program due to the diverse and extensive needs of many individuals. Therefore, a team approach to service delivery is harder to develop and coordinate with an interagency team than when all caregivers are employed within the same agency. Interagency team structures are required, in particular, for older students and adults, who may be living and receiving programming in community-based facilities (e.g., group homes), performing work, or attending school or other programs provided through multiple agencies. Those individuals with special health care needs may receive additional and often essential medical services through hospitals, multiple physicians, or other health providers, requiring coordination with yet other agencies.

Processes for coordination of different professional disciplines vary within agency structures. Some agencies use a consultant or transdisciplinary model for coordinating education and related services, while others may use a multidisciplinary approach. Each agency may function under a different set of standards and guidelines. Translation of these standards into assessment procedures, individual program planning, and monitoring may result in differences that hinder interagency coordination.

Use of an integrated programming approach provides one mechanism through which agency differences can be accommodated (Campbell, 1987a). In this approach, one caregiver is designated as the team leader. He or she is responsible for coordinating and overseeing programming that is to be provided for a student (or group of students). This team leader is typically the student's teacher or case manager; however, another professional, such as a therapist, may also function as a team leader. Team members agree on the type of programming approaches that will be used with infants, school-age students, and adults. By operating under the principles of this jointly developed programming philosophy, difficulties are avoided that can occur when various professionals (or agencies) approach programming from widely varying perspectives. The team leader is the key person responsible for instituting communication between school and home, for providing information about other community resources for families, and for ensuring that child and family needs are met through appropriate school and community services.

Other approaches employ professionals whose specific roles are to ensure that the management of services are coordinated. Case management is often used to run the multiple agencies with which adults may be involved. A transition coordinator or specialist is an individual who coordinates services for students in transition from one service system to another, such as from high school to work (Wehman, Moon, Everson, Wood, & Barcus, 1988) or from infant to preschool programming. The central difference between a team leader in an integrated programming model and case management or transition services is the extent to which a professional performs an exclusive coordination role or assumes this responsibility in addition to other job functions. The important point is that one professional must be designated to assist families of individuals with profound handicaps to access, obtain, and coordinate the diverse services that may be required to enhance overall functioning of the family member with the disability. Families of individuals with profound disabilities also require services that are not specifically directed toward the individual with disabilities but that support a family in the care of that individual. Such services may include respite care, advocacy, information, family support groups, income support, parent training, counseling, or medical services (Salisbury & Intagliata, 1986; Vohs, 1987).

SUMMARY

Secondary physical changes in muscles, joints, and bones are of primary importance for an individual with posture and movement skill disorders. Successful prevention of these changes can occur only when families, caregivers, and professionals collaborate to manage the physical needs of an individual with profound disabilities. Restricted posture and movement abilities negatively influence an individual's opportunities to be independent in skill areas that are dependent on functional use of movement. These restrictions establish a basis for learned helplessness and secondary disabilities in cognition and communication. Impaired cognition and communication cannot be fully prevented in all cases. However, the effect of an impairment in these areas can be alleviated if programming is integrated, systematic, and carried out by all persons who interact with an individual with profound disabilities and across all environmental situations.

REFERENCES

Als, H. (1979). Social interaction: Dynamic matrix for developing behavioral organization. In T.C. Uzgiris (Ed.), *Social interaction and communication in infancy: New directions for child development.* (Vol. 4, pp. 21–41). San Francisco: Jossey-Bass.

Baumgart, D., Brown, L., Pumpian, I., Nisbet, N., Ford, A., Sweet, M., Messina, R., & Schroeder, J. (1982). Principle of partial participation and individualized adaptations in educational programs for severely handicapped students. *Journal of The Association for the Severely Handicapped, 7*(2), 17–27.

Bergen, A.F., & Colangelo, C. (1982). *Posititioning the client with central nervous system deficits: The wheelchair and other adapted equipment.* Valhalla, NY: Valhalla Rehabilitation Publications, Ltd.

Bower, T.G.R. (1982). *Development in infancy.* San Francisco: W.H. Freeman.

Brazelton, T.B. (1961). Psychophysiologic reactions in the neonate, No. 1: Value of observation of the newborn. *Journal of Pediatrics, 58,* 508–512.

Brazelton, T.B., & Als, H. (1979). Four early stages in the development of mother-infant interaction. *The Psychoanalytic Study of the Child, 34,* 349–369.

Bricker, W.A., & Campbell, P.H. (1980). Interdisciplinary assessment and programming for multihandicapped students. In W. Sailor, B. Wilcox, & L. Brown (Eds.), *Methods of instruction for severely handicapped students* (pp. 3–45). Baltimore: Paul H. Brookes Publishing Co.

Bricker, W.A., & Campbell, P.H. (1982). *Individual education planning.* Akron: Children's Hospital Medical Center of Akron.

Campbell, P.H. (1983). Basic considerations in programming for students with movement difficulties. In M. Snell (Ed.), *Systematic instruction of the moderately and severely handicapped* (pp. 168–202). Columbus, OH: Charles E. Merrill.

Campbell, P.H. (1985). *Applications guide for the TA-2 training aid.* Wooster, OH: Prentke-Romich Co.

Campbell, P.H. (1986). *Introduction to neurodevelopmental treatment* (rev. ed.). Akron: Children's Hospital Medical Center of Akron.

Campbell, P.H. (1987a). The integrated programming team: An approach for coordinating professionals of various disciplines in programs for students with severe and multiple handicaps. *Journal of The Association for Persons with Severe Handicaps,* *12*(2), 107–116.

Campbell, P.H. (1987b). Integrated programming for students with multiple handicaps. In L. Goetz, D. Guess, and K. Stremel-Campbell (Eds.), *Innovative program design for individuals with dual sensory impairments* (pp. 159–188). Baltimore: Paul H. Brookes Publishing Co.

Campbell, P.H. (1987c). Physical management and handling procedures with students with movement dysfunction. In M. Snell (Ed.), *Systematic instruction of students with moderate and severe handicaps* (3rd ed., pp. 174–187). Columbus, OH: Charles E. Merrill.

Campbell, P.H. (1987d). Programming for students with dysfunction in posture and movement. In M. Snell (Ed.), *Systematic instruction of students with moderate and severe handicaps* (3rd ed., pp. 188–211). Columbus, OH: Charles E. Merrill.

Campbell, P.H. (in press). Service delivery approaches. In M.J. Wilcox & P.H. Campbell (Eds.), *Communication programming from birth to three: A handbook for public school professionals.* San Diego: College-Hill Press.

Campbell, P., & Bricker, W. (1980). Programming for the severely/profoundly handicapped person. In J.F. Gardner, L. Long, R. Nichols, & D. M. Iagulli (Eds.), *Program issues in developmental disabilities: A resource manual for surveyors and reviewers* (pp. 127–153). Baltimore: Paul H. Brookes Publishing Co.

Campbell, P.H., Cooper, M.A., & McInerney, W.F. (1984). Therapeutic programming for students with severe handicaps. *American Journal of Occupational Therapy,* *38*(9), 594–602.

Campbell, P.H., & Wilcox, M.J. (1987). *Identifying communication cues in students with severe and profound disabilities.* Manuscript submitted for publication.

Campbell, S. (1984). *Pediatric neurologic physical therapy* (Vol. 5). New York: Churchill Livingstone.

Cooper, M.A. (1985). *The impact of individual and group instructional arrangement on skill acquisition by students with severe multiple handicaps.* Unpublished doctoral dissertation, Kent State University, Ohio.

Dunst, C.J. (1981). *Infant learning: A cognitive-linguistic intervention strategy.* Hingham, MA: Teaching Resources.

Durand, V.M., & Kishi, G. (1987). Reducing severe behavior problems among persons with dual sensory impairments: An evaluation of a technical assistance model. *The Journal of The Association for Persons with Severe Handicaps,* *12*(1), 2–10.

Esposito, L.C., & Campbell, P.H. (1986). Computers and the severely and physically handicapped. In J. Lindsey (Ed.), *Computers and exceptional individuals* (pp. 105–124). Columbus, OH: Charles E. Merrill.

Fraser, B.A., Hensinger, R.N., & Phelps, J.A. (1987). *Physical management of multiple handicaps: A professional's guide*. Baltimore: Paul H. Brookes Publishing Co.

Garner, J.B., & Campbell, P.H. (1987). Technology for persons with severe disabilities: Practical and ethical considerations. *Journal of Special Education, 21*(3), 122–132.

Guess, D., Mulligan-Ault, M., Roberts, S., Struth, J., Siegel-Causey, E., Thompson, B., Bronicki, G.J., & Guy, B. (in press). *Implications of biobehavioral states for the education and treatment of students with the most profoundly handicapping conditions*. Manuscript submitted for publication.

Hanson, M.J., & Harris, S. (1986). *Teaching your children with motor delays*. Rockville, MD: Aspen Systems.

Kopp, C.B. (1979). Perspectives on infant motor system development. In M.H. Bornstein & W. Kessen (Eds.), *Psychological development from infancy: Image to intention* (pp.9–35). Hillsdale, NJ: Lawrence Erlbaum Associates.

Landesman-Dwyer, S., & Sackett, G.P. (1978). Behavioral changes in nonambulatory, profoundly mentally retarded individuals. In C.E. Meyers (Ed.), *Quality of life in severely and profoundly mentally retarded people: Research foundations for improvement* (pp. 55–144, monograph of the AAMD, No. 3). Washington, DC: American Association on Mental Deficiency.

Perske, R., Clifton, A., McLean, B.M., & Stein, J.I. (1986). *Mealtimes for persons with severe handicaps*. Baltimore: Paul H. Brookes Publishing Co.

Piaget, J. (1952). *The origins of intelligence in children*. New York: International Universities Press.

Reichle, J., & Keogh, W.J. (1986). Communication instruction for learners with severe handicaps: Some unresolved issues. In R.H. Horner, L.H. Meyer, & H.D.B. Fredericks (Eds.), *Education for learners with severe handicaps: Exemplary service strategies* (pp. 189–219). Baltimore: Paul H. Brookes Publishing Co.

Robinson, C.C., & Robinson, J.H. (1983). Sensorimotor functions and cognitive development. In M. Snell (Ed.), *Systematic instruction of the moderately and severely handicapped* (3rd ed., pp. 227–266). Columbus, OH: Charles E. Merrill.

Sailor, W., & Guess, D. (1983). Severely handicapped preschoolers. *Topics in Early Childhood Special Education, 4*(3), 47–72.

Salisbury, C.L., & Intagliata, J. (1986). *Respite care: Support for persons with developmental disabilities and their families*. Baltimore: Paul H. Brookes Publishing Co.

Scherzer, A., & Tscharnuter, I. (1982). *Early diagnosis and therapy in cerebral palsy*. New York: Marcel Decker.

Seligman, M.E. (1975). *Helplessness: On depression, death and development*. San Francisco: W.H. Freeman.

Smith, M.M. (1984). Sensory-motor facilitation based on the postural reflex mechanism. *Selected proceedings from Barbro Salek Memorial Symposium* (pp. 75–80). Oak Park, IL: Neuro-Developmental Treatment Association, Inc.

Snell, M. (1987). *Systematic instruction of students with moderate and severe handicaps* (3rd ed.). Columbus, OH: Charles E. Merrill.

Staller, J. (1984). An approach to adaptive seating. *Selected Proceedings from Barbro Salek Memorial Symposium* (pp. 223–234). Oak Park, IL: Neuro-Developmental Treatment Association, Inc.

Trefler, E., Tooms, R.E., & Hobson, D.A. (1985). *Seating for cerebral palsied children*. Unpublished manuscript, University of Tennessee Center for Health Science, Rehabilitation Engineering Center, Memphis, TN.

Vohs, J. (1987). *A parent perspective on case management services.* Paper presented at the Surgeon General's Conference on Family-Centered, Comprehensive, Coordinated, Community-based Care for Children with Special Health Care Needs, Houston, TX.

Wehman, P., Moon, M.S., Everson, J.M., Wood, W., & Barcus, J.M. (1988). *Transition from school to work: New challenges for youth with severe disabilities.* Baltimore: Paul H. Brookes Publishing Co.

Wetherbee, R., Campbell, P.H., & Garner, B. (1987). *An analysis for the IEPs of students with physical handicaps.* Manuscript submitted for publication.

Wilcox, M.J., & Campbell, P.H. (in press-a). *Communication programming from birth to three: A handbook for public school professionals.* San Diego: College-Hill Press.

Wilcox, M.J., & Campbell, P.H. (in press-b). Facilitating the emergence of socio-communicative skills. In M.J. Wilcox & P.H. Campbell (Eds.), *Communication programming from birth to three: A handbook for public school professionals.* San Diego: College-Hill Press.

Wilcox, M.J. (in press). Communication and language in infants and toddlers. In M.J. Wilcox & P.H. Campbell (Eds.), *Communication programming from birth to three: A handbook for public school professionals.* San Diego: College-Hill Press.

Wilson, J. (1984). Cerebral palsy. In S. Campbell (Ed.), *Pediatric neurologic physical therapy* (pp. 353–413). New York: Churchill Livingstone.

York, J., Nietupski, J., & Hamre-Nietupski, S. (1985). A decision-making process for using microswitches. *Journal of The Association for Persons with Severe Handicaps, 10*(4), 214–223.

York, J., & Rainforth, B. (1986). *The role of related services in community-referenced instruction.* Manuscript submitted for publication.

York, J., & Rainforth, B. (1987). Developing instructional adaptations. In F.P. Orelove & D. Sobsey, *Educating children with multiple disabilities: A transdisciplinary approach* (pp. 183–217). Baltimore: Paul H. Brookes Publishing Co.

INFLUENCE OF INDICATING PREFERENCES FOR INITIATING, MAINTAINING, AND TERMINATING INTERACTIONS

Joe Reichle, Jennifer York, and Diane Eynon

Keogh and Reichle (1985) describe the population of persons with profound disabilities best as being learners who are "difficult to teach." Difficult-to-teach learners, unlike many persons with severe handicaps, fail to acquire or experience extreme difficulty in acquiring new repertoires in spite of the extensive application of state of the art instructional technology. Among the population described as difficult-to-teach is a small but readily identifiable group of learners who are considered to be passive participants in the educational process. Some passive participants may possess all of the motor competencies required to participate in most activities, but fail to learn because they allow teachers and parents to "put them through" educational tasks and seldom participate actively. Others have such limited movement repertoires or impaired sensory abilities that they are perceived as being uninterested or incapable of interacting with other individuals. Typically, teachers describe passive participants as learners for whom they cannot readily identify likes and dislikes. Additionally, teachers often report that passive participants lack the motivation to learn. Furthermore, they show little interest in interacting with their environment.

Preparation of this work was supported in part by Contract No. 300–82–0363 awarded to the University of Minnesota from the Division of Innovation and Development, Special Education Programs, United States Department of Education. The opinions expressed herein do not necessarily reflect the position or policy of the United States Department of Education, and no official endorsement should be inferred.

191

Watson, 1978; Watson & Ramey, 1969). Perhaps the greatest challenge faced by an interventionist who works with an individual who appears to be passive is in selecting an environmental event that is valued sufficiently by the learner to motivate him or her to acquire an obtaining response.

One strategy used to maximize the available items that might be interesting to learners is to engage him or her in a regular routine of reinforcer sampling. In reinforcer sampling, the learner is exposed systematically to a variety of new objects or events. Some learners may have few reinforcers since the same objects and events are present daily. Often, parents of nondisabled children engage their learners in reinforcer sampling unknowingly. Visits to the toy store to browse, watching toy commercials on television, and playing with novel toys from a neighbor's house all constitute forms of reinforcer sampling. Unfortunately, some of these natural opportunities to sample reinforcers are not made available to persons with severe handicaps. For many learners, watching television may not be a sufficiently direct experience to allow the level of exposure required to determine interest. In other instances, the learner may have relatively few opportunities to sample play environments outside his or her home.

Sometimes learners appear to be somewhat difficult to coax into sampling reinforcers. It may require numerous exposures before a learner shows interest in a new event. It is reasonable to expect that preferences are not established until a history of interaction and experience with a selected item has occurred. Furthermore, until the learner experiences the object or event, it will be impossible to make a judgment regarding his or her preference. An active program of reinforcer sampling requires that the interventionist build into the daily routine numerous opportunities for the learner to be exposed to the items that are being sampled. In the case of learners who are passive, exposure may mean the delivery of fairly intrusive physical guidance in assisting him or her to sample. With learners who appear to be the most passive, reinforcer sampling, interspersed with reinforcer preference probes, are an important use of instructional time. One final consideration is that although a history of experience with a particular item is necessary, it is also important for the interventionist to consistently bring new items into the learner's array to maintain attentiveness and to avoid satiation.

In spite of all of the positive strategies described above, the learner's initial emission of preference responses may seem minimal and inconsistent. If this is the case, the interventionist needs to become more creative in discerning learner preferences while at the same time attempting to identify a voluntary behavior that can be easily executed by the individual or, in some instances, a behavior that has the greatest probability of maintenance after successive prompting. (This is discussed in greater detail in the next section of this chapter.) Another difficulty is found in verifying that a learner actually enjoyed the delivery of a potential reinforcer. Frequently, preferences are observable only in contrast to other behaviors emitted within a similar time frame. For example, some learners may swallow more readily preferred foods than nonpreferred ones. When offered peaches, the learner may open his or her mouth readily, chew quickly and swallow without hesitation. When offered vegetables, the same individual may not open his or her mouth immediately and may allow the food to linger and dribble from the corner of the mouth. Lipsitt (1978) reported an examination of normal infant sucking behavior during feeding episodes. When a sucrose solution was injected into the infants' water, they engaged in more deliberate sucking with shorter rest periods; however, when saline solution was injected into their water, sucking slowed down.

In order to lessen the communicative demand on the learner's partner, it is important that, at some point, more conventional indicating responses be acquired by the learner to obtain his or her desired objects. That is, simply being able to differentiate the learner preferences based upon his or her rate of food intake after the fact does little to actively communicate needs and desires in a timely fashion. Eventually, the learner must come to emit his or her indication of preference prior to the arrival of the reinforcer.

Making Choices among Preferred Items

Some learners who have very severe handicaps may not realize that they can use their own behavior to obtain an object or event of interest without systematic and intense instruction. For example, reaching to obtain a desired object has been described by Piagetian scholars as an exemplar of early means-end competence (Uzgiris & Hunt, 1975). If this is the case, a determination is made as to whether a volitional selecting response should be taught. Chapman and Miller (1980) suggested that until about 8 months of age, nonhandicapped infants are unable to engage in goal directed actions or intentional communicative behavior. However, Keogh and Reichle (1985) pointed out that prior to 8 months of age, infants do exert a significant amount of control over their environment (e.g., most infants cry at birth). Skinner (1957) provided an eloquent description of how a voluntary behavior, such as crying, might come to serve as a social signal. He pointed out that the exact point at which the child's vocalizations become intentional is unclear. However, it does seem clear that the delivery of desirable events contingent on vocal production eventually results in the establishment of a voluntary vocal behavior that can be used to signal preferences. For normal infants, the literature is replete with examples of the influence of reinforcing contingencies on the frequency with which voluntary behavior is emitted (Rheingold, Gewirtz, & Ross, 1959; Weisberg, 1963).

In the realm of motor behavior, Watson (1978) reported a game in which 8-week-old infants could control a crib mobile by putting their head in contact with a pressure transducer. The infants quickly acquired the skill to play the game. More interesting was the observation that the infants' frequency of smiling and cooing also increased significantly, even more than it did for a control group. At ages younger than 2 weeks, investigators have taught contingent head turning responses (Papousek, 1978).

Unfortunately, the voluntary motor behavior available to learners with severe and multiple disabilities may be so limited that it is difficult to observe unless careful and systematic observational procedures are implemented. After extensively observing the learner and interviewing those who are most familiar with him or her, the interventionist seeks a list of discrete voluntary behaviors that are produced by the individual that could be used to approximate self-selecting (e.g., reaching, looking, facial expression, increased body movement, vocalizing). The behavior selected as the target behavior is the one that: 1) is under the most precise voluntary control; 2) is relatively easy to execute, motorically (i.e., does not represent an abnormal reflex or other undesirable topography); and 3) can be physically prompted by the interventionist, if necessary. Next, the interventionist locates specific objects that are potentially reinforcing. Systematically, the interventionist places him- or herself in a position to deliver the object(s) contingent on the emission of a target response.

In addition to the exclusive use of contingent reinforcement, the delivery of a response prompt that ensures the production of the target behavior that serves to signal a preference may enhance intervention efficiency. The use of this strategy requires that the interventionist place the object or event near the learner. Next, the interventionist prompts the emission of the behavior selected as the signaling response. The advantage of this approach is the assurance that an approximation of the target response is emitted. However, the disadvantages are three-fold. First, fading the response prompt may be difficult. Often, learners considered to be passive become very accustomed to allowing others in their environment to do their work for them (Seligman, 1975). Second, the interventionist runs the risk of prompting a simple request signal when, in fact, the learner does not want the available item. Third, if the selected response/signaling mode is vocal or verbal behavior, it may be impossible to find a response prompt that will guarantee the emission of the behavior.

The solution to the first problem is to fade response prompts very quickly even if it means occasionally inducing an incorrect learner response. Another strategy might be to include opportunities for acquisition of the motor behavior at other times during the day. This is highly desirable because movement efficiency requires extensive practice. For example, if elbow flexion is identified as the signaling response, facilitation of arm movement can occur during eating, grooming, and playing activities, as well as to indicate preferences. In the second instance (in which the interventionist may be prompting a request for an undesired item), it may be helpful to frequently sample reinforcers to establish continued interest in the contingent reinforcer. For example, the learner might be offered a very small serving of popcorn (with no response required on his or her part in order to obtain it). If it appeared as though the learner enjoyed the popcorn, an additional quantity may be obtained via the simple signaling response (i.e., an initially prompted response). Finally, in the case of vocal response mode, failing to identify a response prompt may call for the use of an augmentative communication system (e.g., picture, gesture) in addition to a program intervention that leads to the establishment of contingent vocal behavior.

More Sophisticated Ways to Indicate Preference

The act of indicating preference (i.e., making a choice) may or may not involve the emission of a chain of learner responses. For example, if a plate of snack choices is offered to the learner, a simple reaching response in the direction of the desired object is the only one required. However, if a teacher approaches without the plate of snacks and asks if the learner would like one, the learner must signal his or her request and select the item when the plate arrives. In still another instance, the teacher may place a tray of snacks in close proximity, but in a location inaccessible to the learner. In this instance, obtaining the snack would require a chain of behavior in which the individual first obtains his or her listener's attention and then emits a request.

Keogh and Reichle (1985) described an intervention program in which learners are taught initially to extend their hand or arm to reach toward an object that has been established as a reinforcer. Unfortunately, some learners do not have sufficient control of their hand, arm, foot, eye gaze, or other voluntary behavior that can be used to point at a specific desired object or event. In this instance, indicating preference must be handled a bit differently.

For individuals who are unable to select stimuli differentially, a scanning mode of communication is a viable alternative. The simplest application of scanning requires that the learner's speaking partner sample the array of available referents. For example, the interventionist might point to the initial object in an array as he or she asks "Do you want this?" The interventionist then waits a brief period of time for the emission of a voluntary behavior predetermined as the signaling response to be emitted by the learner (i.e., vocalization, eye blink, arm movement). If the learner emits the predetermined voluntary behavior, he or she has communicated selection of a particular referent to his or her listener. If no voluntary response is produced, the interventionist moves to the next object in the array and continues this process until the learner signals that he or she has arrived at the desired object.

In a communication system that relies on scanning, the mere presence of the object is no longer the discriminative stimulus for indicating a preference. Instead, the discriminative stimulus consists of the presence of the desired object among an array of other objects paired with the communicative partner touching the relevant object. In scanning, the learner must refrain from emitting the signaling response until the relevant object is shown by his or her partner. Early in the intervention process, it is important to deliver response prompts that result in the emission of the learner's signaling response immediately after the relevant object is offered. To ensure that the learner's attention is not directed exclusively at the teacher's "scanning finger" (at the sacrifice of attending to the symbol display), it is important that on some occasions the teacher touches his or her finger to other objects in the stimulus array in which the learner might be less interested. During these occasions, the learner should refrain from responding (i.e., responding to the teacher's finger touching an object should occur only when the teacher selects the most desired object).

Generalization Issues in Indicating Preference

One generalization issue to consider during the initial stages of intervention requires a decision about the number and type of items to include in the array. Reichle and Piche-Cragoe (1986) suggested pairing the presentation of a potentially desired object with the presentation of a nonpreferred object to more easily establish the rule that one member of an array is selected during an indicating preference opportunity. Once the learner has a history of selecting a single desired object from a larger array, members that are chosen for the array can be of more equal reinforcement value. Although there are data to support the efficiency of this strategy in teaching learners to select one member of an array without acting on the remaining members, there is some question as to what degree this selection behavior generalizes.

Results of several investigations (Reichle & Piche-Cragoe, 1986; Sigafoos & Reichle, 1987) suggest that for some learners with the most severe handicaps, the ability to choose a preferred from a nonpreferred object does not generalize to making a choice between two preferred items. Learners in these studies attempted to obtain both preferred items or discriminatively selected items that did not correspond to their preceding requests. It appears to be very important to the intervention that as soon as the learner reliably chooses a preferred object over a nonpreferred object that the array should quickly begin to introduce choices among the more preferred items.

Alternatively, it might be more fruitful to begin indicating preference selections using two highly preferred objects and to be committed to the use of more intrusive response prompts during the initial phase of the intervention program. The generalization problems described by Reichle and Piche-Cragoe (1986) elicit interest in whether learners who have been taught to indicate preferences among preferred items generalize this skill to indicating preferences among less preferred items (e.g., choosing between corn or spinach when neither is particularly preferred). It is possible that indicating preferences encompasses several different response classes depending on the reinforcement value of items in the stimulus array and that training "sufficient exemplars" (Stokes & Baer, 1977) across a wide variety of these arrays is a necessary intervention strategy. Thus far, the authors' discussion has focused on the establishment of selecting reinforcers as a method of indicating preferences. However, preferences may also be indicated by refusal to accept offered objects or events or by signaling a desire to leave or exit events (i.e., leavetake) in which one has become satiated.

Indicating Dislikes

Rejecting objects or events that are disliked can be conceptualized as the result of a negative reinforcement paradigm (i.e., the learner produces a generalized rejecting signal in order to escape or avoid undesired objects or events).

Just as the establishment of choosing desired objects from an array begins with the establishment of reinforcer preferences, indicating dislikes begins with the establishment of objects or events that the learner dislikes or objects or events for which he or she becomes either satiated or habituated quickly. The initial step requires caregivers to formulate a list of objects and events for which the learner has demonstrated a dislike or reluctance to participation. Included in this list should be a description of any behaviors emitted that suggest that the learner is disinterested in the identified objects or events.

Identifying dislikes for a passive learner may require subtle observational skills. For example, a learner's desire to end his or her mealtime may be indicated via an increasingly slower rate of food intake accompanied by more spillage. In other instances, a learner's dislike for a particular item may surface only when a desired object is clearly available but a nonpreferred item is offered. For example, the learner may usually accept spoonfuls of peas; however, when peas are offered in the presence of pudding, avoidance behavior related to the peas is emitted. Task variables that typically influence the probability of rejecting or leavetaking attempts involve the length of an activity; the difficulty of an activity; or the quantity of consumption, if food is involved. Once episodes or items are identified that provoke attempts to reject or leavetake, an effort can be made to select stimulus events to use during intervention as well as a form of behavior to be used as a rejection signal.

Members of the learner's instructional team select stimulus items or events that they would be willing to allow the learner to use to escape or avoid a situation if he or she produced a consistently observable rejecting response. This can be a difficult task since the learner may exhibit dislikes or desire to leave activities in which he or she must participate. For example, a learner who experiences extreme difficulty eating may prefer not to participate in mealtimes. Obviously, this cannot be allowed; however, breaks within the meal may be desirable to the learner and acceptable to the caregivers. The learner's instructional team must identify items or events for which a rejecting response is acceptable and can be consistently reinforced. In addition, items or events that may be rejected under certain conditions can be identified. For example, after participating in an activity for a specified period of time or after producing a specified quantity, a rejecting response could be honored.

Because rejecting responses may not be readily generalized, the interventionist should select initial intervention targets across a variety of objects and activities. Additionally, the interventionist should consider selecting teaching instances that comprise a full range of existing behaviors that may be used by the learner to display his or her dislikes. For example, during some instances a learner might turn his or her head away from an offered object but, during other episodes of rejecting different items, might whine. Unless teaching instances include the learner's range of existing response forms, the generalized effects of the program may be minimized.

Having identified potential items for a generalized rejecting response program, the interventionist implements opportunities for the learner to access the targeted objects and events. Systematically, the interventionist observes the learner's behavior for evidence of his or her dislikes just as the reinforcer preference sampling stage was observed for evidence of enjoyment. Specifically, the types of behavior emitted to indicate dislike are identified. After the initial implementation, an acceptable topography of motor behavior that will communicate a generalized rejecting response is selected. Obviously, selecting a behavior that is currently in the learner's repertoire, and strengthening it, is easier than selecting a brand new topography. Several considerations are addressed in making this decision.

First, the interventionist must determine whether the behavior under consideration for use as a generalized rejecting response is socially acceptable. For example, pushing offered objects out of the hands of the person making the offer and onto the floor or sticking out one's tongue represent socially unacceptable response forms. Second, the interventionist must determine whether the behavior is apt to be produced by the learner consistently to indicate rejection (i.e., Are there other competing behaviors used by the learner? This will be particularly important if competing behaviors are excess behaviors that must be targeted for deceleration). Third, for individuals with neuromotor difficulties, the behavior should be an efficient motor response that does not reinforce deleterious movement patterns. Finally, any existing behavior used to mark rejection must be readily understood in the community. For example, gazing at the floor may be used to signal rejection. Unfortunately, only those individuals who are familiar with the learner or who have been provided with a dictionary with entries that correspond to the learner's gestures will be in a position to understand his or her communicative attempts.

Obviously, the conditions that we have just described will be difficult to meet. Typically, when teaching rejecting responses, the learner is confronted with only one potentially undesirable object rather than an array. Consequently, initial rejection intervention need not address choicemaking directly.

Implementing Generalized Rejection

Once the topography to be used by the learner as a rejecting response is chosen and specific naturally occurring opportunities for training have been selected, intervention may proceed. In the case of the learner producing a rejecting response to avoid the offer of an undesired object, the interventionist approaches the learner with the object in question. As soon as the offer of the object is made, the interventionist prompts the learner to produce the targeted rejecting response behavior. Immediately after the delivery of the response prompt, the undesired object is withdrawn. With consecutive teaching opportunities, the level of prompt delivered to the learner is reduced systematically.

Unlike implementation in the generalized requesting response program, the interventionist must consider more carefully the maximum number of teaching opportunities that can be introduced on a given day. Care must be taken to ensure that the learner's day is sufficiently positive to accommodate approaches by interventionists who are bearing objects and events that the learner does not enjoy (i.e., the learner must avoid equating the presence of the interventionist with the occurrence of undesired events).

Generalization Issues in Teaching Generalized Rejection

The situations that serve to prompt a learner to emit a signal indicating that he or she wishes to escape or avoid contact with presented persons or objects differ greatly. For some events, a child's rejection may be based upon seeing a particular object (e.g., medicine bottle) regardless of presented circumstances or objects. For other events, a child's escape or avoidance response may be based upon the length of exposure to the provoking event. For example, a learner may readily approach and engage in a work activity. As the activity continues, the learner begins to habituate. Eventually, the learner is provoked sufficiently to emit a generalized leavetaking response. Finally, some events that set the occasion for a generalized rejecting response signal may involve items that under most circumstances serve as reinforcers. For example, while dining at a restaurant, a waitress repeatedly offers refills of coffee. At some point, the learner becomes satiated and emits a generalized rejecting response (i.e. no thanks) in the presence of usually reinforcing coffee.

Because the characteristics in the preceding tasks differ greatly with respect to the conditions of reinforcement for each of the provoking events, it is reasonable to assume that the use of a generalized leavetake, exit, or rejecting response may not generalize across exemplars of each of the three types. Consequently, the authors believe that if the intent of the interventionist is to establish completely generalized use of a symbol, then the professional must incorporate teaching instances for each of the preceding types of functions.

Requesting and Rejecting: Which to Teach First

Both requesting and rejecting responses are viable initial intervention targets. If the topography selected to signal requesting and rejecting responses are different, learners may more readily acquire competence in these areas. For example, a learner might communicate requesting via a graphic symbol and rejecting using a headshake (for a discussion of *mixed mode systems* involving both gestures and graphics, see Reichle & Keogh, 1986).

There are some instances in which it may be counter productive to attempt

the concurrent implementation of generalized requesting and rejecting responses. Some learners who readily select objects or events may not be particularly discriminating; they may select virtually anything offered. Other
learners may show "whopping" dislikes but may fail to make overtures toward
any objects, persons, or events. In these instances, intervention to establish the
communication function that appears to be of the greatest immediate use to the
learner may be most desirable.

If a learner is a candidate for both requesting and rejecting intervention
but, for whatever reason, only one program can be implemented, the authors
recommend implementing the requesting response as the initial target behavior.
A request program presents the interventionist as a deliverer of reinforcers
rather than bad tidings, as is the case during instances of generalized rejecting
intervention. With learners who show little interest in other individuals, attempting to establish caregivers and teachers as conditioned positive reinforcers may be useful.

An initial repertoire of indicating preference via the application of the requesting and rejecting intervention must be considered in the context of daily
interactions. All daily activities have a point of initiation and termination. Additionally, most activities require the emission of socially acceptable behavior
to maintain participation in the activity. One way to view the social validity of
requesting and rejecting intervention lies in the influence of these programs on
the learner's ability to use these skills to initiate, maintain, and terminate social
interactions in the context of daily routines.

INITIATING INTERACTIONS

Determining What Constitutes Initiation

Attempting to separate instances of strategies that are used to initiate social
interactions from those that are used to maintain social interactions represents
less than a straightforward task. Many child behaviors are interpreted by parents as initiations, regardless of the child's intention. For example, around
mealtime, children as young as 12 weeks of age typically cry and fuss. Parents
interpret these cries as rudimentary requests for nutriment even though 12-
week-old infants are still unable to regulate their vocal behavior to be used as a
function for their listening audience. Keogh and Reichle (1985) observed that,
over time, instances such as the preceding example form an opportunity for the
child to learn that he or she can actually manipulate the actions of others
through the initiated use of his or her vocal behavior. In this instance, initiated
social behavior is established via a history of reinforcement.

Other initiated behavior may be taught in a slightly different manner. For
example, at approximately 7–8 months of age, many children become interested in the game of "patticake." Typically, the caregiver sings as he or she

dutifully guides the child's hands through the appropriate motions. Over time, the need to assist the child in producing the appropriate hand motions decreases. At some point the child's actions come under instructional control of the song itself (i.e., the motor component of the game becomes self-initiated in that the learner is no longer dependent on an explicit prompt from another in order to engage in the game). In the preceding instance, a system of response prompts paired with reinforcement resulted in initiated learner behavior, given a natural cue.

In the area of communicative behavior, initiation has often been characterized as the emission of language in the absence of a verbal cue from another. However, more recently, other antecedent stimuli have been addressed in the analysis of self-initiated communication (Simic & Bucher, 1980). Halle (1987) characterized initiated social-communicative behavior as that which is uncued by another individual. Any definition of initiated communicative behavior must consider a number of critical variables. Among those are the proximity of the learner to others in the environment, the proximity of the learner to objects of interest, and the familiarity of the activities in which the learner is engaged.

In the area of establishing communicative behavior, there is a limited literature that addresses initiating. Carr and Kologinsky (1983) examined the use of initiated requests by three persons with autism. These learners had sign repertoires that ranged between 25–50 expressive signs (used as requests). Carr and Kologinsky (1983) believed that the learners' requests were prompted by the sight of the objects. During initiation intervention, no verbal prompts were used by interventionists, and objects were not visible during the procedures. At the conclusion of the investigation, the learners' rate and variety of spontaneous signs had increased. Carr and Kologinsky (1983) concluded that initiated signing was facilitated as a result of a shift in stimulus control from imitative prompting to the simple presence of an attending adult.

Halle, Baer, and Spradlin (1981) taught six individuals with mental retardation to request the assistance and materials that were required to participate in a variety of daily activities. A constant 5-second time delay was used to fade the use of a verbal instructional prompt. Charlop, Schreibman, and Thibodeau (1985) also utilized a constant 2-second time delay procedure in teaching seven verbal individuals with autism to spontaneously request desired objects. These researchers reported that spontaneous requests generalized across settings, persons, and objects that had not been originally taught. Gobbi, Cipani, Hudson, and Lapenta-Neudeck (1986) implemented a procedure that they described as "quick transfer" to establish spontaneous requesting responses between two learners with severe handicaps. The instructional procedure consisted of the use of a 30-second time delay procedure that was incorporated with the use of graduated levels of stimulus prompts. Gobbi et al. (1986) reported high rates of spontaneous requesting responses as a result of the intervention procedure. Further, they reported that spontaneous requesting responses generalized to other settings and to individuals who did not serve as teachers in the original procedural implementation.

For some learners, initiating a request in the absence of either a verbal cue or the presence of the requestable item seems to be an insurmountable obstacle. Some requesting response intervention procedures rely heavily on the immediate prior experience of the learner with regard to a reinforcer. For example, suppose that at snack time a learner requests juice and is offered a small quantity that is subsequently consumed. In this case, the absence of the reinforcer may serve as the discriminative stimulus for another request for juice. Initially, juice may have to be present as part of the discriminative stimulus. Across successive opportunities, the serving pitcher of juice may be absent and only the consumption of juice by peers (who are also seated at the table) serves as the discriminative stimulus. The systematic removal of these antecedent events may result in the presence of a cup without juice that serves as the discriminative stimulus for a juice requesting episode. In these examples of recurrence (i.e., a request for a greater quantity or another instance), the probability of a self-initiated response is enhanced by the potential for repeated trials over a relatively short period of time. That is, an immediately preceding request may come to serve as part of the discriminative stimulus for the emission of a subsequent request.

Goetz, Gee, and Sailor (1985) suggest the use of an interrupted chain of actions within a routine as an opportunity for a learner to engage in a request. Opportunities for communicative emission are embedded in the context of daily routines. For example, a learner may be engaged in a breakfast routine in which toast is being made. Just after the the toast has been buttered, the interventionist may interrupt the routine to ask the learner what he or she wants or needs. In order to resume the routine, the learner must provide a correct approximation of the targeted response. Interrupted chain training is hypothesized to be efficient because it uses naturally occurring events that are part of a chain of discriminative stimuli to reach the targeted communicative behavior. That is, buttering toast becomes the discriminative stimulus to talk about buttering toast. These investigators caution that in order for interrupted chain training to be effective: 1) the learner must be highly motivated to complete the task that has been interrupted, and 2) the level of anxiety created by interrupting the task must not be great.

Inviting assistance is a type of requesting behavior that allows the natural application of an interrupted chain procedure. Specifically, the learner comes to the portion of a task that he or she cannot independently complete. This problem creates a natural interruption in the task that could be used for teaching a generalized requesting assistance symbol. The authors' experience suggests that many individuals who are considered to be passive engage in substantial repertoires of idiosyncratic behavior that could be interpreted by others as requests for assistance. For example, when an individual gets his or her finger stuck in the small opening of a toy, twists him- or herself into an uncomfortable position in bed, or finds that his or her head has fallen forward out of a stabilized position, the result may be an instance of crying or fussy behavior. In these instances, a request for assistance, similar to the request for desired objects, may be taught. The main difference is that requests for assistance typically occur with less frequency and require the use of a more incidental teaching paradigm because the conditions that require assistance are less predictable and more difficult to engineer than opportunities to request objects.

Combatting Learned Helplessness
via Communicative Initiations

One of the primary rationales for teaching a learner to initiate communicatively is to minimize the influence of learned helplessness (discussed earlier). Unfortunately, unless this is done carefully, the interventionist's plans may result in strengthening the helplessness. The learner may fail to discriminate between refraining from use of communicative behavior and requesting in lieu of independent acting.

Typically, in order for a learner to communicatively request objects, he or she should be taught that the available object choices should be visible and in fairly close proximity to him or her. With this in mind, an intervention history may be established in which the learner acquires the rule that "whenever you see the object and you want it—emit a communicative request." Although adherence to this rule results in the establishment of desirable behavior, it does not necessarily lead to normalized social behavior. For example, while eating family style, serving yourself a food item that is nearby without requesting it is considered socially acceptable. When the food item is beyond reach, a request is required. An extreme example of the failure to engage in the "conditional," more normalized use of an established repertoire occurs with a learner who requests food between each successive spoonful.

The need to establish the conditional use of behavior is not limited to requests for objects. For example, if a learner is taught to request assitance in order to remove a tightly affixed lid on a peanut butter jar, it is unlikely that he or she will independently remove the jar lid unless that condition is addressed directly. Reichle, Schermer, and Anderson (1987) taught a learner with severe handicaps to remove a twist tie from a loaf of bread. On some occasions the twist tie was very loosely affixed, in which case the learner was reinforced for continuing on in the task without making a request. On other opportunities after trying to remove a tightly affixed twist tie, the learner was reinforced for emitting a generalized requesting assistance symbol.

Establishing initiated indicating preference skills clearly comprises one important aspect for making choices. That aspect is that choices are not always made from a learner's preferred alternatives or determined by the initiated involvement in an activity. A generalized choicemaking competency also involves determining which activity might be the most beneficial for the learner or when he or she should maintain or exit an activity. Indicating the desire to maintain involvement in an activity might also include a preference paradigm response.

MAINTAINING INTERACTIONS

In the simplest sense, reacting to an environmental event represents an initial instance of maintaining an environmental interaction. In other words, the learner has simply taken his or her turn participating in an environmental interaction. For many persons who appear to be passive, documenting awareness of environmental events represents the initial objective in establishing interactional maintenance. Typically, changes in the learner's visual tracking and his or her localization (e.g., tactual, auditory, visual) prior and subsequent to the presentation of a stimulus have been used as indices of environmental awareness. Home and educational environments provide a wealth of visual and auditory events to attract a learner's attention (e.g., pots and pans bang in the kitchen, televisions and stereos droan, siblings yell, toilets flush, doorbells ring). There are many environmental events in which the learner can participate.

For learners who often fail to respond to their surroundings, several instructional strategies are available. The first involves enhancing the saliency of the stimuli to which the interventionist wishes the learner to respond. The second involves the assumption that the learner is aware of the antecedent event but simply fails to respond and requires the use of a response prompt that is faded systematically.

A number of examples of rudimentary interactive exchanges have been reported between mothers and their infants. Brazelton, Koslowski, and Main (1974) reported rhythmic cycles of attention and nonattention during face-to-face interactions between mothers and their children. Piaget provided a very exacting description of the emergence of vocal and verbal imitation. He noted that very early in children's development, the probability that they would vocalize was influenced by surrounding events. Specifically, if others in the learner's environment were vocalizing, he or she was more apt to also talk. This phenomenon has been referred to as vocal contagion. Within the child's first years, he or she comes to engage in "child-initiated turntaking." During these episodes, the child produces a vocal behavior and waits for the adult to vocalize before producing his or her next vocalization. It is at this level of social interaction maintenance that persons with the most severe handicaps meet reasonable objectives.

Several intervention procedures can be used to establish vocal turntaking routines; however, all procedures begin with attempts to increase the instances of the learner's vocal behavior. Increasing vocal frequency involves the delivery of a reinforcing event contingent on the production of vocal behavior. Once the learner is vocalizing frequently, a condition is added to the reinforcement contingency. The interventionist then reinforces only the vocal behavior that is produced immediately after the speaking partner's responses. Effectively, this strategy places a portion of learner-produced vocal behavior on extinction. In order to continue getting reinforced, the learner must begin to adhere to the rule, "Vocalize right after you hear someone else vocalize."

In the mid-1980s, the establishment of interactive vocal behavior has been the focus of several communication interventionists. J. MacDonald (personal communication, November, 1987) has indicated that establishing interactive exchanges represents the cornerstone in the establishment of a communicative repertoire. MacDonald's intervention procedures rely heavily on shaping existing exchanges between children and those around them into more sophisticated communicative events. Initial efforts to establish communicative exchanges may require the interventionist to address motor topographies of exchange as well as vocal exchanges.

The motor domain is replete with examples of social exchanges. Games such as "peek-a-boo" and "I'm gonna get you" require topographically easy responses from the child and can be repeated often in a game-like format. Consequently, the routine is quite easy but because of the redundant nature of the game, the learner receives experiences in maintaining an interaction over trials (or time).

The identification of age-appropriate routines for adolescents that have the same simplicity as the routines described above presents a challenge to the prospective interventionist. Similar routines, observed regularly in junior high and high school settings include: 1) "give me five," 2) playing catch, and 3) waving "hello." Among younger nonhandicapped children, it is quite common to see exchange games that involve a child who is taking, showing, and giving his or her collection of toys to a friend. Games that involve the emission of taking, showing, and giving behavior were of particular interest to Reichle and Yoder (1979). They described assessment and intervention strategies for each of these classes of social exchange.

The bulk of communicative maintenance reported in the literature focuses around its function of providing information (i.e., tacting) rather than indicating preference. However, among persons with the most severe handicaps who may show a greater inclination to request than to provide information, opportunities to indicate preferences that involve conversational maintenance are quite plentiful. For example, indicating preferences as a variety of different foods are passed family style at mealtime represents extended opportunities for communicative exchange.

Terminating Interactions

When a learner terminates an interaction, it usually means that he or she wishes to either avoid the presentation of an object or event, or end an ongoing experience with a particular object or event. The need to engage in a terminating response may be because an aversive object or event is being offered (e.g., a mosquito has landed on one's arm), the learner has simply grown tired of a particular object or event (i.e., has become satiated), a neutral event (e.g., eating a meal) has been completed, or a still reinforcing event must end to move to another scheduled event.

Terminating responses are not emitted exclusively in the presence of undesired objects and events. Sometimes neutral stimulus events (i.e., events that are not particularly liked but also not particularly disliked) are thrust upon the learner. If the learner is required to continue to participate, he or she may begin to habituate in the activity. Examples of this phenomenon include slowed production during a vocational activity throughout the day, and, at mealtime, engaging in a slower rate of consumption with increased dribbling. Another application of a terminating social competency involves a signal to a communicative partner that a task has been completed. This terminating response may be interpreted by the learner's listener to have at least several distinct intents depending on the context in which it is emitted. For example, upon completing a meal program in which the learner was required to eat independently, the learner's indication of "finished" might actually mean "I'm done, check my work and deliver a reinforcer," or, "I'm full," or, "I'm done eating but would like a drink." Conversely, for a learner who does not understand the daily routine, an indication of "finished" might mean "what do I do now?"

At the start, the interventionist must determine which of these situations is important to emphasize as a teaching instance. There is a modicum of evidence to suggest that learners with severe handicaps do not generalize across the breadth of different stimulus situations (Reichle, 1987). Because these learners seem to rarely generalize across all of the preceding stimulus dimensions, two separate communication objectives were chosen to be focused on: 1) the establishment of a generalized rejecting response to be used whenever undesired or usually desired objects that are currently in a state of satiation are offered, and 2) the termination of an ongoing activity (i.e., I'm done) that the authors refer to as the social function of leavetake or exit.

Establishing generalized rejecting can be extended to instances in which the learner has become satiated on a known reinforcer. That is, under some circumstances it is appropriate to use a generalized rejecting response in the presence of an object or event that would normally serve as a reinforcer. If the interventionist wishes to extend the use of a rejecting response to the multiplicity of situations displayed by that of a nonhandicapped individual, teaching opportunities must include situations in which items are offered to the learner that are in a state of satiation. Some objects and events better lend themselves to repeated exposure than others. For example, at mealtime, the interventionist can continue to offer to fill a learner's drinking cup after a beverage has been consumed in an attempt to elicit a request to terminate the activity.

At some point, a decision must be made on whether the generalized rejecting response can also be used as a "leavetaking (i.e., I'm done)" symbol in which the learner will be allowed to exit events in which he or she has been participating (e.g., mealtime, work). This issue addresses the question of whether the interventionist wishes to include all of the examples that we have given of termination in a set of exemplars used to teach generalized rejecting responses, or whether the interventionist wishes to create two separate classes of stimuli in which one set involves the offer of disliked items (i.e., generalized rejection), and a second set of exemplars of objects or activities that the learner completes, satiates on, or habituates in (generalized leavetake [i.e., "I'm done."]). Choosing both generalized rejection and generalized leavetake symbols is most informative to the learner's listener but involves teaching a relatively sophisticated discrimination between rejecting and leavetaking symbols.

Once the symbol(s) have been selected, the interventionist creates a schedule that coincides with a daily routine. The initial objective of assessment opportunities is to determine what repertoire might be exhibited by the learner to terminate or avoid the presentation of an object or activity. Additionally, evidence of satiation during repeated access to known reinforcers (and if so, approximately how many stimulus presentations are required) and habituation to events that are of limited interest to the learner can be determined.

During the intervention procedure, it is important to determine at approximately what point the learner is apt to wish to leavetake. Initially, the interventionist should deliver a prompt for a leavetake response as close to the point of satiation or habituation as possible. Doing so minimizes the possibility that the learner might emit some socially unacceptable behavior in an effort to leave. In order to be most successful, it is important that the desired leavetake response be prompted prior to the emission of the socially unacceptable topography; otherwise, the interventionist runs the risk of establishing a chain of behavior that includes that unacceptable response (e.g., tantrumming, hitting).

SUMMARY

The purpose of this chapter is to address indicating preference as an instrumental social skill that can be taught in the context of initiating, maintaining, or terminating interactions during daily routines. With individuals who are considered to be passive and who also have the most severe handicaps, the establishment of indicating preference responses involves a careful delineation of those objects, persons, and events that spark either interest or dislike in the learner. For some learners, establishing likes and dislikes represents an aggressive instructional effort. However, the authors believe that such programming efforts serve as the foundation for communication intervention procedures to establish requesting and rejecting responses (including leavetaking). Furthermore, the authors believe that requesting and rejecting responses represent viable communicative functions that are needed in order to establish socially desirable communicative initiation, maintenance, and termination strategies that are useful in many daily routines.

In developing functional contexts in which to teach communicative behavior to persons who have the most severe handicaps, it is exciting to embark on intervention efforts that attempt to coordinate the use of instrumental communicative functions (e.g., requesting and rejecting responses).

REFERENCES

Brazelton, T., Koslowski, B., & Main, M. (1974). The origins of reciprocity: The early mother-infant interaction. In M. Lewis & L. Rosenblum (Eds.), *The effects of the infant on its caregiver* (pp. 49–76). New York: John Wiley & Sons.

Carr, E., & Durand, V.M. (1985). The social-communicative basis of severe behavior problems in children. In S. Reiss & R.R. Bootzins (Eds.), *Theoretical issues in behavior therapy* (pp. 219–254). Orlando, FL: Academic Press.

Carr, E., & Kologinsky, E. (1983). Acquisition of sign language by autistic children II: Spontaneity and generalization effects. *Journal of Applied Behavior Analysis, 16,* 297–314.

Chapman, R., & Miller, J. (1980). Analyzing language and communication in the child. In R.L. Schiefelbusch (Ed.), *Nonspeech language and communication: Analysis and intervention* (pp. 159–196). Baltimore: University Park Press.

Charlop, M., Schreibman, L., & Thibodeau, M. (1985). Increasing spontaneous verbal responding in autistic children using a time delay procedure. *Journal of Applied Behavior Analysis, 18,* 155–166.

Gobbi, L., Cipani, E., Hudson, C., & Lapenta-Neudeck, R. (1986). Developing spontaneous requesting among children with severe mental retardation. *Mental Retardation, 24,* 357–363.

Goetz, L., Gee, K., & Sailor, W. (1985). Using a behavior chain interruption strategy to teach communication skills to students with severe disabilities. *Journal of The Associations for Persons with Severe Handicaps, 10,* 21–30.

Guess, D., Benson, H., & Siegel-Causey, E. (1985). Concepts and issues related to choicemaking and autonomy among persons with severe disabilities. *Journal of The Association for Persons with Severe Handicaps, 10,* 79–86.

Halle, J. (1987). Teaching language in the natural environment: An analysis of spontaneity. *Journal of The Association for Persons with Severe Handicaps, 12,* 28–37.

Halle, J., Baer, D., & Spradlin, J. (1981). An analysis of teachers' generalized use of delay in helping children: A stimulus control procedure to increase language use in handicapped children. *Journal of Applied Behavior Analysis, 14,* 389–409.

Keogh, W., & Reichle, J. (1985). Communication intervention for the "difficult to teach" severely handicapped. In S. Warren & A. Rogers-Warren (Eds.), *Teaching functional language* (pp. 157–194). Austin, TX: PRO-ED.

Lipsitt, L. (1978). The pleasures and annoyances of infants: Approach and avoidance behavior of babies. In E.B. Thoman & S. Trotter (Eds.), *Social responsiveness of infants* (pp. 22–26). New York: Johnson & Johnson.

MacDonald, J. (1985). Language through conversation: A model for intervention with language-delayed persons. In S. Warren & A. Rogers-Warren (Eds.), *Teaching functional language* (pp. 89–122). Austin, TX: PRO-ED.

Meyer, L., Reichle, J., McQuarter, R., Cole, D., Vandercook, T., Evans, I., Neel, R., & Kishi, G. (1985). *Assessment of Social Competence (ASC): A scale of social competence functions.* Minneapolis: The University of Minnesota.

Monty, R., & Perlmuter, L. (1975). Persistence of the effects of choice on paired associate learning. *Memory and Cognition, 3,* 183–187.

Newhard, M. (1984). *Effective of student choice of materials on learning and stereotypical and effective behavior.* Unpublished master's thesis, University of Kansas, Lawrence.

Papousek, H. (1978). The infant's fundamental adaptive response system in social interaction. In E.B. Thoman & S. Trotter (Eds.), *Social responsiveness of infants* (pp. 27–37). New York: Johnson & Johnson.

Perlmuter, L., & Monty, R. (1977). The importance of perceived control: Fact or fantasy. *American Scientist, 65,* 759–765.

Reichle, J. (1987, October). *Stimulus control procedures used to establish communicative repertoires among persons with severe handicaps.* Paper presented at the annual convention of The Association for Persons with Severe Handicaps, Chicago.

Reichle, J., & Keogh, W.J. (1986). Communication instruction for learners with severe handicaps: Some unresolved issues. In R.H. Horner, L.H. Meyer, & H.D.B. Fredericks (Eds.), *Education of learners with severe handicaps: Exemplary service strategies* (pp. 189–219). Baltimore: Paul H. Brookes Publishing Co.

Reichle, J., & Piche-Cragoe, L. (1986). *Teaching learners with severe handicaps to correspond their requests to reinforcer selection.* Unpublished manuscript, University of Minnesota, Minneapolis.

Reichle, J., Schermer, G., & Anderson, H. (1987). *Teaching the discriminative use of a requesting assistance symbol to an adult with severe handicaps.* Unpublished manuscript, University of Minnesota, Minneapolis.

Reichle, J., & Yoder, D. (1979). Communication behavior of the severely and profoundly mentally retarded: Assessment and early stimulation strategies. In R. York & E. Edgar (Eds.), *Teaching the severely handicapped* (Vol. 4, pp. 180–218). Seattle: American Association for the Education of the Severely/Profoundly Handicapped.

Rheingold, H., Gewirtz, J., & Ross, H. (1959). Social conditioning of vocalizations in the infant. *Journal of Comparative and Psychological Psychology, 52,* 68–73.

Seligman, M. (1975). *Helplessness: On depression, development and death.* San Francisco: W.H. Freeman.

Sigafoos, J., & Reichle, J. (1987). *Teaching valid and explicit requesting to a severely intellectually delayed learner experiencing a vision deficit.* Unpublished manuscript, University of Minnesota, Minneapolis.

Simic, J., & Bucher, B. (1980). Development and spontaneous manding in language deficient children. *Journal of Applied Behavior Analysis, 13,* 523–528.

Skinner, B.F. (1957). *Verbal behavior.* New York: Appleton-Century-Crofts.

Stokes, T., & Baer, D. (1977). An implicit technology of generalization. *Journal of Applied Behavior Analysis, 10,* 349–367.

Uzgiris, I., & Hunt, J. McV. (1975). *Assessment in infancy: Ordinal scales of psychological development.* Urbana: University of Illinois Press.

Watson, J. (1978). Perception of contingency as a determinant of social responsiveness. In S. Trotter & E. Thoman (Eds.), *Social responsiveness of infants.* New York: Johnson & Johnson.

Watson, J., & Ramey, C. (1969, March). *Reactions to response contingent stimulation in early infancy.* Paper presented at biennial meeting of the SRCD, Santa Monica, CA.

Weisberg, P. (1963). Social and nonsocial conditioning of infant vocalization. *Child Development, 34,* 377–388.

EDUCATIONAL PROGRAMMING FOR YOUNG CHILDREN WITH THE MOST SEVERE DISABILITIES

Donna H. Lehr

Most, although not all, children with the most severe handicaps are disabled due to congenital abnormalities of a biological, physical, or genetic basis and acquire their disabilities during the fetal period, birth process, or newborn period. Their disabilities are often easily identifiable very early in infancy (Bricker, 1986). This being the case, health professionals are enabled the opportunity to provide early intervention to these children and their families sooner than with other children who possess less obvious disabilities. The severity of these children's disabilities makes very early intervention critical for both the children and their families (Bricker, 1986). Such children often have serious medical conditions that require specialized care as well. The birth of a child with severe disabilities is often devastating to families, and generally necessitates family support and/or counseling. Infants with the most severe disabilities require care beyond that which most parents are equipped to provide, making instruction about care providing necessary. Infants with the most severe disabilities require more systematic instruction to develop than do nonhandicapped children or those with handicaps who sometimes seem to develop despite their environment.

While these may be compelling reasons for providing early intervention to children with the most severe disabilities and their families, the fact is, educational programs for these individuals have not been prevalent (Gentry & Olson,

Preparation of this work was supported in part by Grant No. G 0083-02248 awarded to the University of Wisconsin-Milwaukee by the United States Department of Education, Office of Special Education Programs. The opinions expressed herein do not necessarily reflect the position of the United States Department of Education and no official endorsement should be inferred. Special thanks to Penny Urben, Nadine Schatz, Karen Clemens, and Kristen Peppey for their participation in the development of the model program described in this chapter.

1985). Reasons include lack of previous emphasis on education for young children with any degree of handicap, and, where there has been a focus on programs for young children with handicaps, lack of emphasis on those with severe disabilities (Bricker & Kaminski, 1986).

The passage of federal legislation, such as the Handicapped Children's Early Education Assistance Act (PL 90-538), can be seen as encouraging for individuals with severe disabilities. In 1968, Congress enacted PL 90-538 providing discretionary monies to establish program models for serving young children with handicapping conditions. Since that time approximately 100 programs have been funded annually to develop and disseminate those models as a way of assisting in the establishment of new programs to serve this population; however, few of the programs focused on the needs of students with severe handicaps (Bricker & Kaminski, 1986). The Education for All Handicapped Children Act of 1975 (PL 94-142) mandated that programs be established for children between ages 3 and 5, but only when compatible with state law. The Education of the Handicapped Amendments of 1986 (PL 99-457) required that states establish educational programs for all eligible handicapped children between the ages of 3 and 5 by the 1990-91 school year and provide encouragement to states to develop programs for children between the ages of birth through 2.

However, despite this increased emphasis on the needs of young children with handicapping conditions, current data indicate that a low proportion of children with handicaps are actually being served and inequities exist in the service provision (Peterson, 1987). Variability exists throughout the country regarding the ages of students who are eligible for educational programs and the types of children served, relative to their handicapping conditions (Peterson, 1987). The consequence of this lack of consistent availability of programs for some children can be extremely serious for those not receiving services. For some individuals, 6 years can pass before the children or their families receive any assistance. The effect of this latency can be understood by considering the program goals for very young children with the most severe disabilities.

PROGRAM GOALS

The program goals for young students with severe handicaps have been described as being similar to those for the population of students considered to be at-risk or to have mild handicaps, but only at a global level (Weatherford, 1986). Weatherford (1986) states that the primary goal should be that of "facilitating growth in all realms of development to the maximum degree possible determined by genetic and organic limitations." (p. 8) However, for the student with more severe handicaps, goals must also focus on: helping these individuals to adapt to their handicaps (Weatherford, 1986), preventing secondary negative behaviors (see Chapter 7), training the individual to perform self-care skills, and avoiding regression (Weatherford, 1986). When describing specific goals for early intervention services for students with severe handicapping conditions, Bricker and Kaminski (1986) identify such primary goals as: 1) enhancing developmental growth, 2) increasing behavioral repertoires, 3) preventing or minimizing secondary disabilites, 4) providing parental support, 5) maintaining the child in less restrictive educational and residential environments, and 6) reducing the cost of service provision and increasing human productivity. Bricker and Kaminski (1986) emphasize that "the more disabled the child, the more costly the programs over time; therefore, any early habilitative efforts that lead to the placement of children in a less restrictive environment . . . potentially save finite educational resources." (p. 59)

It should be noted that the previous discussion focuses on program goals for students with severe disabilities. For those children with the most severe disabilities, the program goals can be seen as being similar to those with less severe disabilities. However, differences may exist when considering curricular goals for individual children. Once again, it must be pointed out that little attention has been given in the literature to curricular goals for the students with the most severe disabilities. The following section includes a discussion of this area.

HISTORIC CURRICULA BASES

When looking specifically for descriptions of what should be taught to very young students with the most severe disabilities, confusion can, and does, result. Much of the literature on instructional goals for similar students focuses on either young students with mild or moderate disabilities (Bricker, 1986; Cook, Tessier, & Armbruster, 1987; Neisworth & Bagnato, 1987; Thurman & Widerstrom, 1985), or students with severe disabilities who are middle school and high school age (Brown, Nietupski, & Hamre-Nietupski, 1976; Gaylord-Ross & Holvoet, 1985; Snell, 1987). For these students, the normal developmental model (Bailey & Wolery, 1984; Bricker, 1986) or the functional model (Brown et al., 1976) and its extension, the criterion of the next environment (Vincent et al., 1980) are the predominant models used. While these models may be appropriate for some students, difficulties are encountered when applying these approaches to young children with the most serious disabilities.

Normal Developmental Model

Traditionally, the underlying theoretical basis for the education of all young children with and without handicaps has been developmentally oriented (Bailey & Wolery, 1984; Bricker, 1986). With this model, students are assessed according to identified sequences of normal development, and the results are used to generate curricular content for individual students. That is, the behaviors that the child does not demonstrate are taught in the sequence in which they appear in individuals who are developing normally. Such a model is inappropriate for students with severe handicaps for the following reasons:

1. Use is based on the assumption that the sequences in which nonhandi-capped students acquire skills are the same as the sequences in which students with severe and profound handicaps acquire skills. However, students with severe and profound handicaps often develop skills in different sequences (Brown, 1987).
2. Assessment based upon normal developmental sequences may result in the identification of skills for instruction that are inappropriate for students with severe handicaps within their chronological age and not essential to them for independent functioning (Brown, 1987). For example, a normally developing 3-month-old mouths objects; however, would it be appropriate to teach a 4-year-old who has not learned to mouth objects to do so? Mouthing objects is considered inappropriate for a normal 6-year-old and although it is demonstrated by all normally developing infants, it is not seen as being a necessary skill to increase the child's ability to function independently.
3. Use of the developmental model results in the identification of individual skills that are often taught in isolation, rather than in an integrated fashion that serves to provide essential meaning to the performance of the task (Brown, 1987).
4. Curriculum development is usually based on assessments that utilize normal developmental scales. The skills that make up such scales may be important in terms of assessing developmental levels; however, they may not be appropriate to translate into curricular objectives (Brown, 1987).

As a consequence of the failure of the normal developmental model when applied to students with severe handicaps, the human services professionals instituted the functional curricular approach.

Functional Curricular Model

The concept of functional curriculum has been discussed extensively as being the most appropriate approach for teaching students with severe disabilities (Brown et al., 1976; Gaylord-Ross & Holvoet, 1985; Snell, 1987; also see Chapter 10). The Criterion of Ultimate Functioning (Brown et al., 1976) served as the basis for this model. By utilizing this criterion, program planners can identify and teach those skills that are essential in allowing an individual to function as productively and independently as possible in adult integrated environments. When using this approach, predictions are made about possible future living and working environments for each individual. The skills that are needed in order to participate in these environments become the curricular content.

The emphasis of the functional curricular approach is placed on teaching only those skills that are critical to adult functioning and can be used in the natural environments. Also emphasized is the selection of age-appropriate skills for instruction, using as a reference point students of the same age who do not have handicaps.

While this model clearly revolutionizes instruction for students with severe handicaps, most often the functional curricular approach, as discussed in the literature, has focused on the elementary, middle, and high school age students with moderate to severe handicaps. This model has been extended to students with more severe handicapping conditions and younger children but only with difficulty (Ferguson, 1987). A study conducted by Brown, Helmstetter, and Guess (1986) revealed a lack of empirical justification for applying this concept to individuals with profound disabilities. Furthermore, when considering very young children, many professionals are uncomfortable with attempting to predict possible adult environments for a child who is 20 years away from adulthood. As Vincent et al. (1980) pointed out, many skills that could be identified as being essential to the functioning of an adult in an integrated environment would be inappropriate to teach very young children (e.g., teaching a 10-month-old child with profound handicaps to learn to shop in community stores or order lunch at McDonalds). Clearly these are not age appropriate skills; other children the same age are not yet learning these skills.

Criterion of the Next Environment Model

Vincent et al. (1980) suggest focusing on students' "next," rather than "ultimate," educational environments to determine what skills will be needed. Vincent et al. (1980) proposed that for all preschool children, the curriculum should be designed to facilitate movement into environments that include non-handicapped peers. Consequently, skills taught using the criterion of the next environment should be those that lead to "survival" in least restrictive environments, such as kindergarten. For example, for preschool children about to enter kindergarten, Vincent et al. (1980) identified a group of social and behavioral "survival skills" that were found to be more critical for success than academics. These skills then became the focus of the curriculum for individual students.

The emphasis of the Vincent et al. (1980) article and the subsequent implementation of this approach was based upon students who were receiving regular education curriculum. Again, difficulties are encountered when attempting to apply this approach to young students with profound disabilities. The most frequent next educational environment is not a kindergarten; it is more likely a class for primary age individuals, also with profound disabilities. When looking ahead to such an educational environment, it is difficult to use this approach as a reference for skill identification. The curriculum in such classes is based on each student's individual needs, and, consequently, no specific required skills can be identified.

CURRICULAR BASES FOR YOUNG
CHILDREN WITH THE MOST SEVERE DISABILITIES

The basic developmental model for instruction is based upon the assumption that learners of these basic skills will eventually be able to apply them in different environments and situations. That is, if a student develops a pincer grasp, it is assumed that he or she will eventually be able to use clothespins to hang up clothes. However, this model's failure rests on the fact that while acquisition of some tool skills may occur, students do not automatically transfer the skills to applied settings (Brown et al., 1976). The models that utilize the criteria of ultimate functioning (functional curricular) and next environment are based upon independence in the future. These models are also unsuccessful for individuals with the most severe disabilities because teachers fail to consider degrees of independence, in spite of the fact that they are explicitly proposed (Baumgart et al., 1982). "As teachers measure this future vision [of ultimate or next environments] against some students' present skills, . . . they find only large, seemingly untenable discrepancies" (Ferguson, 1987, p. 68). The consequence is that either instruction occurs on less complex skills (Baumgart et al., 1982) or no curricular decisions are made for such students (Ferguson, 1987).

Goal Continuums

It may be more helpful for teachers of students with the most severe disabilities to consider several goals, each on a continuum. Figure 9.1 presents suggestions of such goals (see also Chapter 4 for a discussion of meaningful outcomes for such individuals). The following section offers suggestions for establishing goals for the youngest children with the most severe disabilities.

A continuum of independence related to functional tasks can be viewed in two ways: 1) independence on some substeps of tasks, and 2) less dependence on other tasks. For example, it may be appropriate to set the goal of having a student independently hold a toothbrush; however, the rest of the task may have to be done for the students. Similarly, it may be appropriate to set the goal of having a student bear some weight to assist in transferring him- or herself from one seat to another, resulting in less dependency on the caregiver.

The principle of partial participation refers to the process of considering that an individual may be able to participate in activities in other ways than through independent functioning (Baumgart et al., 1982; Brown, Evans, Weed, & Owen, 1987). Consequently, by considering partial participation as a goal,

Dependence <----------> Independence
No participation <----------> Full participation
Difficult to care for <----------> Easy to care for
Unpleasant <----------> Pleasant

Figure 9.1. Curricular goal continuums.

individuals may gain access to many more activities and environments. For example, 2–3-year-olds often show great interest in participating in snack and meal preparation. Children with the most severe disabilities are often automatically eliminated from such activities since it is thought they could never learn to make the meal themselves. Positioning the child so the activity can be observed, involving him or her in stirring, and/or adapting a blender so that it can be activated by an easy-to-operate switch, all have the effect of increasing a child's participation in normal daily routines (see Chapter 10 for more examples of application of this concept).

The two other goals in Figure 9.1, making the child easier or more pleasant to care for, may also be helpful to consider. These both may result in improvements in the quality of an individual's life. It is recognized that many individuals with very severe disabilities might always be cared for, often in group settings. While quality care for all residents of such programs is expected, it is also likely that variations in the nature, quality, and quantity of the interactions between the resident and caregivers will occur and may be a function, in part, of the behaviors that are displayed by the residents. Simply stated, the "cuter" or more attractive the resident, the more frequent the contact; the easier the resident is to care for, the more positive the interactions during the provision of care. Consequently, identifying goals for students that result in them being more engaging or easier to care for may be very appropriate. For example, setting the goal of having a very young disabled child raise his or her arms to be lifted when the mother approaches may result in it being easier to lift the child. More importantly, this action may also result in the mother experiencing that most rewarding feeling of responsiveness. Such responses clearly have potential for changing the nature of the interactions between the caregivers or parents and child.

Criterion of Importance and Appropriateness

Questions of the importance of certain skills can be asked of not only students with severe handicaps, but also young children with the most severe disabilities. Questions such as, "Is learning this skill going to result in the student doing something that previously had to be done for him or her?" must be asked. Even though stacking blocks and putting pegs in peg boards are standard activities in all programs for young children without handicaps, these activities clearly do not pass the test of importance for young children with the most severe handicaps. Another method of determining a targeted skill's value is by determining how often the activity is performed by the caregiver or adult.

Skills and materials are also selected according to their age-appropriateness for students with severe handicaps (Brown et al., 1976; Gaylord-Ross & Holvoet, 1985; Snell, 1987). This refers to the selection of skills based upon whether other children the same age are demonstrating the same skills. It has been necessary to emphasize such a concept since past reliance on the normal developmental model for curriculum resulted in the identification of skills demonstrated by children at a much younger chronological age than the actual age of the child. According to this model, a 21-year-old student who has been identified as functioning developmentally at 3-month-old level might be taught to bat at a mobile; however, if that same person, through various norm referenced tests, was identified as functioning at the 6-month developmental level, he or she would then be taught to play with a busy box. Critics of this model question the necessity of such skills in relation to the individual's ultimate functioning and the possible detrimental effects that they may have on the individual over an extended period of time. As for the materials used, people tend to judge individuals' capabilities by their amount of participation in a given activity and the materials that they used. For example, Bates, Morrow, Pancosfar, and Sedlak (1984) found that university students ascribed higher competency to students who were observed engaged in functional age-appropriate activities than to those who were observed in nonfunctional, age-inappropriate activities. For this reason, the emphasis for students with severe disabilities has been placed on not using peg boards and busy boxes.

Children with the most severe disabilities are first of all children and do need to play with toys, such as peg boards, busy boxes, rattles, and dolls; however, instructional priorities should not primarily address how to use these toys. Such a goal is time limited. That is, those skills are age-appropriate for a short period in an individual's life. Given the difficulty with which children with the most severe disabilities have in acquiring new skills, in some cases, by the time a student learns the skill, it might be inappropriate for his or her age. It would be much more efficient to provide instruction on skills that will continue to be age-appropriate throughout a lifetime. It is more appropriate to focus on critical skills that could be used with various materials and that may change as a function of age. An example is teaching a child to push the lever on a busy box when the child is very young and using that same skill to push tape recorder levers as the child gets older.

EDUCATIONAL SERVICE DELIVERY

The previous sections have presented considerations in developing goals and establishing curricular priorities for young children with the most severe disabilities. Such goals may be met through a variety of approaches differing according to the setting (e.g., home, school, center), the target of instruction (e.g., parent, child), the instructor (e.g., educator, therapist, nurse) and the methodologies used. Throughout the country many such differences can be observed (Hanson, 1982). There is no research available that could provide information regarding the "best" model. Peterson (1987) points out that flexibility in service delivery may not only be necessary but is essential. The most important reason for its flexibility may be the fact that no single approach can be considered to be the best for all students. Flexibility, based upon the individual needs of students, may be optimal. Program variation may also be necessary due to a number of reasons: 1) geography may make center-based instruction inappropriate for young children who live two hours from the nearest center, and 2) an agency's theoretical and philosophical beliefs will determine if the program is parent-centered, child-centered, family systems oriented, or didactic instructionally orientated.

To reiterate, no one model can be said to be the best; however, considering a variety of models may be helpful. For this reason the Handicapped Children's Early Education Program (HCEEP) was enacted by federal legislation in 1968. The HCEEP set its goal at attaining the development, demonstration, and dissemination of a variety of educational models for young children with handicapping conditions. However, as was previously mentioned, few of these programs have focused specifically on the education of young children with very severe disabilities. Project SPICE (Special Program for Infant and Child Education), an HCEEP funded program, is one of the programs that has focused on those children with the most severe disabilities. The remainder of this chapter is designed to focus on that program's model for providing a center-based educational program for children between the ages of birth to 3 who have the most severe disabilities.

Project SPICE goals and objectives were based upon the following needs and assumptions regarding young children with the most severe handicapping conditions:

1. These children have learning and behavioral characteristics that interfere with their ability to acquire and generalize skills without the benefit of highly structured systematic instruction and data-based decisionmaking.
2. Such children require a unique curricular approach that recognizes their limitations to the normal developmental approach and their need for a functional curriculum that considers the utility of skills taught.
3. Children with very severe handicaps may be in families that need quality center-based care. It is believed that such care should not detract from, but rather could be combined with, instruction to maximize the instructional time available, and offer care providing opportunities in which to facilitate generalization of skills across settings and people.
4. These children may have health-related needs that must be met during school hours. Furthermore, these needs must be met in a manner that places an emphasis on the student as a child, and not as a patient.
5. These children need related services such as occupational, speech/language, and physical therapy to facilitate total development; however, such services must first be determined to be an integral part of the student's educational program.
6. These children are seen as part of a family unit, be it a natural, foster, or

adoptive family; therefore, an equal emphasis must be placed not only on the fostering of positive interactions between that child and other members of the family unit but also on the specific educational interventions for the child.

A number of components were considered essential to meet the unique needs of this population of students. Some of these components are explained in the following sections.

Program Location

Greater variability exists in program locations for young children with severe disabilities than for older children because of: 1) the unique needs of the children due to their age; 2) the lack of public school program mandates and, consequently, the variety of responsible agencies (contrasted with mandated local education agency responsibility for school-age children); 3) the philosophical orientation of the program's agency; and/or 4) the logistic considerations (i.e., where there is space available). Programs may be located in neonatal intensive care units, a child's home, school, and centers (Filler, 1983). Project SPICE was designed to be a center-based program, located in an agency serving children with mild to moderate disabilities. The justification for the center location was based on the community needs at the start of the program. At that time, there were no programs with a primary focus on the provision of education that also provided full-day programming. Working parents of children with severe disabilities were provided with opportunities for full-day child care; however, it was provided in a center with a student-teacher ratio higher than optimal for structured educational interventions. A full-day center-based educational program provided parents with an additional option.

Locating the program in a center with more mildly handicapped children represented a compromise. The desired goal was integration into a program with young children without disabilities. However, this area, like many others, was experiencing extreme shortages in programs for this nonhandicapped population due to the lack of available space, caregivers, and funding. No program could be located that could assist in meeting those goals. An existing program operated by the Easter Seal Society of Milwaukee County was interested in working together with the project staff in order to develop a model that would meet the goal of integration and that was able to provide the project with space in their building. Consequently, the classroom was located there.

Combining Care and Instruction

Staff that work in center-based educational programs for young children with severe disabilities find themselves engaged in two primary activities: caregiving and instruction. Careful attention must be paid to the manner in which these two activities are delivered to ensure that quality, hygienic care is provided and to guarantee that caregiving does not detract from instructional time.

Historically, an entrance requirement for school admission was bladder and bowel control—children had to be toilet-trained. That is no longer a prerequisite. Very often, children attending school programs require extensive care similar to that provided in daycare centers. Educational institutions that are not accustomed to attending to such needs as diaper changing and feeding have not adequately addressed methods for meeting these needs in a manner that ensures hygienic group care (Wood, Walker, & Gardner 1986). This can be contrasted with the tremendous emphasis on hygienic caregiving procedures and contingent licensing of daycare programs (Lawton, 1988; Marotz, Rush, & Cross, 1985).

Regardless of the quality of caregiving, it was reported by McCormick, Cooper, and Goldman (1979) that attention to the care needs of children with severe disabilities results in a decrease in available instructional time. McCormick et al. (1979) also showed that instructional time could be increased by teaching instructional staff to combine care with instruction.

Project SPICE was designed to provide education to children with the most severe disabilities using a center-based model. It was structured to incorporate hygienic caregiving procedures into the educational program. This was accomplished through a zoned staffing approach, the uses of instructional and caregiving routines, and the establishment of structured scheduling and monitoring of the students.

Zoned Staffing Approach   The classroom and daily structure of Project SPICE was based upon the recognition that young children primarily participate in four activities: eating, sleeping, eliminating, and playing. Consequently, Project SPICE uses the zoned staffing approach that is used with non-handicapped infants (Herbert-Jackson, O'Brien, Porterfield, & Risley, 1977). Modifications were made to meet the unique needs of the specialized population of infants and young children that are served by Project SPICE.

The physical space in the classroom was divided into three functional zones through the use of low barriers: activity, eating/napping, and diapering/toileting. Each of three staff members (i.e., a teacher and two instructional aides) was assigned to a specific zone for a period of one hour. Hourly rotations to other zones occurred as specified on a posted schedule (see Figure 9.2). Such a staffing pattern had advantages such as: 1) all staff were involved in instruction as well as caregiving, 2) all staff became knowledgeable of specific instructional objectives that they could then incorporate into caregiving, and 3) all staff worked with each child in every setting facilitating generalization of skills across persons, places, and materials.

Instructional Procedures   Instruction was organized based upon an individualized curriculum sequence (ICS) (Guess et al., 1978; Helmstetter,

Project SPICE

STAFF				STUDENTS							
ACTIVITY	EAT/NAP	TOILET	TIME	Kim	Don	Terry	John	Karl	Allison	Lori	Sue
KC	P	K	9:30		Drink	Drink	O.T. / Drink	Drink	Drink	Nap	Drink
K	KC	P	10:30		Eat	Eat	Drink	Eat		Drink	
P	K	KC	11:30	MEDS / Eat		Nap	Nap	Nap	Eat	MEDS / Eat	Eat
KC	P	K	12:30	Nap			Eat		Nap		Nap
K	KC	P	1:30		Drink	Drink	P.T.	Drink			
P	K	KC	2:30							Drink	Drink

Figure 9.2. An example of a master schedule that reflects zoned staffing. (KC = staff person one; P = staff person two; K = staff person three; O.T. = occupational therapy; P.T. = physical therapy.)

Murphy-Herd, Roberts, & Guess, 1984; Holvoet, Guess, Mulligan, & Brown, 1980). The ICS incorporates a number of components that reflect the current best practices in the area of education of students with severe handicaps (Bambara, Warren, & Komisar, 1988). The components, as described by Holvoet, Mulligan, Schussler, Lacy, & Guess (1982), include:

1. Use of functional materials and activities
2. Use of functional settings and cues
3. Use of varied materials
4. Incorporation of behavioral checks
5. Distribution of practice
6. Incorporation of instruction on communication, motor, and social goals with other instructional programs
7. Group instruction

Considering the usual activities of young children, it was decided that unless the children's care needs were being attended to, they should play. Thus, all students were scheduled to use the activity area of the room as a "home base." In this zone, students were offered structured learning opportunities, but only within the context of play. Targeted skills in each area of development were clustered together and sequenced as they would naturally occur. A skill cluster was described by Mulligan Ault (1988) as:

> . . . a group of two to five educational objectives that, when sequenced together, produce a functional unit of behavior for the student when interacting with the environment. Examples may be reach and grasp, maintaining visual fixation, auditory localization, and maintaining head in midline. The opportunity to practice these objectives may be sequenced so as to not only teach the individual skills to the student but to teach the relationship between the skills. (p. 251)

This cluster of skills could then be taught across materials in the activity area and all other zones of the room, whenever natural opportunities occurred or could be arranged.

The activity zone manager had the responsibility of implementing the specific instructional strategies stated as a written instructional program and prepared for each objective included in the sequence. The specific student actions in the sequences were specified on a data sheet along with cues and correction procedures for quick reference. An illustration of a data sheet is provided in Figure 9.3. Data were recorded concurrently with instruction.

Routine Caregiving Procedures The managers of the other zones followed the procedures as illustrated in Figure 9.4. Additionally, specific procedures for feeding, sleeping, awakening, and diapering a child were delineated and posted in each zone.

Since each staff member rotated through every zone of the program, they were all knowledgeable of instructional and caregiving priorities for each child.

DATA SHEET

Special Program for Infant and Child Education

Objective No. 2.1

Name __Jeffrey__

Objective: __head control, localizing sound, obtaining Objects__

Materials

__age-appropriate toys which produce sound__

__tumble form chair__

Behaviors

Cue/Prompt	Student Actions
	3. Get it, Jeffrey holds/touches obj. momentarily full phys.
	2. produce sound 30° turns head 10 sound w/in 10sec
side of midline	
	1. hold toy midline; hold's head slightly forward
produce sound   for 5 seconds at midline

Corrections

Date: 4/10, 4/10, 4/10, 4/11, 4/11, 4/12, 5/1

Time: 10:15, 10:28, 11:45, 11:20, 10:30, 10:15, 10:30

Initials: KPB KPB KPB KK BB

Reinforcers __Verbal praise__

Schedule __1:1__

0 = correct response
X = incorrect or no response

● = % correct

Figure 9.3. An example of an individualized curriculum sequence data sheet.

DIAPERING PROCEDURE CHECKLIST
Step 1: Check every child as they arrive in the morning
Step 2: Check any child who is scheduled to leave within half an hour
Step 3: Check any child who is scheduled to eat soon
Step 4: Check any child who will soon be put down to nap
Step 5: Diaper any child who another caregiver tells you is wet or soiled
Step 6: Check any child who has not been checked or changed in your hour
For each child:

Getting ready
Step 1: Get the child's diaper bin, read the notes above the diapering table, and set the bin on the diapering table
Step 2: Take the materials needed for diapering out of the diaper bin
Step 3: Get the diaper ready

Diapering
Step 1: Go get the child or have someone bring him to you and put him gently on the diapering table
Step 2: Remove the child's diaper, clean the child, and apply powders and ointments as the above diapering table indicates
Step 3: Diaper the child
Step 4: Dress the child
Step 5: Be sociable while you are changing diapers
Step 6: Take the child to their designated area when completed

Cleaning up
Step 1: Take care of the diaper
Step 2: Clean up the other supplies used
Step 3: Clean the diapering table with the spray disinfectant
Step 4: Wash your hands

Recording
Step 1: Record the diapering on the child's daily schedule and note whether he or she was wet or had a bowel movement
Step 2: Move the clipboard to the same area as the child

Making daily health checks
Step 1: Look at the child from head to toe
Step 2: Have the coordinator look at anything unusual
Step 3: Diaper the child and return him or her to another area
Step 4: Record anything unusual on the daily schedule

SLEEPING PROCEDURE CHECKLIST
Step 1: Plan ahead so that the children are put down for a nap before they become overtired
Step 2: Check the child's diaper
Step 3: Get a crib ready by lowering sides and placing blankets down
Step 4: Bring the child to the sleep area and put him or her in a crib
Step 5: Raise the side of the crib and fasten it securely
Step 6: Place the child's clipboard next to his or her crib
Step 7: Attend to individual children according to special sleep instructions

GETTING CHILDREN UP FROM SLEEPING
Step 1: Attend to any child that is standing up either crying or quiet in his or her crib
Step 2: If his or her nap is over, lower sides of crib and lift child out
Step 3: Check clipboard—mark length of time child has slept
Step 4: Take child and clipboard to staff in diaper changing zone
Step 5: Remove that child's blankets from the crib and store them for use next time

Figure 9.4. Examples of care providing procedures. (Adapted from Herbert-Jackson, E., O'Brien, M., Porterfield, J., & Risley, T. R. [1977]. *The infant center.* Baltimore: University Park Press; reprinted with permission.)

(continued)

Figure 9.4. *(continued)*

FEEDING PROCEDURE CHECKLIST
Step 1: Plan ahead by looking at the master schedule board
Step 2: Wash your hands
Step 3: Read the feeding instructions on the feeding chart
Step 4: Take the child's food storage tray out of the refrigerator and set it on the counter
Step 5: Remove the child's feeding supplies from the food storage tray and put the tray back in the refrigerator
Step 6: Prepare the amount of food suggested on the feeding chart near the refrigerator
Step 7: Place prepared food and feeding supplies on a serving tray
Step 8: Decide where the child will eat, place the serving tray and clipboard on a table nearby, and get the child's chair ready
Step 9: Check the time of feeding on the daily schedule and note the amount of food that the child ate during his or her meal. Also note any other observations regarding mealtime that should be communicated to the parent/guardian

The importance of teaching across "zones" was emphasized. That is, the diapering zone managers were encouraged to incorporate the ICS into their diapering routine as appropriate. Eating area managers were similarly encouraged to use that method. The consequence was the opportunity for students to demonstrate skills across people, places, and materials; a strategy essential to facilitating generalization. Data on the children's responses in these settings were taken periodically to determine if, in fact, generalization did occur.

Structured Scheduling and Monitoring A schedule posted on a classroom wall, large enough to be seen throughout the room, ensured that: 1) each staff member knew their zone assignment, and 2) each student's schedule for eating, napping, or medications was clearly specified and understood by all staff members (Figure 9.2). This schedule was modified daily to reflect changes in the students' needs or staff and student absences. The Velcro-backed cards made such changes easy to accomplish.

Each zone manager was responsible for recording both specific program data on the data sheets (Figure 9.3) and general information on each student's daily schedule (Figure 9.5). One copy of the daily schedule form was retained at school and the other was sent home to the parents to inform them about their child's day. Space was included on the form for return messages. Such a monitoring system facilitated the communication of information across staff and families while minimizing the amount of time spent in recording information.

Providing for Special Health Care Needs

Many young children with the most severe disabilities have accompanying special health care needs including the need for apnea monitoring, tube feeding, and mechanical suctioning (McDonald, Wilson, Turner, & Mulligan Ault, 1988; see also Chapter 6, this volume). To enable these students to attend and

DAILY SCHEDULE

Special Program for Infant and Child Education

Name Jeffrey

D.O.B. 6/5/83 Age 2 Date 10/10/85

TIME	*ACTIVITY E	S	D/T	A	COMMENTS
9:00-9:30			✓		wet
9:30-10:00	✓				ate all fruit!! meds - P.U.
10:00-10:30			✓	✓	wet
10:30-11:00				✓	rolling went well
11:00-11:30			✓	✓	
11:30-12:00	✓	✓			fell asleep during tube feeding
12:00-12:30		✓			
12:30-1:00			✓	✓	wet
1:00-1:30				✓	liked new playdough
1:30-2:00			✓	✓	suctioned before eating
2:00-2:30	✓				meds P.U.
2:30-3:00			✓	✓	

* Activity Code
E: EAT D/T: DIAPER/TOILET
S: SLEEP A: ACTIVITY

PLEASE SEND MORE:
FOOD fruit DIAPERS ______
CLOTHES ______ OTHER ______

NOTE TO PARENT/GUARDIAN	NOTE BACK TO SCHOOL
J. had a great day! He needed suctioning just once. Tube feeding went fast! He was so relaxed he fell asleep. Is it too cool now for outside trips?	

Figure 9.5. An example of a child's daily schedule.

benefit from the full-day school-based educational programs, specific health-related procedures had to be administered at school. While various models exist for meeting the health-related needs of such students (Sirvis, 1988; see also Chapter 6), in Project SPICE, the educational staff were responsible for administering the procedures in the classroom.

It is easier to educate students when their health-related needs are implemented in the classroom by instructional staff rather than having the school nurse provide the care. When students are in the classroom, educational programs can be continued with minimal interruptions. The health-related procedures can be incorporated into the daily routines and not viewed as an "intrusion" in the student's instructional day. Similarly, instruction on priority objectives can occur simultaneously as health care is being provided. The "down time" for these students is also decreased since students do not need to sit and wait for their medications or feedings; nor, as previously stated, must the caregiving be accomplished without instruction. Some of the methods used for meeting the health-related needs of students with severe disabilities include staff training, communications assistance, and implementing emergency procedures.

Staff Training Procedures   The staff at project SPICE participated in a number of different training experiences to gain the necessary skills that were needed to provide appropriate physical and health-related care to the students. All staff completed standard American Red Cross first aid courses that included training in cardiopulmonary resuscitation (CPR) for adults and infants. Special training sessions were arranged for the staff to teach them: the correct procedures for using the apnea monitors, feeding tubes, and suctioning instruments; the proper care of tracheotomies; and the various methods of feeding, positioning, and/or handling disabilities and handicapping conditions by instructional nursing staff at a local hospital. Additionally, specific information regarding procedures for meeting the children's unique medical needs was gained through written and oral contact with each child's physician. Demonstrations were then provided by the parents to ensure specificity and consistency for each child. If questions or major differences regarding variations in the procedures occurred, the child's physician was contacted to resolve the inconsistencies.

Communicating with Parents and Involved Professionals   Communicating with other people involved with the students was very important to ensure that the best care was given and to establish consistent daily routines. This communication occurred daily with the family by use of the daily schedule (Figure 9.5) form that was sent home from school with the child. Any unusual behaviors, problems, or new skills were noted on the form, as well as documentation of medication administration, seizures, or monitor alerts. Reviews of instructional data enabled the team of professionals to see if there were patterns that were developing with specific behaviors or conditions. If there were, immediate appropriate action could then be taken. If any serious problems occurred or questions arose, the family and/or physician were contacted immediately.

Emergency Procedures   While the need for the administration of emergency procedures is always possible in any program serving children, it is inevitable in programs that serve infants with severe multiple handicaps and special health care needs. Since "no practical plan can assure that health professionals can arrive within the critical minutes in which definitive action is required" (McDonald et al., 1988, p. 96), school personnel must be prepared to respond immediately. Consequently, a clear delineation of emergency procedures is essential. The plan used in Project SPICE specified:

1. How to alert others in the room that assistance is needed
2. Who should assume primary responsibility to providing emergency care
3. Who should contact the rescue squad
4. Who should contact the family
5. Who would accompany the child to the hospital, if necessary
6. How will other children be treated

Family Involvement

The family becomes involved in the child's intervention through home-school communications efforts and joint planning sessions.

Home-School Communication   Young children, both with and without disabilities, are continually growing, changing, and participating in new events and activities. Therefore, the child's parents, whether natural, foster, or adopted, want to be aware of these changes. This is especially true when parent and child are not together all the time. When a child is in an early childhood program of any sort and away from his or her mother and/or father, it becomes very important for the staff of the program to communicate with the parents and to inform them of the child's general and daily events. If the child has developmental or medical problems it becomes imperative that critical information be shared daily.

Project SPICE built into its program a structured system for communicating with the families of its students. One part of the system utilizes the aforementioned form called the daily schedule (Figure 9.5). Every staff person was assigned the responsibility for recording his or her pertinent information for the day. At the end of the day, the teacher wrote a brief summative note to the parents and then sent the daily schedule form home with the student. It was then returned to school the next morning with messages from parents.

Joint Planning Sessions   Another component of Project SPICE's interest in family involvement was the biweekly Joint Planning Session with each individual family. The purpose of the biweekly Joint Planning Session was to work with the parents on planning and implementing educational programs for their children. It should be noted that the term "joint planning" is used instead of often-used-terms such as "parent training" or "parent education." The intention was for the staff to work together with the parents rather than having them assume to be experts, imparting knowledge to parents. The parents, considered to be the experts on their child, were considered partners on the educational team. To accomplish this most effectively, the *Early On Home Intervention Program* (Early on Staff, 1978) was used. Each Joint Planning Session was begun by discussing the activity that was jointly prepared at the last session. A sample activity can be viewed in Figure 9.6. In this example, the teacher observed the parent implementing a specific activity with the child and determined possible plan modifications, if needed. Summarized information was recorded on the Joint Planning Session Form (Figure 9.7). If the child had not completed an activity successfully, the teacher and parent might have decided to modify the activity, continue to work on it, or suspend work on it and begin a new one.

If satisfactory progress had been made by the child in the activity, the teacher and parent discussed ideas for new activities. The teacher often came to sessions with ideas of future activities; however, the goal of the Joint Planning Session was to have the parents generate ideas for themselves. For any activity that was agreed upon, it was considered important to discuss the reasons behind the activity and what skills would be developed when the activity was learned. Once the activity had been agreed upon, the teacher wrote out the steps to be followed by the family members to ensure consistency by staff at school and family at home. The teacher then used a *model, lead, and test* sequence with the parent for clarification of that activity. Below is a description of each step:

Model: After explaining the activity to the parent, the teacher demonstrates implementation of the activity with the child. During this modeling step, the teacher also records data on the student's performance, thus gaining baseline data and serving as a model of how to collect data.

Lead: After the teacher has modeled the activity, he or she leads the parent in implementing the activity with the child. He or she offers suggestions and makes corrections regarding how the parent presented the activity.

Test: To ensure that the parent fully understood the activity, the teacher asks the parent to implement the activity independently. The teacher also checks the parent's understanding of data collection by having him or her record the data.

At the end of the session the parents and teacher engaged in a general conversation regarding the child's progress in school; situations that needed to be problem-solved were discussed, and new resources or materials were shared.

SUMMARY

While children with the most severe disabilities are often identified at birth, gaps in mandates may result in no programs being offered to such children. Due to the complexities of their needs, serious complications and consequences

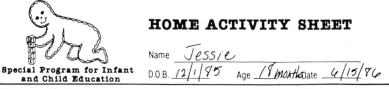

HOME ACTIVITY SHEET

Special Program for Infant
and Child Education

Name _Jessie_

D.O.B. _12/1/85_   Age _18 months_ Date _4/15/86_

The activity is: Program Planner _Penny_

Moving her head trward the sound & holding the
noise producing object.

The reason for this activity is:

To increase motor skills and participation in
functional activities

The materials needed are:

Household materials - see procedures below

The way to record is:

O each time she moves head & touches
   and holds object momentarily
X if she does not

The procedures to follow are:

When ever you are doing household chores
that lend themselves ...

1. position Jessie in wheelchair
      near you
2. produce a sound with the object
      (hit side of pan with spoon;
      shake cleaning solution in
      container, etc.)
3. Observe to see if J moves
      head forward and arm forward.
      Physically assist if necessary

Figure 9.6. An example of a child's home activity sheet.

may result for these children and their families. Very early intervention is necessary to facilitate development, prevent further disabilities, provide support to the families, and reduce the future costs of care by providing less expensive early intervention.

Despite this critical need, few descriptions of educational programs exist that specifically address students with the most severe disabilities. Usual prac-

JOINT PLANNING REPORT

Name ___Tim___

Special Program for Infant and Child Education

D.O.B. _10/2/83_ Age _1 ½_ Date _7/25/85_

Activity Summary	Met Criteria yes no	Suspended yes no	Continued yes no	Parent Generated yes no	Data Taken yes no
#1	X			X	X
#2	X		X	X	X

Previous Activity	Curricular Area	Activity Description	Baseline	Post Baseline
	Soc/Lang/ motor	extends hands to " Let's get up "	10%	80%

Current Activity	Curricular Area	Activity Description	Baseline
	eating	Goal: increase rate to ½ cup in 20 min	½ c. in 30 min.

Log Information (Appointments, schedule changes, medical update, general comments.)

- Shorten naps - 45-1 hr max.
- Copies of IEP should be sent to therapists, pediatrician
- blood work shows everything OK.
- observe therapy 7/30

Figure 9.7. An example of a Joint Planning Report Form.

tice is to borrow appropriate examples of educational programs from literature addressing the needs of individuals with severe handicaps or young children with mild and moderate handicaps. Teachers who attempt to apply this literature to their programs often have difficulties. Use of these models does not always result in meaningful goals and objectives for students. Alternative goals and objectives placed along a continuum may be appropriate to consider with developing curricular priorities for infants with the most severe disabilities.

Young children with the most severe disabilities require special considerations in the delivery of educational programs. Their very young age, their need for routine caregiving, and their probable need for specialized healthcare dictate the inclusion of particular program components that address the needs that are related to the children and their families. Models such as the one presented in this chapter must be considered.

Increases can be seen in the number of infants with the most severe disabilities; however, little research exists that provides us with clear direction. Much additional attention must be paid to this population of students to ensure that their very critical early start is optimal.

REFERENCES

Bailey, D. B., Jr., & Wolery, M. (1984). *Teaching infants and preschoolers with handicaps.* Columbus, OH: Charles E. Merrill.

Bambara, L. M., Warren, S. F., & Komisar, S. (1988). The individualized curriculum sequencing model: Effects on skill acquisition and generalization. *Journal of The Association for Persons with Severe Handicaps, 13*(1), 8–19.

Bates, P., Morrow, S. A., Pancosfar, E., & Sedlak, R. (1984). The effect of functional vs. non-functional activities on attitudes/expectations of non-handicapped college students: What they see is what they get. *Journal of The Association for Persons with Severe Handicaps, 9*(2), 73–78.

Baumgart, D., Brown, L., Pumpian, I., Nisbet, J., Ford, A., Sweet, M., Messina, R., & Schroeder, J. (1982). Principle of partial participation and individualized adaptations in educational programs for severely handicapped students. *Journal of The Association for Persons with Severe Handicaps, 7*(2), 17–27.

Bricker, D. (1986). *Early education of at-risk and handicapped infants, toddlers, and preschool children.* Glenview, IL: Scott, Foresman.

Bricker, D., & Kaminski, R. (1986). Intervention programs for severely handicapped infants and children. In L. Blickman & D. L. Weatherford (Eds.), *Evaluating early intervention programs for severely handicapped children and their families* (pp. 51–78). Austin, TX: PRO-ED.

Brown, F. (1987). Meaningful assessment of people with severe and profound handicaps. In M. E. Snell (Ed.), *Systematic Instruction of Persons with Severe Handicaps* (pp. 39–63). Columbus, OH: Charles E. Merrill.

Brown, F., Evans, I. M., Weed, K. A., & Owen, V. (1987). Delineative functional competencies: A component model. *Journal of The Association for Persons With Severe Handicaps, 12,* 117–124.

Brown, F., Helmstetter, E., & Guess, D. (1986). *Current best practices with students with profound disabilities: Are there any?* Unpublished manuscript, Institute of Professional Practice, New Haven.

Brown, L., Nietupski, J., & Hamre-Nietupski, S. (1976). The criterion of ultimate functioning and public school services for severely handicapped students. In M. Thomas (Ed.), *Hey, don't forget about me: New directions for serving the severely handicapped* (pp. 2–15). Reston, VA: Council for Exceptional Children.

Cook, R., Tessier, A., & Armbruster, V. B. (1987). *Adapting early childhood curriculum for children with special needs.* Columbus, OH: Charles E. Merrill.

Early On Staff. (1978). *Early On Home Intervention Program.* San Diego: San Diego State University, Department of Special Education.

Ferguson, D. (1987). *Curriculum decision making for students with severe handicaps.* New York: Teacher's College Press.

Filler, J. (1983). Service delivery model for handicapped infants. In G. Garwood & R. Fewell (Eds.), *Educating handicapped infants* (pp. 369–386). Rockville, MD: Aspen Publishers Inc.

Gaylord-Ross, R. J., & Holvoet, J. F. (1985). *Strategies for educating students with severe handicaps.* Boston: Little, Brown.

Gentry, D., & Olson, J. (1985). Severely mentally retarded young children. In D. Bricker & J. Filler (Eds.). *Severe mental retardation: From theory to practice* (pp. 50–75). Reston, VA: Council for Exceptional Children.

Guess, D., Horner, D., Utley, B., Holvoet, J., Maxon, D., Tucker, D., & Warren, S. (1978). A functional curriculum sequencing model for teaching the severely handicapped. *AAESPH Review, 3,* 202–215.

Hanson, M. J. (1982). Issues in designing intervention approaches from developmental theory and research. In D. Bricker (Ed.), *Intervention with at risk and handicapped infants* (pp. 249–268). Austin, Texas: PRO-ED.

Helmstetter, E., Murphy-Herd, M.C., Roberts, S., & Guess, D. (1984). *Individualized curriculum sequence and extended classroom models for learners who are deaf and blind.* Unpublished manuscript, University of Kansas, Department of Special Education, Lawrence.

Herbert-Jackson, E., O'Brien, M., Porterfield, J., & Risley, T. R. (1977). *The infant center.* Baltimore: University Park Press.

Holvoet, J., Guess, D., Mulligan, M., & Brown, F. (1980). The individualized curriculum sequencing model (II): A teaching strategy for severely handicapped students. *Journal of The Association for the Severely Handicapped, 5,* 325–336.

Holvoet, J., Mulligan, M., Schussler, N., Lacy, L., & Guess, D. (1982). *The KICS Model: Sequencing learning experiences for severely handicapped children and youth.* Unpublished manuscript, University of Kansas, Department of Special Education, Lawrence.

Lawton, J. T. (1988). *Introduction to child care and early childhood education.* Glenview, IL: Scott, Foresman.

Marotz, L., Rush, J., & Cross, M. (1985). *Health, safety and nutrition for the young child.* Albany: Delmar Publishers.

McCormick, L., Cooper, M., & Goldman, R. (1979). Training teachers to maximize instructional time provide to severely and profoundly handicapped children. *AAESPH Review, 4,* 301–310.

McDonald, P.L., Wilson, R., Turner, R., & Mulligan Ault, M. (1988). Classroom-based medical interventions. In L. Sternberg (Ed.), *Educating students with severe or profound handicaps* (pp. 53–100). Rockville, MD: Aspen Publishers Inc.

Mulligan Ault, M. (1988). Curriculum development. In L. Sternberg (Ed.), *Educating students with severe or profound handicaps* (pp. 219–266). Rockville, MD: Aspen Systems.

Neisworth, J. T., & Bagnato, S. J. (1987). *The young exceptional child.* New York: Macmillan.

Peterson, N. L. (1987). *Early intervention for handicapped and at-risk children.* Denver: Love Publishing Co.

Public Law 90-538, *Handicapped Children's Early Education Assistance Act,* 1968.

Public Law 94-142, *Education for All Handicapped Children Act of 1975,* § 121, 1975.

Public Law 99-457, *Education of the Handicapped Amendments of 1986,* §§ 619, 676, 1986.

Sirvis, B. (1988). Students with special health care needs. *Teaching Exceptional Children, 20*(4), 40–44.

Snell, M. E. (1987). *Systematic instruction of persons with severe handicaps.* Columbus, OH: Charles E. Merrill.

Thurman, S. K., & Widerstrom, A. H. (1985). *Young children with special needs.* Newton, MA: Allyn & Bacon.

Vincent, L. J., Salisbury, C., Walter, G. Brown, P., Gruenwald, L. J., & Powers, M. (1980). Program evaluation and curriculum development in early childhood/special education: Criteria of the next environment. In W. Sailor, B. Wilcox, & L. Brown (Eds.), *Methods of instruction for severely handicapped students* (pp. 303–328). Baltimore: Paul H. Brookes Publishing Co.

Weatherford, D. L. (1986). The challenge of evaluating early intervention programs for severely handicapped children and their families. In L. Bickman & D. L. Weatherford (Eds.), *Evaluating early intervention programs for severely handicapped children and their families* (pp. 1–20). Austin, TX: PRO-ED.

Wood, S. P., Walker, D. K., & Gardner, J. (1986). School health practices for children with complex medical needs. *Journal of School Health, 56*(6), 215–217.

CURRICULUM FOR SCHOOL-AGE STUDENTS
The Ecological Model

Edwin Helmstetter

Instructional practices with persons with severe disabilities have shifted from a basic skills model to an ecological approach that emphasizes the preparation of students to function in domestic settings that are located in the community; in integrated competitive work and recreational/leisure environments; and in other generic service environments such as transportation systems, stores, and restaurants. Unfortunately, with only a few exceptions, this model has seen little use with those students with the most severe disabilities. Specifically, these students include those who have inconsistent or no motor movement, who appear to possess very low IQs (e.g., below 15), or who are referred to in such denigrative terms as "medically fragile" (Brown, Helmstetter, & Guess, 1986).

ECOLOGICAL MODEL

Although the ecological model is rarely used with students with the most severe disabilities, it is appropriate for this group of individuals. The ineffectiveness of basic skills training, limited exposure to normal experiencing and every individual's right to equality are three reasons why this is true.

Ineffective Basic Skills Training

Research and practice with students with the most severe disabilities has traditionally emphasized training on basic skills such as bearing weight, reaching, activating a microswitch connected to an attention-getting signal, visual attention, and head control. The rationale for this approach appears to be that basic skills training, while it rarely leads to full independence, will presumably allow

and general community use areas (e.g., stores, restaurants, transportation systems, healthcare services).

2. Select specific current and future least restrictive environments in which a student might participate (e.g., corner market, movie theater).

3. Conduct ecological inventories of the current and future environments for the purpose of delineating their subenvironments (e.g., the kitchen is a subenvironment of the home), and for identifying the activities that typically occur in the subenvironments (e.g., washing dishes occurs in the kitchen subenvironment).

4. Establish priorities among the activities and select the highest ranking ones for instruction. The activities selected will constitute the goals of the student's individualized education program (IEP).

5. List the sequence of skills for each activity that was selected that nondisabled persons typically use in order to complete the activity.

6. Conduct a discrepancy analysis for each activity in order to identify how the individual's present skills compare to the skills that nondisabled persons use in completing the activity.

7. Develop individualized adaptations for those skills that the student lacks and is unlikely to learn quickly.

8. For each activity, develop an IEP objective that takes into consideration the results of the discrepancy analysis and the individualized adaptations.

9. Address implementation issues such as scheduling, staffing, transportation, and locating monetary resources.

The remainder of this chapter briefly describes each of the above steps and illustrates how the process might be extended for use with students with the most severe disabilities. The following points are stressed when the ecological model is implemented with persons who are the most severely disabled:

1. There is greater emphasis on partial participation in activities (Baumgart et al., 1982) than on no participation at all. For example, a student who is unable to independently use a vending machine to purchase a snack can partially participate by pushing the selection button after a companion deposits money in the machine. Furthermore, partial participation is interpreted to mean not only active motor involvement in an activity (e.g., pushing a vending machine button, signing a prewritten check with a name stamp), but also relatively passive behaviors that enable the individual to obtain information about the environment (e.g., visual or auditory attending, tolerating noisy or novel settings).

2. The use of adaptations is emphasized (Step 7 of basic steps from the previous section). Adaptations make it easier for students to fully or partially participate in activities, and reduce the need for extensive skill training. For example, for a student with poor motor control, the buttons on a remote control for a television could be covered, a hole cut out for the channel

change button, and the device fastened to a surface. These adaptations would eliminate the need for lengthy training on the motor skills needed to hold the remote control and to touch only one button at a time. Furthermore, it would provide the student with immediate control over one aspect of his or her environment.

3. More attention is given to how students respond to settings and activities. This information is then used to identify student preferences. A student's response might consist of minute responses that previously may have gone unnoticed (e.g., change in muscle tone, averting the eyes), or were observed but regarded as noncommunicative (e.g., tantrums, stereotyped behavior) (See Chapter 7, this volume, for a detailed discussion of identifying communicative responses). Information on the student's preferences with regard to settings and activities should be considered when establishing priorities for selecting various activities for instruction. It is also useful information for parents and residential staff who can then provide the individual with at least access, if not training, to his or her preferred settings and activities. It is recommended that this important process of identifying student responses become a new step in the ecological model (see previous section of this chapter), inserted between the ecological inventory (Step 3) and establishing priorities (Step 4).

Underpinning the first and second adaptations that were just described (i.e., partial participation and the use of technology) is the assumption that partial participation, regardless of its amount, is a valid educational goal. Underpinning the third adaptation (i.e., assessment of student preference for settings and activities) is the assumption that improving one's quality of life is a valid educational outcome, and that quality of life is improved when an individual gains access to situations that he or she prefers, even if participation in these situations is extremely limited.

Identifying Settings in the Community

The first step of the ecological model is to identify the integrated settings that are available in the community. Table 10.1 lists examples of the types of environments that exist in many communities. Resources to identify specific community settings (e.g., French's Cafe, Acme Movie Theater, Supported Living Alternatives) include local newspapers; telephone books; entertainment guides; parent or professional organizations; publications of the state Developmental Disabilities Planning Council; the Chamber of Commerce business directories; the United Way's directory of funded agencies; and directories compiled by state vocational, educational, health, and social service agencies. In addition, a drive or walk through the community is a very useful way to identify businesses, industries, recreational settings, and other community environments in which students might participate.

Table 10.1. Examples of types of environments

Domestic	*General community environments*
Natural homes	Transportation systems (e.g., bus, subway, taxi)
Adoptive homes	
Trained foster families with no other disabled persons	Intersections (e.g., controlled, uncontrolled)
Shared apartments or homes with non-disabled adults	Restaurants (e.g., fast food, sit down/order, cafeteria)
Supervised apartments or homes with 1–2 disabled persons	Grocery stores (e.g., supermarkets, small convenience stores)
Group homes with five or fewer persons	Merchandise stores (e.g., clothing, general merchandise, sports, hardware, pet, pharmaceutical)
Work	
Stores: grocery, clothing, general merchandise, sports, music, hardware, pharmaceutical, pet	Service locations (e.g., doctor, dentist, hairstylist, post office, bank)
Industries	*Community recreational/leisure*
Libraries	Arcades
Courthouses	Nature centers and trails
Employment agency buildings	Arts and crafts classes
Public health buildings	Libraries
Mental health buildings	Cultural centers
United Way offices	Shopping centers
American Red Cross facilities	Parks
Service organization facilities (e.g., Lions, Rotary Club)	Movle theaters
Parks and Recreation facilities	Bowling alleys
Fire and police departments	Fishing ponds
Universities and colleges	Boating areas
Hospitals	Horseback riding stables
Churches and synagogues	Beaches
Laundromats	Swimming pools
Housekeeping services	Skating rinks
	Spectator sports arenas

Selecting Specific Current and Future Environments

For 5–10-year-olds, more emphasis is placed on current domestic, recreational/leisure, and community use environments and activities, as well as on opportunities for students to make friends at school and in their home communities. As the student approaches 10 years of age, more and more of what is needed in the current environments should overlap with what will be needed in future environments as well.

For 11–21-year-olds, the major emphasis is on what is needed for postschool domestic, recreational/leisure, work, and community use settings, as well as on opportunities to form friendships at school that will carry over into the student's life as an adult.

When selecting an appropriate, specific current or future environment for an individual, the interventionist must take into account that person's domestic, recreational/leisure, work, and general community environments.

Domestic Environment Least restrictive living situations for 5–10-year-old children include the natural or adoptive home, or a foster home in which the parents are trained and have few, if any, other disabled foster children. Unfortunately, many 5–10-year-old children with the most severe disabilities reside away from their home communities, in institutions or other congregate living arrangements. These congregate care programs are inappropriate targets as current environments. Instead, the teacher, social worker, or case manager should identify the least restrictive residential options in the student's home community as the current placement to be inventoried, and advocate for the individual who is most severely disabled to move to such homes. The preferred residential options are the natural home or an adoptive home. For persons who are 11–21 years old, the preferred future living environments are shared apartments or homes with nondisabled persons, supervised apartments, or homes with five or fewer disabled persons.

Recreational/Leisure Environments Recreational/leisure settings exist at home, at school, and in the community. Recreational/leisure environments for 5–10-year-old children are age-appropriate settings in the current home and school, as well as community recreational/leisure settings currently frequented by the students' families. For the 11–21 age group, emphasis is placed upon the recreational/leisure subenvironments found in those individuals' future residential settings, and the environments in his or her community. Also emphasized are the recreational/leisure settings at school that maximize social integration and the development of friendships that might last into adulthood.

Work Environments Future work settings are referenced beginning at age 11 and include: 1) actual community competitive employment sites; and 2) other work situations, such as school jobs and community volunteer work, where students can learn general work skills (e.g., travel using public transportation, maintaining balance while seated in a car enroute to work), and can obtain extra practice on skills required in competitive employment settings (e.g., moving a lever to dump items during a packaging activity) (cf. Chapter 11, this volume).

General Community Environments General community environments for 5- to 10-year-old children should be those settings that the individual can visit from his or her current living environment. For the 11–21 age group, community environments should include those that will likely be visited from the future domestic setting.

Identifying Subenvironments and Corresponding Activities

After the specific current and future environments are identified for a student, the settings are visited, and the subenvironments are delineated. For example, the current recreational/leisure environments that a fictitious student uses or might use would be the Cinerama and Twilight movie theaters, and Eastside park. Future leisure environments might be the Cinerama and Twilight movie theaters, the YMCA swimming pool, and Metro Public Library. Future work environments for this individual could include the Metro Public Library and the Memorial Hospital. Each of these environments would be visited in order to identify their subenvironments. Examples of subenvironments of the Cinerama theater are the parking lot, entrance, ticket booth, refreshment area, restroom, and seating area. Subenvironments of the library are the entrance, reference desk, checkout desk, work room, reading area, book shelf area, and current periodicals room.

In addition to listing the subenvironments of each setting, the activities that typically occur in each subenvironment are also delineated. One approach for generating the list of activities is to observe nondisabled persons, and to note the activities in which they typically participate. For example, possible activities that may be conducted in the parking lot subenvironment of the library are entering and exiting an automobile, using sidewalks and crosswalks, locating the library entrance, and placing books in the overnight deposit box.

An activity should not be excluded on the assumption that a student is too disabled to participate in it. For example, in order to return a library book, an individual need not be able to accomplish all of the activities in which his or her nondisabled peer participates (e.g., exiting a car, traveling to the entrance of the library while carrying a book, and placing the book in the deposit box). Instead, the individual can partially participate by holding the book while being taken in a wheelchair to the deposit box, or by indicating the book that he or she wants to return by looking at one of several books held up by a companion.

Further examples of ways in which a student with the most severe disabilities can partially participate in common activities are shown in the following tables. Table 10.2 contains examples of activities (e.g., toileting) that typically occur in some subenvironments (e.g., bathroom) of a domestic setting. The parenthetic information for each activity illustrates how an individual with the most severe disabilities might partially participate if he or she was unable to acquire all of the skills that comprise the activity. For example, the grooming activity of brushing one's hair typically occurs in the bathroom subenvironment of the home. An individual with the most severe disabilities could partially participate in brushing hair by holding his or her head motionless and by not resisting having the hair brushed (see Table 10.2). Other examples are relaxing one's jaw in order to partially participate in tooth-brushing, and learning to tolerate water in order to participate in bathing. Such partial participation is not unlike present instruction in classes for students with the most severe disabilities. The difference here is that learning is validated against what is needed in real-life settings, and instruction occurs in the natural settings.

Table 10.3 contains examples of recreational/leisure activites that might occur in the subenvironments of the home, in community settings, and at school. Ways in which persons with the most severe disabilities might partially participate in these activities is once again illustrated by the parenthetic infor-mation. For example, at a sports facility in the community (see Table 10.3, Community), partial participation could involve handing an admission ticket to

Table 10.2. Examples of activities in domestic subenvironments

Bathroom

Toileting (e.g., indicate need by vocalizing or touching self, maintain balance on toilet)

Brush hair (e.g., hold head motionless while hair is brushed, tolerating having hair brushed)

Brush teeth (e.g., relax jaw while teeth are brushed)

Bathing (e.g., increase tolerance of water or of hair blower, bear weight during dressing, turn water on or off)

Clean mirror or other surface (e.g., turn water on and off, pour soap into water, wipe mirror or surface)

Pick up clothing (e.g., open or close hamper lid)

Kitchen or dining room

Eat (e.g., assist with holding food, cup, utensil, or napkin; tolerate different textures of foods; select food or drink by turning head toward items offered)

Wash dishes (e.g., push food off plates, turn food disposal on or off, push tray into dishwasher, turn on dishwasher)

Put tableware away (e.g., open or close cabinet doors and drawers, push tableware into sorted piles)

Prepare meal (e.g., empty contents of packets; activate blender, food processor, can opener, or timer; turn stove or oven on or off)

Living room or recreational area

Recreational/leisure activities (see Table 3)

Bedroom

Dress (e.g., assist with dressing by lifting head, relaxing arm, bearing weight, flexing ankle, opening or closing drawer, removing items from or placing items in drawer)

Use alarm clock (e.g., awaken to alarm, push alarm button)

Make bed (e.g., pull sheets or bedspread to top of bed)

Straighten room (e.g., open or close hamper lid or dresser drawer, close closet door)

Utility area or work room

Wash clothes (e.g., push clothes into sorted piles, place clothing in or remove from washer or dryer, turn appliances on or off)

Care for tools (e.g., put tools away, wipe work surfaces)

General housekeeping

Clean surfaces (e.g., wipe surface, pour soap into water, turn water on or off)

Empty garbage (e.g., turn trash compactor on or off, push trash into container)

Vacuum (e.g., turn vacuum cleaner on or off)

Care for plants (e.g., tip watering container to water plants)

Outdoors

Plant flowers (e.g., drop seed or plants into holes)

Care for plants (e.g., pull weeds, water plants, snip flowers)

Rake leaves (e.g., turn leaf blower on or off)

the ticket collector, increasing the amount of time a person is able to sit at the event, or increasing the individual's visual or auditory awareness of environmental events. Tables 10.4 and 10.5 are similarly structured, but with reference to the work and general community use domains, respectively.

As discussed earlier, active partial participation in activities (e.g., dropping a book in a library's deposit box) need not be the only goal; the quality of an individual's life can be improved by participating at whatever level is possible, providing that he or she is willing to participate. This means that for some students it may be appropriate to emphasize visual or auditory attending and tracking behaviors so they can gain more information from the activity and benefit more from being in the settings. For example, a student could learn to visually attend to a mirror placed above an arcade game being played by a compan-

Table 10.3. Examples of recreational and leisure activities for home, community, and school

---

Home: Current and future environments

Living room, den, recreation room, bedroom
 Play board and table games, such as checkers and foosball (e.g., watch game, move game pieces, move handle of foosball)
 Play cards (e.g., watch card game, activate electronic card shuffler, look at cards and signal if a card matches another)
 Play computer game (e.g., signal choice of games, activate controls for computer games, watch as sibling plays game)
 Read books and magazines (e.g., look at book or magazine, indicate choice of books by looking, activate electronic page turner, activate tape recorder for recorded book, listen to audiocassette of book)
 Photography (e.g., operate switch activated shutter, look through camera, look at photograph album, activate electronic page turner with photograph album)
 Use home entertainment equipment (e.g., select by smile or by looking at a record, audiocassette, or videocassette; activate controls for on or off, loudness, channel selection, forward or reverse; watch or listen to television, record player, radio, or tape player)
 Play a musical instrument (e.g., use keyboard with hands, head, or foot; blow a wind instrument)

Kitchen
 Cook (e.g., watch cooking activity; activate blender, food processor, popcorn popper, can opener, timer)

Outside
 Care for pet (e.g., accompany animal on walks, pet animal, brush animal, watch animal, move lever to release animal food into dish or tank)
 Care for plants (e.g., water or mist plant, turn plant to face sunlight)
 Gardening (e.g., pull weeds, drop seeds into holes, water plants with can or hose)

Swimming pool and side of pool
 Swim (e.g., tolerate water, remain on or in a flotation device, splash water, bear weight, maintain balance while sitting on side of pool)

Yard
 Use playground equipment (e.g., watch other children play, remain in swing, maintain an erect posture while on slide)

Community: Current and future environments

Arcade at shopping center: Game area
 Use computer and arcade games (e.g., watch as peers play, move controls)

Library: Magazine and tape browsing area
 Read magazines or listen to tapes (see Home section of this table for examples of partial participation with books or tape equipment)

Park: Pathways and picnic areas
 Cycling (e.g., tolerate riding in child's seat, maintain balance)
 Take nature walk (e.g., accompany peer or adult on walks, look through binoculars or telescope)
 Picnic (e.g., assist with eating, choose food or drink)

Theater or playhouse: Entrance, audience, refreshment, and restroom areas
 Attend cultural events (e.g., watch event, hand ticket to usher, indicate choice of events, select refreshments, use restroom)

Shopping center or shopping district
 Watch people, window shop

(continued)

Table 10.3. (*continued*)

Swimming pool: Pool, locker room, and refreshment areas
  Swim (e.g., assist with showering, assist with dressing, tolerate water, use flotation device, bear weight, maintain balance)
  Purchase refreshments (e.g., select refreshment by looking at picture, hand money to cashier)

Bowling alley: Bowling lanes, restroom, refreshment, and game entertainment areas
  Bowl (e.g., watch bowling, push ball off bowling ramp)
  Purchase refreshment (e.g., select refreshment by looking at picture, hand money to cashier)
  Use restroom (e.g., indicate need to use restroom, assist with dressing, bear weight, maintain balance on toilet)
  Play video games (e.g., watch peers play, place coin in machine, move video game controls)

Skating rink: Rink, restroom, and refreshment areas
  Skate (e.g., watch skaters, support weight on skates)
  Purchase refreshment (e.g., select refreshment by looking at picture, hand money to cashier)
  Use restroom (e.g., indicate need to use restroom, assist with dressing, bear weight, maintain balance on toilet)

Pond or lake: Shore area
  Fish (e.g., hold fishing pole, pull in fish, open or close fishing tackle or bait box)

Sport facility: Entrance, audience, restroom, and refreshment areas
  Enter facility (e.g., hand ticket to usher)
  Watch spectator sports (e.g., increase the time that one can watch an event)
  Purchase refreshment (e.g., select refreshment by looking at picture, hand money to cashier)
  Use restroom (e.g., indicate need to use restroom, assist with dressing, bear weight, maintain balance on toilet)

Stable: Barn and trail areas
  Horseback riding (e.g., maintain balance on horse)
  Animal care (e.g., dump water into trough, brush horse)

School: Current environment
See Home and Community sections of this table for examples of ways in which students can participate in activities in each of the following subenvironments:
  School library
  Kitchen or home economics area
  Photography laboratory
  Greenhouse
  Theater
  Sport facility
  Playground

ion, or to listen to a bowling ball advancing toward its target. For other students, being able to sit for longer time periods at a basketball game or tolerating the noise at a hockey match may be important.

Assessing Student Responses to Environments and Activities

Emphasis up to this point has been on the activities that the student should learn in order to participate in current and future environments. A further consideration is a student's preference toward particular settings and activities. Because

Table 10.4. Examples of activities in work subenvironments

Stores (e.g., grocery, general, clothing, sports, music, hardware, pharmacy, pet)

Sales and stockroom areas

Stock shelves (e.g., push on stamp to price cans, boxes; push items into alignment on shelves)

Bag items (e.g., move lever to dump nuts, beans, pills, and other items for bagging; slide items to companion who bags them)

Display cases, restrooms, and break areas

Clean surfaces (e.g., wipe windows, mirrors, or counters; add soap to water; turn water on or off)

Break and lunch areas

Eat snack or lunch (e.g., select refreshment in vending machine, place money in vending machine, assist with eating)

Look at magazine (e.g., choose magazine, use page turner)

Listen to tape (e.g., choose tape, tolerate headphones, use microswitch to turn on or off)

General work skills

Clock in or out (e.g., remove card from holder, hand card to coworker who clocks in the disabled person)

Use restroom (e.g., assist with toileting, grooming, dressing)

Industries

Work area

Packaging (e.g., move lever to dump contents for packaging, activate switch to seal package)

Break area

(see the Stores section for examples)

General work skills

(see the Stores section for examples)

Offices

(Examples of community sites with offices: stores, industries, libraries, courthouses, employment services, social services, public health, legal services, mental health, Council on Aging, universities and colleges, fire department, religious organizations, United Way, American Red Cross, Lions Club, Rotary Club)

Storage and work areas

Stock shelves with paper, pencils, paper clips, and other office material (e.g., push items into alignment on shelves)

Photocopy (e.g., push copier button)

Shred paper (e.g., release paper into shredder)

Staple (e.g., move papers on paper holder to activate electronic stapler)

Collate (e.g., activate electronic collator)

Sharpen pencils (e.g., activate electronic pencil sharpener)

Date documents received (e.g., push stamp to date materials)

Libraries

Check out desk

Process returned materials (e.g., push stamp to cancel books, push books onto cart for reshelving)

Book and magazine shelves

Reshelve materials (e.g., push materials to align on shelves, hand items to coworker who places them on shelves)

Clean shelves (e.g., wipe low shelves)

(*continued*)

Table 10.4. (*continued*)

Restaurants
(Types of restaurants: fast food, cafeteria, sit down/order)

Eating area
Fill sugar or creamer bowls (e.g., wipe bowls, slide sugar or creamer packets into bowls, slide bowl into position on table, hand materials to coworker who fills bowls)
Clean (e.g., wipe showcase or table tops, pour soap into water, turn water on or off)

Kitchen
Fold cloth napkins (e.g., slide napkin to coworker, stack napkins on tray)
Wash dishes (e.g., pick silverware off of plates, turn dishwasher on)
Stock shelves (e.g., push items to straighten on shelves)
Clean (e.g., wipe shelves and counters, pur soap into water, turn water on or off)

Motels/hotels

Rooms
Clean bathrooms (e.g., wipe mirror or sink, take supplies to coworker)
Make beds (e.g., pull sheet or bedspread to top of bed, straighten pillows

Animal shelters

Animal quarters
Feed animals (e.g., dump food into bowl or tank)

---

persons with the most severe disabilities have little control over their lives, it is imperative that educators closely observe individuals for behaviors that indicate preference, dislike, or indifference toward environments or activities.

Assessing reactions to environments and activities is a simple task when students make such overt and typical responses as smiling, frowning, crying, increasing attention or active involvement in an activity, and increasing motor movement in anticipation of an activity. However, for many students, the responses may be less obvious. For these students, teachers and parents must be keen observers and interpreters of student behavior. For example, a student might indicate pleasure or displeasure for a particular activity or person by changing his or her body tone, through subtle changes in the level and type of motor activity, or by changes in vocalizations. More specific examples of expressions of displeasure include averting the eyes or head, tightening the lips, becoming increasingly passive, refusing to maintain the head in an erect position, deep sighing, or maintaining an "empty" or "looking through you" gaze. Other examples include refusing to open the mouth for feeding, increasing the frequency of tongue thrusts when disliked foods are introduced, or refusing to free the grip on a wheelchair armrest when being transferred to a low preference activity. Examples of specific behaviors in the presence of preferred events include attempting to make visual eye contact with persons or objects, leaning forward in anticipation, expressing positive affect or vocalizations, and struggling to participate as evidenced by straining to look, touch, or cooperate.

In order for educators to recognize these behaviors, they must first regard all student behavior as potentially communicative. In addition, they must repeatedly observe the student in integrated settings in order to accurately inter-

Table 10.5. Examples of activities in community use subenvironments

Transportation (e.g., bus, train, taxi)	Cashier
Ticket booth/machine	Pay (e.g., hand money, push on name
Purchase ticket (e.g., hand money to	stamp for check signature)
attendant or insert coin)	

Transportation (e.g., bus, train, taxi)

Ticket booth/machine
Purchase ticket (e.g., hand money to attendant or insert coin)

Turnstile/vehicle entrance
Pay (e.g., hand ticket or money, place money in machine)
Board/disembark (e.g., assist by bearing weight or stepping)

Passenger area
Find seat (e.g., look toward empty or preferred seat)
Ride (e.g., maintain balance, hold on, look at scenery)

Intersections (e.g., controlled, uncontrolled)

Crosswalk
Obey signal (e.g., push walk button, attend to walk light)
Walk (e.g., assist with walking or moving wheelchair, assist with stepping up or down)

Restaurants (e.g., fast food, cafeteria, sit down/order)

Table or counter
Order (e.g., look at picture held by peer, hand picture of choice to waiter)
Eat (e.g., assist with eating)

Restroom
Toileting (e.g., assist with dressing, maintain balance on toilet)
Wash (e.g., turn water on or off, push dryer button)

Cashier
Pay (e.g., hand money, push on name stamp for check signature)

Grocery stores (e.g., small convenience, supermarket)

Aisles
Shop (e.g., look at choice, drop item into cart, push cart)

Counter
Purchase (e.g., place items on counter; hand money, credit card, or purchase order to clerk)

Merchandise stores (e.g., clothing, general, sports, music, hardware, pharmacy, pet)
(see Grocery stores section for examples)

Services (e.g., doctor, dentist, hairstylist, post office, bank)

Waiting room
Entertain self (e.g., choose magazine, turn pages, tolerate tape recorder headphones)

Lobby
Wait in line (e.g., bear weight)

Counter
Pay (e.g., hand money or credit card to pay, push on name stamp for signature)

pret the function of the behaviors displayed. In some cases, such behaviors may have been extinguished in the classroom because they were previously regarded as meaningless and ignored by others. Therefore, repeated experiences in new environments or with new activities may be necessary in order for the behaviors to emerge again.

Observations of students could be conducted by including them in visits to inventory the subenvironments and activities of various environments. Another context for observation is during the discrepancy analysis stage (discussed later in this chapter) of the ecological model at which point the student's skills in performing activities are assessed. A third option is to have parents or residential staff observe the student during visits to settings identified as current or future environments.

Since many persons who have the most severe disabilities have been exposed to a limited number of environments, it is appropriate to also provide them with access to situations that have not been targeted as current and future environments, and to gauge their reactions to the experiences in these settings. If preference is shown for a particular setting, then that locale should be inventoried for activities in which the student can participate.

Finally, information about a student's responses to environments and activities is important not only for educators, but also for parents, roommates, and residential staff. Such information can be used by these individuals to improve the quality of a student's life through access to places and activities that the student enjoys.

Establishing Priorities and Selecting Activities

One approach to selecting an activity from the large number of potential ones that could be taught is to establish criteria and a rating system. Figure 10.1 provides several possible criteria and a sample rating system for setting priorities among the activities. After rating each activity using the 20 criteria, a total sum is computed for each. Activities with the highest sums are given the highest priority for instruction. This procedure gives equal weight to each criterion. An alternative is to differentially weight the criteria so that items regarded by parents and professionals as more important are assigned greater value. For example, the least important items would be given a weight of one, the items with the next higher level of importance would be weighted with a two, and so on. Then, the rating (e.g., a rating of "somewhat agree with the statement" is worth 2 points) for an item would be multiplied by the weight assigned to that item to obtain a weighted score.

Listing Skills that Comprise Each Activity

A task analysis process is used to identify the skills that comprise each of the activities for the student that are selected for instruction. A task analysis is completed by either observing someone who is performing an activity or by completing the activity him- or herself. In both cases, the steps (i.e., skills) needed to complete the activity are listed in the order in which they occur. As an example, a task analysis of checking out a book at the library would consist of the following:

1. Scan the library to find the librarian's desk.
2. Go to the librarian's desk.
3. Hand the book to the librarian.
4. Remove wallet or purse.
5. Remove library card.
6. Hand card to librarian.
7. Receive card from the librarian.

Criteria	Activity											
	1	2	3	4	5	6	7	8	9	10	11	12
1. Can be used in current environments	—	—	—	—	—	—	—	—	—	—	—	—
2. Can be used in future environments	—	—	—	—	—	—	—	—	—	—	—	—
3. Can be used in four or more different environments	—	—	—	—	—	—	—	—	—	—	—	—
4. Affords daily opportunities for interaction with non-disabled persons	—	—	—	—	—	—	—	—	—	—	—	—
5. Increases student independence	—	—	—	—	—	—	—	—	—	—	—	—
6. Helps maintain student in, or promotes movement to a least restrictive environment	—	—	—	—	—	—	—	—	—	—	—	—
7. Is chronologically age-appropriate	—	—	—	—	—	—	—	—	—	—	—	—
8. Student will acquire in 1 year the necessary skills to participate in the activity	—	—	—	—	—	—	—	—	—	—	—	—
9. Parents rate as a high priority	—	—	—	—	—	—	—	—	—	—	—	—
10. Promotes a positive view of the individual	—	—	—	—	—	—	—	—	—	—	—	—
11. Meets a medical need	—	—	—	—	—	—	—	—	—	—	—	—
12. Improves student's health or fitness	—	—	—	—	—	—	—	—	—	—	—	—
13. If able, student would select	—	—	—	—	—	—	—	—	—	—	—	—
14. Student shows positive response to activity	—	—	—	—	—	—	—	—	—	—	—	—
15. Advocacy, training, and other support can be arranged so that student can participate in the activity in the absence of educational services	—	—	—	—	—	—	—	—	—	—	—	—
16. Related service staff support selection of activity	—	—	—	—	—	—	—	—	—	—	—	—
17. Transportation is no barrier	—	—	—	—	—	—	—	—	—	—	—	—
18. Cost is no barrier	—	—	—	—	—	—	—	—	—	—	—	—
19. Staffing is no barrier	—	—	—	—	—	—	—	—	—	—	—	—
20. Environments are physically accessible	—	—	—	—	—	—	—	—	—	—	—	—
TOTAL	—	—	—	—	—	—	—	—	—	—	—	—

Figure 10.1. Twenty examples of criteria used for setting priorities (Rating of: 3 = strongly agree with statement, 2 = agree somewhat with statement, 1 = disagree somewhat with statement, 0 = disagree strongly with statement) for 12 different activities. (Adapted from Dardig, J.C., & Heward, W.L. [1981]. A systematic procedure for prioritizing IEP goals. *The Directive Teacher, 3,* 6–7.)

8. Place card in wallet or purse.
9. Receive book from the librarian.

Conducting the Discrepancy Analysis

After the activities are task analyzed, the student's ability to perform each activity is assessed in the environments where the activities naturally occur. Discrepancies are noted between the skills used by a nondisabled person in carrying out an activity, and the student's skills. Table 10.6 (York & Rainforth, 1987) illustrates the discrepancy analysis process with a student who is very severely disabled. The example involves the recreational/leisure domain, the environment is the public library, and the subenvironment is the library's browsing area that contains magazines and tapes. A nondisabled person's behaviors in performing the activity are listed in the first column. Column two contains the results of assessing the student's status on each behavior comprising an activity, with notes on the assistance required in order for the student to perform each behavior.

Developing Individualized Adaptations

The next step in the ecological model is the development of adaptations. For example, the last column of Table 10.6 contains notations as to whether to teach (T) the student on the actual behavior, or whether it should be adapted (A) in some way. Adaptations are very important if students with the most severe disabilities are to participate in integrated settings. Baumgart et al. (1982) have identified five categories of adaptations.

The first type is the provision of personal assistance. In order for a student to participate in an activity, it may be necessary to have peer or adult assistance. Examples are physical assistance such as pushing a student's wheelchair, holding up pictues of menu items for an individual from which he or she can make a selection, or supporting a student's weight during a transfer from a wheelchair to a bench. A second form of personal assistance is a gestural or verbal aid such as a peer pointing the way to the playground or pointing to the controls of a computer game. If a student is unlikely to learn the behavior and personal assistance is available, then this adaptation may be appropriate. In Table 10.6, personal assistance is in the form of pushing the student to areas, positioning the tape recorder, holding objects up for selection, pointing to areas to which the student must go, and adjusting the volume of the tape recorder.

A second type of adaptation is the modification of the sequence of skills. For instance, a student who must be fully supported when boarding a bus and whose balance is poor, could board the bus, sit in the front seat, then hold the bus ticket out. This varies from the typical sequence of boarding, giving the ticket to the driver, and then finding a seat.

A third adaptation is the modification of rules. For example, if one nondisabled employee typically completes an entire work task, then the rules might

Table 10.6. Example of a partial assessment conducted at a public library

Nondisabled person inventory	Student with disabilities inventory (assessment)[a]	Instructional solutions (teach directly or adapt)[b]
ACTIVITY: Choosing a tape		
Skills:		
Locate tape section.	− T pointed to audiovisual section, then to tapes.	T: S will look in direction of tape area once in visual field (T/peer push wheelchair).
Browse through tapes.	− T located age-appropriate tapes, then selected four.	A: S will look at tapes pulled from stack by T/peer.
Select one tape.	+ S looked at one tape after T presented four.	
ACTIVITY: Listening to tape		
Skills:		
Locate tape.	+ S scanned then located after T pointed to picture of recorder on communication board	
Position self.	− T wheeled and positioned S.	A: S will be pushed by T/peer to tape section.
Open tape player lid.	− S initiated move toward eject button; T relaxed S's arm then primed reach for and push button.	A: S will push on lever extended from eject button; T/peer positions tape recorder.
Insert tape.	− S pushed tape into place with back of wrist after T aligned tape in track.	A: S will push in tape after T/peer places recorder close to S's wrist and aligns tape.
Close lid.	− S initiated move toward lid; T relaxed S's arm then assisted reach down and push closed.	T: S will push lid closed with forearm after T/peer places recorder near forearm.
Put on headphones.	− T places earphones on S's head.	A: T/peer will perform.
Turn on tape.	− S was unable to reach and exert enough pressure; T turned on.	A: S will turn on tape with hand/head using microswitch.
Adjust volume.	− T moved volume dial; S frowned then smiled.	A: S will smile when appropriate volume dialed by T/peer.

(continued)

Table 10.6. *(continued)*

Nondisabled person inventory	Student with disabilities inventory (assessment)[a]	Instructional solutions (teach directly or adapt)[b]
ACTIVITY: Choosing a magazine Skills:		
Locate magazine section.	− T pointed to magazine section.	T: S will look in direction of magazines once in visual field (eventually S will choose between tapes and magazines).
Locate preferred magazines.	− T located age-appropriate and preferred content magazines.	T: S will scan magazine section with T/peer guide by pointing.
Select one magazine.	+ S looked at one magazine and smiled after T presented three.	
ACTIVITY: Browsing through magazine Skills:		
Locate an area to sit.	− T pointed out several open spots then decided to go near window.	T: S will choose where to sit by looking at one area (window or lounge) pointed out by T/peer.
Position self.	− T wheeled and positioned S.	A: S will be positioned by T/peer (consider getting S out of chair to sit on carpet).
Hold magazine.	− T positioned and held magazine on wheelchair tray.	A: T places magazine in book holder adaptation.
Read articles/ look at pictures.	+ (S looked at pictures.)	
Turn pages.	− S initiated reaching to page but required T's assist to relax, reach, turn pages.	A: S will turn pages with hand/mouth using dowel rod with Plasti-Tac on end.

[a] T = teacher, S = student. + indicates independent and acceptable performance; − indicates assistance was required to achieve acceptable performance.
[b] T = teach directly, A = adapt.

be altered to permit two persons, one with severe disabilities and the other who is nondisabled, to work together to complete the entire task. Similarly, a disabled employee might be allowed to complete only part of a task. For example, in operating a dishwasher, an employee with a disability could add soap to the washer and then turn it on, rather than completing the entire job that involves bussing tables, cleaning tableware, loading and unloading the dishwasher, and measuring the correct amount of soap.

A fourth adaptation is the modification of the social environment or the changing of attitudes that interfere with student involvement in activities. Thus, teachers, peers, and others who might be uncomfortable with persons with disabilities could be provided with information about disabling conditions. More importantly, they could learn ways to interact with persons who are disabled. For example, at school, classmates could learn to interpret the eye movements of the student with the disability to indicate his or her choice of areas to be taken to during recess. Similarly, the cashier at the grocery store might be taught to assist a student, who has difficulty releasing items, to loosen his or her grip on the money that is held out in payment for the purchases.

A fifth adaptation involves using special equipment to assist a student in completing an activity. Creative use of adaptations is necessary if persons with the most severe disabilities are to participate in domestic, recreational/leisure, work, and other community settings. In Table 10.6, adaptive equipment is in the form of a lever extended from the eject button of the tape recorder, a hand or head activated microswitch to turn on the recorder, and a dowel rod that is operated by the hand or mouth to turn pages in a magazine.

Numerous other adaptive devices are also available. For eating, there is an electric self-feeder that is controlled by a slight body movement. There are also sandwich holders, grips and splints to help an individual grasp utensils and cups, and no-tip drinking glasses.

Adaptive devices used for dressing include one-handed belts, large handled zippers, and buttoning aids. Examples of equipment to aid meal preparation are one-handed openers for plastic bags, jars, cans, and boxes; and grips to reduce the strength required for removing lids. For obtaining water from a faucet, there is a pressure switch attached to the facet that turns water on when a cup is held against it. Door opening is made easier with a foot activated opener or a door knob extension. Aids for hygiene include levers that assist an individual in flushing toilets and obtaining toothpaste from a tube, and extended or enlarged grips for brushes.

For recreational/leisure activities, available adaptive devices include switch activated page turners; microswitch controlled computer software; one-handed card shufflers; a fishing aid to support line casting by those with some shoulder and elbow movement; and specially designed grips for pool cues, table tennis paddles, and other recreational equipment.

Adaptive equipment has seen extensive use in work settings. Jigs that obviate the need for an individual to be able to count or to have sophisticated manual dexterity skills are common. York and Rainforth (1987) describe a stapling adaptation used in a community setting by a student with no purposeful arm movement other than occasional random movements. The student moved a sliding tray, containing papers that were inserted by another worker, into the mouth of an electric stapler.

In another example by York and Rainforth (1987), a student who lacked sufficient strength to stamp brochures at a travel agency was provided a hinged Plexiglas apparatus with adjustable positions for the stamp on the upper plate, and with space on the lower plate for the material to be stamped. A third example involved a student maintained in a reclined position in a wheelchair, who had limited movement of his upper extremities (York & Rainforth, 1987). This individual performed a collating activity in a community setting. The task was adapted by using a sticky, putty material on the tip of his hand splint, thereby enabling him to move one paper at a time from a pile to a device that was controlled by a microswitch activated by the worker's elbow. The device, when activated, collated the papers.

Developing Instructional Objectives

The results of a discrepancy analysis can be directly translated into instructional goals and objectives. The goal consists of the activity to be learned. The objective states the unacquired skills that will be taught, as well as any necessary adaptations. For example, using the discrepancy analysis and instructional solutions in Table 10.6, the goal and objectives for choosing and listening to a tape might consist of:

Goal: George will choose and listen to a musical tape at the public library.

Objective 1: When taken to the browsing area in the Metro Public Library, George will locate the tape section by looking in its direction for 3 seconds duration, on five of seven consecutive trips to the library.

Objective 2: In the browsing area at Metro Public Library, when a teacher or peer holds four tapes in front of him, George will choose one by looking at it for 3 seconds duration, or indicate disapproval of options by looking at his lap, for eight of ten consecutive opportunities.

Objective 3: In the browsing area at Metro Public Library, George will complete 80% of the following steps involved in listening to a tape, for 5 consecutive opportunities:

1. Push the tape recorder eject lever after the tape recorder is positioned in front of his hand on his wheelchair tray.
2. Push tape into recorder lid after tape is aligned by a teacher or peer.
3. Push lid closed after recorder is positioned in front of his arm.
4. Turn on the tape recorder using microswitch.
5. Indicate desired volume by smiling at person adjusting it.

Addressing Implementation Issues

A number of issues concerning scheduling, staffing, transportation, and monetary resources may arise during the implementation stage. Some suggested solutions to these issues are shown in Table 10.7. These suggestions are taken from Baumgart and Van Walleghem (1986), Ford and Checkosky (1984), Hamre-Nietupski, Nietupski, Bates, and Mauer (1982), and Sailor et al. (1986). In regard to scheduling, Table 10.7 provides guidelines for the amount of time spent in various types of community environments versus classroom and other school settings (Ford & Checkosky, 1984; Sailor et al., 1986). Generally, time in the community increases as students become older. Time at school is dedicated to: 1) additional training on skills needed in community settings, 2) social integration with nondisabled peers, and 3) specialized therapies that cannot be trained within the context of community activities.

Staffing patterns for implementing the ecological model include utilizing a consultant, staggering implementation of the model across students, teaming less skilled students with higher skilled ones during community training, and arranging for support staff to train or consult in community settings (Baumgart & Van Walleghem, 1986). Other approaches include having support staff train groups of students at school in order to free other staff for community-based training, team teaching, using computers as a more efficient approach to administrative tasks, and utilizing volunteers (Baumgart & Van Walleghem, 1986).

Transportation is frequently a barrier to implementing the ecological model. Transportation demands can result from the model's emphasis on instruction in a variety of community settings. In addition, normalization principles would dictate against traveling in large groups and having a disproportionate number of persons with disabilities in the same place at the same time (e.g., one individual with a disability per setting would be optimal). Some possible solutions include having school buses take students to community sites the first thing in the morning, walking to sites, using public transportation, reimbursing staff and volunteers for use of personal vehicles, and using public school cars (Hamre-Nietupski et al., 1982; Sailor et al., 1986).

Another common issue concerns funding. Possible sources of funds include using classroom material funds for community training costs, having parents pay a nominal amount, conducting fund raising events, and having students shop for groceries for parents or staff (Hamre-Nietupski et al., 1982; Sailor et al., 1986).

SUMMARY

The ecological model for developing curriculum content describes and explains how the model can be extended to students with the most severe disabilities. Use of the model with students with the most severe disabilities requires: 1) an

Table 10.7. Suggested solutions to implementation issues

Scheduling
—Proportion of time in different environments for various age groups

Environments	Age			
	6–9	9–12	12–16	16–21
Classroom	40%	25%	10%	—
School	35	25	15	15%
Community	25	50	75	85

—Number of training opportunities in different domains for various age groups

Environments	Age				
	6–10	11–21	11–17	18–19	20–21
Community					
street crossing (times/wk)	2–3	5	—	—	—
transportation (times/wk)	2–3	5	—	—	—
store shopping (times/wk)	.5	1	—	—	—
restaurant use (times/wk)	2–3	1	—	—	—
Recreation and leisure (times/wk)	.5	1	—	—	—
Competitive employment (half days per week)	—	—	2–3	4–5	Full-time

—Classroom instruction should consist of extra training related to skills and activities needed for nonclassroom settings and specialized therapies that cannot be incorporated into school or community activities
—School settings should focus on social contact with peers and on involvement in typical age-appropriate school activities

Staffing
—Use a consultant to assist during the planning stage
—Stagger implementation where the number of students or amount of community-based training increases gradually
—Use heterogeneous groupings so that a student with the most severe disabilities accompanies a student with a lesser disability
—Restructure related services to permit support staff to train or consult in community environments
—Restructure related services so that support staff teach groups of students for longer periods of time at school, while other students are in the community
—Procure temporary paraprofessional staff
—Team teach, with one teacher instructing a large group while the other teacher conducts community-based training
—Make more efficient use of time by using computers to manage data and other administrative tasks
—Use volunteers, such as parents, college students, and senior citizens; and peer companions or tutors
—In terms of liability, staff and volunteers are usually covered if the school district carries insurance, if the community training is approved by a school official, and if the school district's policies regarding use of volunteers are followed

(continued)

Table 10.7. *(continued)*

Transportation
—Public school vehicles
—Have school bus take student to a
community site first thing in the
morning
—Driver's education vehicles
—Walk to sites

—Volunteers' or parents' cars
—Public transportation
—Reimburse school staff for using
their cars
—University cars

—Whenever staff or volunteer cars are used, district policies must be followed in terms of minimal insurance coverage, written permission by a school official, and other district rules

Monetary resources
—Use the money designated for classroom materials for community training costs
—Pay restaurant meals by transferring money from the school lunch program
—Have parents pay a nominal amount to help offset costs
—Conduct fund raising events
—Request funds from parent groups or student government
—Establish a purchase order account between merchants and the school
—Run a school soup and salad bar to raise money
—Have students shop for groceries for parents or teachers
—Use vocational education money

From Baumgart and Van Walleghem (1986), Ford and Checkosky (1984), Hamre-Nietupski, Nietupski, Bates, and Mauer (1982), and Sailor, Halvorsen, Anderson, Goetz, Gee, Doering, and Hunt (1986).

emphasis on the concept of partial participation and an interpretation of that concept that allows passive engagement in activities; 2) greater dependence on technological adaptations that permit an individual to participate in activities; and 3) assessing the communicative intent of students' behavior, including very subtle responses, and interpreting the meaning of those behaviors in regard to preferences for environments and activities.

REFERENCES

Baumgart, D., Brown, L., Pumpian, I., Nisbeth, J., Ford, A., Sweet, M., Messina, R., & Schroeder, J. (1982). Principle of partial participation and individualized adaptations in educational programs for severely handicapped students. *Journal of The Association for the Severely Handicapped, 7*(2), 17–27.

Baumgart, D., & Van Walleghem, J. (1986). Staffing strategies for implementing community-based instruction. *The Journal of The Association for Persons with Severe Handicaps, 11*(2), 92–102.

Brown, F., Helmstetter, E., & Guess, D. (1986). *Current best practices with students with profound disabilities: Are there any?* Unpublished manuscript, The Institute of Professional Practice, Inc., New Haven.

Brown, L., Branston, M., Hamre-Nietupski, S., Pumpian, I., Certo, N., & Gruenewald, L. (1979). A strategy for developing chronological age appropriate and functional curricular content for severely handicapped adolescents and young adults. *Journal of Special Education, 13*(1), 81–90.

Brown, L., Branston-McLean, M., Baumgart, D., Vincent, L., Falvey, M., & Schroeder, J. (1979). Utilizing the characteristics of current and subsequent least restrictive environments as factors in the development of curricular content for severely handicapped students. *AAESPH Review, 4*(4), 407–424.

Brown, L., Falvey, M., Vincent, L., Kaye, N., Johnson, F., Ferrara-Parrish, P., & Gruenewald, L. (1980). Strategies for generating comprehensive, longitudinal, and chronological age appropriate individualized education programs for adolescents and young adult severely handicapped students. *Journal of Special Education, 14*(2), 199–215.

Brown, L., Shiraga, B., York, J., Zanella, K., & Rogan, P. (1984a). Ecological inventory strategies for students with severe handicaps. In L. Brown, M. Sweet, B. Shiraga, J. York, K. Zanella, P. Rogan, & R. Loomis (Eds.), *Educational programs for students with severe handicaps* (Vol. XIV, pp. 33–41). Madison, WI: Madison Metropolitan School District.

Brown, L., Shiraga, B., York, J., Zanella, K., & Rogan, P. (1984b). The discrepancy analysis technique in programs for students with severe handicaps. In L. Brown, M. Sweet, B. Shiraga, J. York, K. Zanella, P. Rogan, & R. Loomis (Eds.), *Educational programs for students with severe handicaps* (Vol. XIV, pp. 43–47). Madison, WI: Madison Metropolitan School District.

Dardig, J. C., & Heward, W. L. (1981). A systematic procedure for prioritizing IEP goals. *The Directive Teacher, 3,* 6–7.

Falvey, M. A. (1986). *Community-based curriculum: Instructional strategies for students with severe handicaps.* Baltimore: Paul H. Brookes Publishing Co.

Ford, A., Brown, L., Pumpian, I., Baumgart, D., Nisbet, J., Schroeder, J., & Loomis, R. (1984). Strategies for developing individualized recreation and leisure programs for severely handicapped students. In N. Certo, N. Haring, & R. York (Eds.), *Public school integration of severely handicapped students: Rational issues and progressive alternatives* (pp. 221–244). Baltimore: Paul H. Brookes Publishing Co.

Ford, A., & Checkosky, D. (1984). *A community-based curriculum guide for moderately and severely handicapped students.* Syracuse: Syracuse City School District.

Hamre-Nietupski, S., Nietupski, J., Bates, P., & Mauer, S. (1982). Implementing a community-based educational model for moderately/severely handicapped students: Common problems and suggested solutions. *The Journal of The Association for the Severely Handicapped, 7*(4), 38–43.

Nietupski, J., & Hamre-Nietupski, S. (1987). An ecological approach to curriculum development. In L. Goetz, D. Guess, & K. Stremel-Campbell (Eds.), *Innovative program design for individuals with dual sensory impairments* (pp. 191–223). Baltimore: Paul H. Brookes Publishing Co.

Sailor, W., Halvorsen, A., Anderson, J., Goetz, L., Gee, K., Doering, K., & Hunt, P. (1986). Community intensive instruction. In R. H. Horner, L. H. Meyer, & H. D. B. Fredericks (Eds.), *Education of learners with severe handicaps: Exemplary service strategies* (pp. 251–288). Baltimore: Paul H. Brookes Publishing Co.

Wehman, P., Renzaglia, A., & Bates, P. (1985). *Functional living skills for moderately and severely handicapped individuals.* Austin, TX: PRO-ED.

York, J., & Rainforth, B. (1987). Developing instructional adaptations. In F. Orelove & D. Sobsey, *Educating children with multiple disabilities: A transdisciplinary approach* (pp. 183–217). Baltimore: Paul H. Brookes Publishing Co.

VOCATIONAL TRAINING FOR PERSONS WITH PROFOUND DISABILITIES   ⑪

Paul Bates

Vocational training for persons with profound handicaps is a challenging and provocative topic for educators, consumers, parents, employers, rehabilitation professionals, and others. Until the late 1980s, people with severe and profound handicaps were excluded from vocational training programs due to perceived lack of potential to benefit from such involvement (Bellamy, Horner, & Inman, 1979; Wehman, Renzaglia, & Bates, 1985). This exclusion has been evident in both public school and adult service rehabilitation programs. A lively debate still exists regarding the appropriateness of including vocational objectives for people who appear to have limited potential for performing meaningful work or attaning gainful employment. While most professionals have recognized the value of training vocational skills to individuals with moderate mental retardation and some persons with severe retardation, considerable controversy continues to surround the question of vocational potential involving persons with profound handicaps, including mental retardation, physical disabilities, and sensory impairments.

In many public school programs, vocational objectives are not included for students with profound handicaps. When vocational objectives have been incorporated into a student's individualized education program (IEP), seldom are community-based employment experiences used as instructional activities. The cumulative effect of these practices is that many students have been denied the opportunity to receive vocational training in settings where most adults eventually work. As a result, vocational skills for community employment are not developed, "normal" expectations and aspirations regarding employment beyond high school are discouraged, and employers are denied the opportunity to experience the benefits associated with the meaningful work contributions of individuals with profound mental retardation.

The failure of public schools to more fully involve persons with profound mental retardation in vocational training and community employment experiences has made it too easy for adult services to continue their exclusionary practices. In many cases, persons with profound handicaps are relegated into nonvocational day activity programs, and/or they are excluded from available community programs. For individuals with profound handicaps, exclusion is the all-too-common postschool experience. Exclusion typically means that young adults remain in their homes after their public school eligibility is exhausted and are forced into life-styles of isolation, dependence, and minimal community participation. In these situations, family resources and supports are taxed to the point that institutionalization and further isolation from the mainstream of community life are likely results.

Will (1985), the Assistant Secretary of the Department of Education and Director of the Office of Special Education and Rehabilitative Services (OSERS), made the following comment: "I firmly believe that all youth with disabilities enrolled in our nation's schools are capable of moving from school to employment with the provision of necessary support services tailored to the needs of those individuals" (p. 1). If Will's optimism is to be fulfilled, radical changes in the existing special education and rehabilitation services will be required. Furthermore, equally dramatic changes will be required in the cultural values regarding meaningful productivity and independence, and with the rights of persons with profound handicaps to participate in all aspects of community life. Several issues that are related to these needed changes are developed in this chapter, including the meaning of work to the individual and society, vocational curriculum in the public schools, employment services for adults, and progressive vocational training practices for enhancing participation in community work settings.

MEANING OF WORK

The value of work to the individual and society is a basic assumption that underlies the development of this chapter. Meaningful work can take many forms and fulfill varying functions. Work is a very broad concept, referring to actions that contribute in one or more ways to a person's self-sufficiency, the welfare of one's household, and the benefit of society. Some of these actions are performed for pay, while others are not.

This broad interpretation of work expands the range of meaningful outcomes that can be obtained through vocational training. Work should be valued for its contributions to an individual's self-sufficiency and for its benefit to the individual's community, regardless of the level of pay or the nature of the work itself. By placing greater value on work as a personal and social contribution, there is less chance that the status of various jobs becomes stratified and there is a greater likelihood that a system that values the unique contributions of all citizens will be created.

Advocates for reform of vocational training and rehabilitation services have emphasized that persons with disabilities can be productive, independent citizens capable of participating in complex, integrated community settings. Although such advocacy is intended to emphasize the abilities of persons who experience handicaps, it may inadvertently contribute to a value system that rejects individuals who are not as productive or independent as others (Ferguson & Ferguson, 1986). If society differentially values people on the basis of productivity and independence, does that mean that society rejects those individuals who are not as productive as others and who are dependent on others for food, shelter, clothing, and other necessities of daily living? The value system that rigidly stratifies individuals' worth based upon arbitrary and narrow definitions of productivity and independence will continually discriminate against people with disabilities who are not as productive or independent as others.

People who experience profound handicaps may or may not attain levels of productivity that cause industry to make radical changes in the availability of employment opportunities. If individuals with profound handicaps do not attain such levels of productivity that are valued by industry, should these persons be denied the opportunity to contribute vocationally? If individuals with profound handicaps do not attain independence in basic feeding, toileting, and dressing skills, should they be denied the opportunity to live in a personalized community residence? Rather than focusing on arbitrary achievement levels in productivity and independence, the emphasis in this chapter is placed on the development of practices that nurture individual growth and enhance participation in meaningful work. These practices must focus simultaneously on the individual and societal variables that enhance vocational participation by persons with profound handicaps.

According to Ferguson and Ferguson (1986):

> Understanding the integration of adults with severe disabilities into the workplace is no longer simply a clinical training issue. It is a social, economic, political, and historical issue; but it is not—or should not be—a debate over individual abilities. (p. 335)

The implication of the Ferguson and Ferguson observation is that the focus of intervention in vocational training must expand beyond the individual and encompass the complexity of societal influences that make it possible for persons with profound handicaps to experience the personal and social benefits associated with performing meaningful work in community settings. The development of supported employment (discussed later in this chapter) as a viable employment outcome is an example of a shift in focus from an individual's "readiness" or "ability" to work to a focus on the services or supports that enable individuals to contribute vocationally. To enable the potential benefits of supported employment to be more fully extended to persons with profound handicaps. additional changes in the sophistication of vocational curriculum and training technology must be accompanied by radical changes in the receptivity of community employers to the expansion of vocational opportunities. Undoubtedly, these changes will require a more indepth focus on the values that support inclusion and integration rather than isolation and segregation.

The importance of vocational training can be traced directly to a person's development of self-esteem and his or her perceived value to society. The personal satisfaction and respect that a person receives as a result of his or her vocational contributions are related closely to most conceptualizations of "quality of life." However, it must be emphasized that vocational contributions vary widely, including activities that are performed for pay and on a voluntary basis. Due to the lack of employment opportunity and/or the combinations of profound handicaps (e.g., comatose condition, frequent seizure activity, severe self-abuse, and aggressive behavior), some individuals will not work for pay outside of the home in an integrated community employment situation. However, it should be possible to attain a dignified life-style that does not include paid employment. Furthermore, even though society acknowledges that it is acceptable not to work for a wage, it is imperative that every effort be put forth to give all persons the opportunities and training experiences that could possibly enable them to develop the adult life-style of their choice. These opportunities and training experiences include expanded vocational curriculum during the public school years, supported employment beyond school, and innovative training strategies such as systematic behavioral interventions and rehabilitation engineering.

Vocational Curriculum in the Public Schools

Given the importance of work and vocational training to the concept of "quality of life," it is imperative that researchers, practitioners, and consumers examine methods by which these activities can be enhanced for all people. Decreasing deviance, increasing competence, and expanding choices are broad programmatic goals that have been associated with initiatives in the vocational curriculum area. An examination of these broad programmatic goals appears to be critical in obtaining a clearer understanding of purpose in developing vocational training programs for persons with profound handicaps.

Decreasing Deviance Decreasing deviance refers to interventions that are intended to reduce differences between nonhandicapped individuals and persons with disabilities. In these interventions, behavioral deviations from the norm are identified and training is focused on reducing or eliminating these differences. For example, high-rate stereotypical behaviors, loud vocalizations, and self-abuse would be identified as such target behaviors pinpointed for correction. Although it is easily understood how the presence of certain behaviors interferes with a person's community life-style, it is important to emphasize that the rationale for "decreasing deviance" intervention should not be based upon the assumption that all differences or deviance between nonhandicapped students and individuals with disabilities are bad. Disability, difference, and deviance are facts of life. The elimination of all disabilities, differences, and deviance is not possible, nor desirable. In situations where discrepancies between workers who are handicapped and those who are not contribute directly to limitations on a person's vocational choices, these differences may warrant programmatic attention. However, in many situations, intervention may be more profitably focused on increasing an environment's tolerance for deviance and/or support for individuals who exhibit atypical behavior patterns.

Increasing Competence Programmatic goals for increasing competence may be viewed as the alternative of decreasing deviance goals. With the focus more squarely on increasing skills, a more positive view of intervention and persons with disabilities is encouraged. In the vocational curriculum, work and work-related competencies should be identified and vocational intervention should be directed toward establishing behaviors that are to be judged as important in determining meaningful vocational involvement. The rationale for vocational intervention, which is focused on increasing competence, is based upon the assumption that the amount of skills in a person's repertoire is directly related to his or her employability.

Expanding Choice Although the importance of increasing the vocational competence of persons with profound handicaps is obvious, it is important not to overemphasize arbitrarily defined skill levels when judging human worth and dignity. "Decreasing deviance" and "increasing competence" interventions need to be viewed from the broader perspective of developing a person's personal control and choice regarding vocational involvement. According to Turnbull and Turnbull (1985), choosing how to live one's life is the "catalytic trigger" of independence. If persons with disabilities were provided opportunities and training experiences that could expand their personal control and choice regarding vocational involvement, a system of individually designed options is likely to emerge as a mechanism for promoting meaningful employment participation for the individuals. Given the expansion of vocational opportunities and training experiences, more people with profound handicaps will be able to choose whether or not to become paid workers as they commence adulthood. Without these opportunities and training experiences, individuals have very little choice or control over their vocational participation.

Providing Vocational Opportunites and Training Experiences Vocational opportunites and training experiences should be available to persons with profound handicaps throughout their public school experience. A publicly supported education is viewed as being the foundation for equitable access to a decent quality of life in society. Vocational training is an extremely important aspect of an appropriate education. Bates and Pancsofar (1981) proposed a model for longitudinal vocational training of persons with severe handicaps. Several components of this model are described below, with specific recommendations regarding the involvement of persons with profound handicaps in vocational training programs. These components include community assessment, job analysis, vocational assessment, selection of vocational objectives, longitudinal vocational training, community training, and transition planning.

Community Assessment   Vocational training activities need to be designed to prepare persons with disabilities for employment opportunities that are available in their home communities. In order to ensure this outcome, personnel who are responsible for vocational programs must continuously assess the availability of jobs locally. By continually collecting information regarding the vocational opportunities for such individuals in a particular community, there is a greater chance that training will be directed in a manner that maximizes successful placement.

Traditionally, community job assessment has relied on analyzing the local job market for high-demand occupations created by expansion or turnover. If a full-employment goal is to be attained, job developers must move beyond an assessment of currently available employment, toward advocacy and related efforts that create expanded opportunity. Work crews, enclaves, and individual work stations in industry are options that have been created to expand opportunity (Mank, Rhodes, & Bellamy, 1986; Rhodes & Valenta, 1985). Also, part-time work and job sharing are arrangements that have been used to increase employment opportunities for more individuals. In combination with varying levels of support that may be required for on-the-job training and continued training/follow-up assistance, innovative employment options may expand the labor market to accommodate a wider range of worker abilities. Without such vigorous job assessment and development activities, persons with profound handicaps have little chance of being employed in traditionally available jobs and supervisory arrangements.

Another possibility for vocational participation in the community is the performance of volunteer work for community agencies and other organizations (Andriano, 1977). Brown et al. (1984) initiated a controversy within the special education and rehabilitation community of professionals by asserting that the Department of Labor should allow for a direct pay waiver to enable people with the most severe intellectual deficits to perform meaningful work in nonsheltered, integrated employment settings. In effect, persons employed under the proposed waiver would be volunteering their time for the opportunity to participate in an integrated community employment situation. Although Brown et al.'s (1984) proposal went well beyond traditional volunteer situations, criticism of the direct pay waiver proposal has led many people to reject the inclusion of persons with disabilities into legitimate volunteer enterprises (e.g., Red Cross, United Way). Criticism of the direct pay waiver proposal and involvement of persons with disabilities in volunteer activities is based upon the position that wages commensurate with productivity should be paid for work completed in integrated settings (Bellamy et al., 1984) and that people who are able to volunteer should also be capable of working for a wage. Both Brown et al. (1984) and Bellamy et al. (1984) provide convincing arguments in support of their positions and concur on the central point that persons with severe handicaps have important vocational contributions to make to their local community. However, an unfortunate result of this debate has been the discrediting of many volunteer contributions and failure to resolve the crisis associated with the sobering realization that few persons with severe mental retardation and virtually no individuals with profound handicaps are involved in integrated community employment. Initiatives that are used to expand meaningful vocational participation for individuals with profound handicaps should comprehensively assess both paid and nonpaid vocational curriculum opportunities. These initiatives should focus on the identification of existing opportunities and on those conditions that are needed to achieve its goal of meaningful vocational participation for such individuals.

Job Analysis Once the availability of vocational opportunities has been determined, the next step in program development is to conduct detailed assessments of the specific skills that are required to succeed in a variety of different vocational situations. Important vocational competencies have been identified by conducting interviews and/or collecting questionnaire responses from employers, supervisors, and others regarding behavior standards for employment success. Mithaug, Mar, and Stewart (1978) and Rusch and Schutz (1982) used similar questionnaire methodologies to identify entry level behavioral requirements for sheltered and competitive employment options. Tables 11.1 and 11.2 provide examples of behavior requirements that are associated with sheltered and competitive employment.

A review of these requirements reveal behavior standards that go far beyond the potential capabilities of individuals with the most profound handicaps. These standards should not be interpreted rigidly or used to exclude persons with profound handicaps from more enhancing vocational opportunities. At best, the behavior requirements identified by Mithaug et al. (1978) and Rusch and Schutz (1982) suggest general vocational competencies that should be approximated in a public school's vocational curriculum. These general competencies also suggest important areas in which partial participation should be developed. To identify the specific purpose of the program planning, interviews should be conducted with employers and questionnaires should be individually administered to provide assistance in identifying important behavioral requirements and possible accommodations or adaptations that may be necessary for someone to contribute meaningfully in a particular setting.

A variety of formats have been proposed for conducting detailed analyses of specific vocational opportunities. Belmore and Brown (1976) proposed the

Table 11.1. Behavior standards in vocational survival skills selected for entry by 90% or more of sheltered workshop supervisors

Employees should be able to:

1. Participate in work environments for 6-hour periods
2. Move safely about the shop by:
   a. Walking from place to place
   b. Identifying and avoiding dangerous areas
   c. Wearing safe work clothing
3. Work continuously at a job station for 1–2 hour periods
4. Learn new tasks when the supervisor explains them by modeling
5. Come to work on an average of five times per week
6. Correct work on a task after the second correction
7. Want to work for money/sense of accomplishment
8. Understand work routine by not displaying disruptive behavior during routine program changes
9. Continue work without disruptions when:
   a. Supervisor is observing
   b. Coworker is observing
   c. Stranger is observing
10. Adapt to new work environment with normal levels of productivity in 1–5 days and with normal levels of contacts with supervisor in 30–60 minutes.

From Rusch, F.R., & Mithaug, D.E. (1980). *Vocational training for mentally retarded adults: A behavior analytic approach.* Champaign, IL: Research Press; reprinted by permission.

"Madison Job Skill Inventory" as a recommended outline for identifying work and work-related behaviors (see Table 11.3). The Belmore and Brown (1976) inventory is developed from direct observations of successful workers and interviews with supervisors at the actual workplace. The emphasis in this method of job analysis is on the skill requirements that workers must fulfill to succeed. Although the Madison Job Skill Inventory is a very useful method for attaining a better understanding of the skills that enable workers to perform more effectively, this method of assessment is not geared toward identifying workplace modification or redesigning job tasks that better accommodate the individual. For workers with profound handicaps, unique modifications of settings and tasks may be necessary to more actively involve these individuals in the work place. Priest and Roessler (1983) recommend the use of an industrial engineer to assist the special education or rehabilitation professional in identifying potential problems in job demands and accessibility that must be addressed. These authors suggest a multilevel analysis of the workplace, including a continuum of macro- to micro-motion assessments. As educators attempt to more fully involve students with profound handicaps in vocational experiences, job analysis will need to be more broadly conceptualized to encompass the realities of the workplace, the unique characteristics of the workers, and the potential accommodations and support services that will be required to enable people to participate in community employment settings.

Table 11.2. Vocational survival skills selected for entry level competitive employment by 90% or more of supervisors

Employee should be able to:

1. Demonstrate basic arithmetic skills to add
2. Tell and follow time
   a. On the hour
   b. On the half-hour
   c. On the quarter-hour
   d. On the five minutes
   e. On the minute
3. Come to work on the average of five times per week
4. Recognize the importance of attendance and punctuality by not being absent from work or late more than an average of three times per month
5. Complete repetitive tasks previously learned to proficiency within at least 0%–25% of average rate
6. Work at the job continuously, remaining on task for at least 30–60 minute intervals
7. Move safely about the work setting by paying attention to obvious obstruction in pathway
8. Understand work routine by not displaying disruptive behaviors when routine task or schedule changes occur
9. Want to work for money
10. Read at least one- to two-word sentences
11. Learn, to minimum proficiency, new job tasks when given a maximum of 6–12 hours of instructions
12. Participate in work environments for periods of at least 3–4 hours

From Rusch, F., & Schutz, R. (1982). *Vocational assessment and curriculum guide.* Seattle, WA: Exceptional Education.

Vocational Assessment Vocational assessment activities should provide information about a person's skills and performance in order to promote appropriate training decisions (Bellamy et al., 1979). The content of vocational assessments should evolve directly from assessment activities that delineate the behaviors associated with participation in community work settings. This method of vocational assessment is termed *criterion-referenced assessment.* In criterion-referenced assessment, vocational behaviors are specified in measurable terms and the person is frequently evaluated regarding his or her progress toward acquiring these skills.

Criterion-referenced assessments should be used for individual comparison purposes regarding a person's present performance level in relation to an established standard. However, it is important to emphasize that the primary purpose of these assessments should be to individualize training and support rather than be used to determine eligibility for vocational involvement (Bates & Pancsofar, 1985).

Traditional vocational assessments, in contrast to criterion-referenced assessment, provide an evaluation of a person's aptitudes and skills in comparison to other workers. Too often, these assessments only confirm that people with

Table 11.3. Madison job skill inventory

General information:
1. Why considered
2. Job description
3. Description of social environment

Specific work skills required:
1. Physical/sensory motor
2. Basic interpersonal
3. Language
4. Functional academic
5. Machine and tool use
6. Hygiene

Supportive skills and other required information:
1. Transportation
2. Work preparation
3. Money management
4. Time telling and time judgment

severe handicaps are not as capable as workers who are nonhandicapped or who have lesser handicaps. The unfortunate result of these assessments is the conclusion that persons with severe handicaps may not be qualified for community employment. For individuals with profound handicaps, this "conclusion of exclusion" is almost inescapable for traditional vocational assessments.

With criterion-referenced assessments, behaviors that are associated with making vocational contributions are identified and personal comparisons are made through frequent evaluations of a person's acquisition of greater competence in their areas of participation. In conjunction with individualized instruction and feedback, modifications of job routines, and use of personalized adaptations to compensate for physical or sensory deficits, criterion-referenced assessments can be used to document the support conditions under which a person's vocational contributions can be maximized.

Selection of Vocational Training Objectives The content of a vocational training program is determined by assessment activities that identify a person's present level of performance in relation to standards for more effective performance in meaningful work activities. Training objectives should represent the discrepancy between what an individual needs to do to succeed more effectively in community employment versus what that person presently does.

Although this recommended procedure for selecting vocational objectives is valid and defensible, a person with profound handicaps typically will experience deficits in virtually all areas. In these situations, the greater challenge will be prioritizing objectives. The prioritization of objectives is inherently subjective to a large degree, involving many of the following considerations: required frequency of the target behavior(s), availability of support services involving specific job demands, consumer (i.e., employer, family, student) interests, physical and sensory disabilities of the worker, physical modifications and/or adaptations of job requirements, and flexibility of the employer or vocational setting. Specific disabilities associated with profound handicapping conditions (e.g., severe spasticity, multiple sensory impairments, high rate self-injurious behavior) may prevent full completion of vocational tasks or job routines. In these situations, partial participation objectives (Baumgart et al., 1982) need to be developed and the value of these "partial" contributions should be recognized and appreciated by employers, consumers, professionals, and others.

Longitudinal Vocational Training   Since individuals with profound handicaps are slow learners and experience problems in skill generalization, it is imperative that vocational education efforts begin at a young age. These efforts should systematically involve the student in a wider range of vocational experiences across several job clusters, vocational supervisors, and training settings. The identification of home-related vocational skills and the development of basic work habits should be considered to be top priorities of longitudinal vocational training efforts within the public schools. Although many of the recommendations provided in this section are derived from work experience and research involving individuals with moderate and severe mental retardation, extensions of these recommendations through "partial participations" should be considered. These extensions can help individuals with profound handicaps to become more meaningfully involved in vocational training.

Several entry level occupations require skills that are necessary for more independent functioning within the home setting. Specific service occupations that overlap with household responsibilities are janitorial/housekeeping, laundry, and food service. Since preparation for a more self-sufficient life in the home and community should begin early in a student's school experience and since the home setting provides a natural environment in which to perform many vocationally related behaviors, students should be prepared to assume increasingly greater responsibility for household tasks. This emphasis on household tasks or chores in the elementary school years may help to offset criticism by teachers or parents that young children should not be involved in vocational education. Most nonhandicapped children are required to do daily or weekly chores from the age of 5 or 6. By encouraging parents to develop creative ways to assist their child to partially participate in household tasks, educators are fostering the development of important vocational competencies and promoting positive attitudes toward work and meaningful participation.

Simplified household chores can be assigned when the child is young and/ or at the beginning skill levels. For example, picking up items from the bathroom floor, unloading the dryer, and sorting silverware are three household skills associated with service industry employment that could be adapted to promote participation across differing ability levels. Cooperative planning with each student's family would contribute toward the identification of individualized vocational objectives and expanded opportunities to perform vocational routines within the home setting. Partial participation in household tasks should be encouraged as a way to involve persons with profound handicaps in meaningful work activities within the home setting.

Vocational training programs for persons with profound handicaps should provide experience that promotes the development of *basic work habits*. Basic work habits are behaviors that contribute to one's productivity and independence in school, home, and community settings, and include paid employment. Training experiences that are designed to improve basic work habits should reflect the behavioral demands of the diverse settings in which these habits are required. As a person progresses through a public school program, the behavioral demands associated with basic work habits may become more complex, duration of work periods may increase, and location of training should shift from school to community settings.

Individuals being trained to work in the community need to learn that they have daily responsibilities that must be fulfilled before they can participate in leisure activities or other special events. Such responsibility can be shaped by scheduling increasingly longer daily work periods for elementary, intermediate, and secondary age students. For students who are younger and/or more profoundly handicapped, these work periods may initially be scheduled for 15-minute time blocks. The duration of daily vocational responsibilities may be increased from 15-minute routines to work periods that approximate work schedules in the community.

Arriving to work on time, wearing appropriate clothing, checking in, going to an assigned work area, and beginning work independently are part of an arrival routine that is performed on a daily basis in most employment situations. Within a school's vocational training program, independence, persistence, productivity, and endurance are vocational competencies that should be developed in order for individuals to participate more effectively in community employment. Independence is a relative criterion that refers to a person's ability to perform various job routines with less supervision or assistance. Persistence may be defined as the percentage of time a worker stays on-task by engaging in actions that are functional to job completion. Productivity refers to the amount of work completed in a given time period and is measured in comparison to individually determined normative standards. Finally, endurance can be measured by the length of time a person works without taking a break and the total amount of time worked in a day. Efforts to assist people in developing greater independence, persistence, productivity, and endurance must begin early in a person's school career.

Independence is best developed by exposing people to a variety of job situations with necessary adaptations/accommodations and individualized instruction for a sufficient length of time to enable them to acquire greater proficiency and to experience success. Independence in vocational skills is made easier by the use of task analyses of required job routines, consistent instruction, and adaptations/accommodations to facilitate effective job performance. As students progress through a school program, their job routines may become more complex, supervision might be reduced to reflect more natural conditions, and location of work experiences should shift from school to community situations. However, some workers may never be independent in the typical sense of the word. For these individuals, unique support services should be orchestrated to enable vocational participation.

Persistence or on-task behavior is best developed by improving a student's independence and increasing his or her productivity. Reinforcement for work productivity will promote the development of greater persistence in vocational situations. For example, early in a student's vocational experience, he or she may be reinforced for each assembly completed or for brief periods of on-task behavior. Later, this student may receive reinforcement less frequently and in less immediately tangible ways (e.g., periodic social praise, paychecks).

It is often assumed that paychecks are reinforcing for all people; however, these payments may not be functionally related to differential productivity records. The traditional 2-week paycheck is too delayed and too indirectly related to work performance to operate as a positive reinforcer for productivity for persons with profound handicaps. However, piece rate payments could be gradually thinned from immediate reinforcement and exchange systems to more intermittent and delayed reinforcement contingencies. As an intermediate step toward establishing more traditional reinforcement and delayed exchange systems for work performance, daily paychecks could be immediately cashed and half of the money made available for purchases of desired items and half made available for savings. To make savings more concrete, bar graphs leading toward the purchase of a desired item could be used to make the abstract nature of savings more concrete. The cooperation of parents is crucial in this effort to make work payment both meaningful and reinforcing. Parents can cooperate by taking their son or daughter to a store, and/or by instituting a simplified "chore" contingent allowance system.

All vocational training programs should emphasize the more naturally occurring, reinforcing aspects of work contributions. For example, parents and teachers or other professionals should verbally connect the person's work contributions with the products produced and/or the changes in an environment that are the result of a vocational effort (e.g., clean table). It may be initially helpful to select vocational tasks that provide a worker with more concrete feedback. For instance, it may be more naturally reinforcing to observe the contrast between a very dirty table and one that has been cleaned. Also, it may be more reinforcing to assemble items that provide differential feedback when completed correctly (e.g., flashlight, ballpoint pen).

In addition to specific vocational skills, time management, social-interpersonal competencies, and community travel are important work-related behaviors that should be emphasized in the development of basic work habits.

Students may benefit from instruction in time management skills to assist them in beginning and terminating work at the appropriate time. Initially, buzzers may be used to provide a more concrete cue that work time should begin or has ended. Socially, students should also be taught skills such as how to act during nonstructured times (e.g., breaks). Finally, travel skills should be developed for employment and other aspects of community participation. Since many people may never travel independently, the importance of appropriate passenger behavior in an automobile or bus (e.g., wearing a seat belt, sitting quietly) should be emphasized. If a person with profound handicaps acquires behaviors that enable him or her to more readily use conventional transportation means and to travel without behavioral disruptions, he or she will have far more opportunities to participate in community activities.

Community Training   It is inappropriate to assume that vocational skills that were acquired in a school setting will generalize to community environments (Bates & Cuvo, 1984). If the goal is to promote community employment, educators must be committed to conducting instruction in those environments where these skills are required. Therefore, schools must establish training sites with community employers. Ideally, throughout a student's secondary education, he or she will have a variety of community employment experiences in different career areas. For individuals with profound handicaps, these community-based training experiences should provide a solid foundation on which to build supported employment opportunities as part of the individual's adult life-style.

Transition Planning   As a student approaches the last years of his or her eligibility for public school services, information from a student's various vocational experiences provides excellent data from which a more permanent career choice can be made as part of a transition plan (Brown et al., 1981). Such a transition plan must involve active input from the student through his or her expressed or observed interests, the student's family, via opinions, and community employers and/or coworkers from their support. A person's transition plan from school to employment must also involve input from school personnel and adult services representatives. The primary objective of such a plan is to assist students in attaining and maintaining a dignified postschool life-style that includes the opportunity to participate vocationally as an adult.

Successful program demonstrations on community employment for people with severe handicaps have usually combined progressive curriculum practices with extended on-the-job training and client advocacy (Rusch, 1986). Unfortunately, these demonstrations are still relatively few in number and many programmatic needs must be addressed before persons with profound handicaps can be served effectively. These needs include a commitment to the philosophy of integration and ongoing skill development for all persons, community-referenced curriculum development, longitudinal training, transition planning, extended on-the-job training, and ongoing follow-up support. One of the most important results of longitudinal vocational training will be the clarification of unique job accommodations and supervisory supports that will be necessary in order to involve persons with profound handicaps in the workplace.

If a school or agency emphasizes the right of all citizens to be included into a sequence of vocational instruction, persons with profound handicaps should receive training that will assist them in working more effectively in such integrated employment settings. Curriculum should be developed through local assessments of employment availability, detailed analyses of requisite vocational competencies, and individualized adaptations to better meet performance demands. Vocational experiences should begin as soon as students enter school and continue through transition planning. These experiences should involve extended community training in a variety of career options. Follow-up support services, cooperative arrangements with family members, and ongoing client advocacy are means through which the benefits of progressive vocational training practices can be maintained and extended throughout a person's adult life.

Although postschool programs have had a degree of success in placing some persons with severe handicaps in competitive employment situations, vocational training in the public schools must be accompanied by a sophisticated system of postschool support services for individuals with profound handicaps. These postschool support services include supported employment for adults and other progressive vocational training practices such as expanded job matching strategies, innovative behavioral interventions, generalization training and rehabilitation engineering.

EMPLOYMENT SERVICES FOR ADULTS

Traditionally, persons with profound handicaps have not been involved in vocationally oriented adult service programs. In fact, such individuals often fail eligibility requirements for most of these programs or find themselves on long waiting lists for services. However, the continuum of vocational training services for adults with disabilities is being reexamined very closely and innovative service options, such as supported employment, are being expanded to more adequately address the needs of all people who want to acquire more meaningful vocational competencies. In this section the traditional continuum of vocational services for adults is examined critically and the development of supported employment is described as a means to more fully realize the potential of persons with profound handicaps to participate in integrated community work environments.

Continuum of Vocational Training Services

In many conceptualizations of the rehabilitation process, the sheltered workshop is viewed as being an intermediate step along a continuum that leads to competitive employment. Within the sheltered workshop facility, many local programs operate work activities or day training programs, work adjustment training, extended sheltered employment, and transitional employment services. This continuum of services is designed, in theory, to meet individual needs and to promote ongoing skill development that results in community employment. However, national placement and movement data within the continuum suggest that an adult with mental retardation has virtually no chance of obtaining competitive employment by progressing through the continuum (Bellamy, Sheehan, Horner, & Boles, 1980).

If the rehabilitation continuum of services is not working, what is the solution? Some people have advocated that the system should be fixed by promoting movement through the continuum; others have suggested that the continuum model is inherently flawed and that it should be abandoned. A major flaw in the continuum model of vocational services for people with disabilities was the development of training settings that were removed physically, socially, and psychologically from the criterion environments of community employment. The nonwork orientation of many of these settings, combined with the handicapped-only coworker environment and lack of individualized instruction, have resulted in a bottleneck in the continuum of vocational training services (Pomerantz & Marholin, 1977). Only the most skilled clients have been able to avoid stagnation within this continuum and to move on to more enhancing employment opportunities in the community. The inadequacies of this continuum are so serious that persons with severe and profound handicaps have virtually no chance of progressing to integrated service settings or community employment.

Abandonment of this continuum model does not mean that all people should be involved in an identical vocational training program, regardless of the severity of their disabilities. As an alternative to the traditional continuum model for providing vocational services, a variety of vocational options varying in intensity of support services should be developed to meet unique training needs. However, these options should emphasize participation in integrated community employment settings rather than preparation for community employment as the primary means of enhancing productivity and independence. Supported employment is a relatively new program initiative of rehabilitation services that has evolved from dual concerns that are related to the value of integration and the need for ongoing support services that may be required for some individuals to participate more effectively in community employment.

Supported Employment

Through the development of supported employment, unprecedented opportunities were created for persons with profound handicaps to perform meaningful work in community employment settings. According to the *Federal Register* (1984), supported employment refers to:

> Paid employment which (i) is for persons with developmental disabilities for whom competitive employment at or above the minimum wage is unlikely and who, because of their disabilities, need ongoing support to perform in a work setting; (ii) is conducted in a variety of settings, particularly work sites in which persons without disabilities are employed, and (iii) is supported by any activity needed to sustain paid work by persons with disabilities, including supervision, training, and transportation. (§ 102)

The target population for supported employment services is intended to be:

> (A) for individuals with severe handicaps for whom competitive employment has not traditionally occurred, or (B) for individuals for whom competitive employment has been interrupted or intermittent as a result of severe disability, and who, because of their handicap, need on-going support services to perform such work. (Supported Employment, 1987, p. 1)

Services authorized under supported employment:

> . . . include but are not limited to an evaluation of rehabilitation potential, provision of skilled trainers who accompany the worker for intensive on-the-job training, systematic training, job development, follow-up services (including regular contact with the employer, trainee, and the parent or guardian), and . . . regular observation or supervision of the individual with severe handicaps at the training site and other services needed to support the individual in employment. (Supported Employment, 1987, p. 1)

Although the supported employment initiative is geared toward individuals with the "most" severe handicaps, there is uncertainty and pessimism among professionals, advocates, and consumers regarding the capability of this initiative to meet the needs of persons with profound handicaps. If supported employment is to successfully involve persons with profound handicaps in community employment, more aggressive and innovative job development strategies will be needed, progressive on-the-job training strategies must be implemented, and ongoing support services must be developed.

In job development, a new relationship between human services agencies (including schools and rehabilitation programs) and employers must evolve. Traditional marketing strategies that support the placement of persons with disabilities in community employment have used advocacy tactics that have promised employers a work-ready, dependable employee who will not require additional supervisory time. Since opportunities and benefits of community employment are being extended to people with more severe disabilities, including those with profound handicaps, innovative job development strategies will be required.

With supported employment, more intrusive means are required to secure and maintain employment. Employers must be willing to work closely with school and/or rehabilitation training staff in job development, training, and ongoing support. Also, since many people who are targeted for supported employment will not attain competitive performance levels, employers must either absorb this loss in productivity or compensate for it with alternative payment mechanisms (e.g., subminimum wage certificates). For people with severe physical handicaps, modifications at the job site may be necessary for accessibility and/or more efficient completion of job duties.

Since the willingness of the private sector to expand available job opportunities and to work closely with human services agencies is pivotal to the expansion of supported employment opportunities, employers must be recruited to assume leadership roles in this process. Employers control the availability of jobs. Therefore, these employers must identify the conditions under which they are more likely to respond favorably to cooperative employment initiatives. In many cases, private employers may reject supported employment arrangements for people with profound handicaps because they see it as being unfeasible or unproductive. If this rejection is widespread, individuals with profound handicaps may be excluded from a program initiative that was originally conceived as a viable means to assist them in attaining and maintaining employment outcomes. Government intervention programs that go beyond present incentives, such as the Targeted Jobs Tax Credit (TJTC) program, may be necessary to offset the reluctance of the private sector to expand employment opportunities through supported employment options for workers who are profoundly handicapped. These intervention programs may include greater economic incentives for employers, more aggressive affirmative action efforts, and publicly supported work opportunities.

The frequency and sophistication of ongoing support services that may be required to maintain persons with profound handicaps in community employment alternatives will soon become more of an issue. The economic cost-benefit of these arrangements varies according to the intensity of support services that are required and the productivity levels of the workers. For example, some workers may only require two to three contacts with a supervisor per month to maintain employment, while others may require constant personalized supervision. As a result, many supported employment alternatives have targeted individuals with milder disabilities rather than those with severe and profound handicaps.

Supported employment must be considered as a viable means to serve all adults who desire vocational participation in community employment settings. However, in addition to the marketing strategies that must be initiated to create greater opportunity for supported employment, government incentives and innovative behavioral training strategies in combination with rehabilitation engineering interventions will be needed to maximize the participation of persons with profound handicaps in community employment.

PROGRESSIVE VOCATIONAL TRAINING PRACTICES

School and adult services are faced with the challenge of matching the philosophy of community employment integration of persons with profound handicaps with an effective technology for facilitating this involvement. In addition to the curriculum recommendations for longitudinal public school preparation and the new opportunities created by the development of supported employment, several extensions and innovations of existing vocational training practices must be explored. These extensions and innovations include: expanded perspective on job matching, increased sophistication and precision in use of behavioral strategies, added generalization training, and increased rehabilitation engineering. Each of these innovations is described as part of an emerging technology for facilitating meaningful participation in community employment.

Job Matching

Many proposals established for use in providing vocational training involving persons with disabilities have emphasized the importance of *job matching*. Job matching typically refers to the compatibility between a person's present skills and interests and the physical and interpersonal demands of the job. Unfortunately, the skill level of individuals with profound handicaps does not match with many, if any, community employment situations. For these individuals, a more expanded and dynamic conceptualization of job matching is needed. This conceptualization should focus on both the worker and the employment situation. Improved curriculum and vocational preparation will result in workers' acquiring more skills that are required in community job situations. Also, employer accommodations (e.g., simplified job routines, flexible schedules) and enhanced coworker/supervisor supports will enable more individuals with significant disabilities to be involved in community employment. Specific job training during an extended period of time, coupled with ongoing supported employment services, should enable an even more diverse and lesser skilled work force to be meaningfully involved in community work situations.

Figure 11.1 provides a diagram of the dynamic nature of the job matching process described above. This diagram illustrates the multiple variables that contribute to a more successful match between a worker's skills and interests and the physical and interpersonal demands of the employment situation. When the employment situations become more accommodating, when the workers are more skilled, and/or when the availability of support services increases, persons with handicaps will become an integral part of the employed work force. By expanding the traditional conceptualization of job matching, the prospects of vocational participation by persons with profound handicaps in the community are increased. The shaded areas of this figure represent the expansion in job matches that are created through an expansion of vocational curriculum and support services.

Behavioral Training Strategies

The use of behavioral strategies in the vocational training of persons with severe handicaps has been documented extensively (Bellamy et al., 1979; Renzaglia, Bates, & Hutchins, 1981; Wehman et al., 1985). These strategies have

Dynamic Match

Worker   Employment Situation

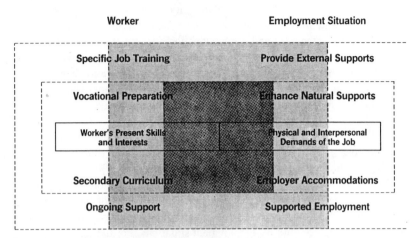

Figure 11.1. A diagram of the dynamic job matching conceptualization that illustrates the multiple variables that contribute to a more successful match.

been empirically validated with acquisition- and production-related target behaviors, as well as work-related social skills. Task analysis, instructional tapes, material arrangement, systematic prompting, response chaining, redundant cues, easy-to-hard sequencing, response feedback, and reinforcement are examples of strategies that have been documented to be effective with persons who are severely handicapped. For more indepth descriptions of behavioral strategies for vocational training, the reader is referred to Bellamy et al. (1979), Renzaglia et al. (1981), and Wehman et al. (1985). Unfortunately, these research demonstrations and programmatic recommendations have not included persons with profound handicaps.

Meaningful involvement of persons who are profoundly handicapped in community employment is hindered by learning problems and physical disabilities that interfere with acquisition and speed of performance. Although not supported by existing literature, these acquisition and production problems can be offset to a certain degree by systematic behavioral interventions. Examples of acquisition- and production-related interventions are presented in the following paragraphs to illustrate programmatic arrangements that meet some of the unique learning needs of persons with profound handicaps.

Bellamy et al. (1979) recommend that task analyses should identify the specific discriminative stimuli that precede each successive step or component behavior of a targeted task. This method for developing task analyses details the specific conditions that a person must discriminate in order to perform his or her duties competently. Assessment data from these detailed task analyses may reveal information that has immediate program utility. If a person exhibits an error pattern that is consistently related to specific stimulus conditions, modifications can be made to highlight the discriminative cue conditions associated with performing specific steps.

In response to a production-related problem, Bates, Renzaglia, and Clees (1980) reported the results of using a changing criterion design to evaluate a systematic strategy for improving the vocational productivity of three workers with severe and profound levels of mental retardation. The one individual in this study with profound mental retardation had been institutionalized most of her life. This individual (Lucy) was 20 years of age, ambulatory, nonverbal, and frequently engaged in off-task competing behaviors such as grabbing materials, flicking her fingers, and staring at other workers.

After several weeks of systematic instruction, Lucy acquired a three-piece drapery pulley assembly; however, her production rate on this task was approximately 1% of the competetive standard and far below the standard established by the local sheltered workshop for admission to their program.

Due to Lucy's low production rate, a program was developed to specifically address this deficit in her vocational repertoire. This program initially consisted of teaching her to self-administer reinforcements (e.g., one penny after completing every two drapery pulleys). After Lucy was self-administering reinforcements consistently on the FR-2 schedule, changing criterion contingencies were initiated. The initial criterion contingency was determined by calculating Lucy's average production rate during baseline and requiring her to meet or exceed this rate to keep her money so that she could purchase snacks in the workshop store. The criterion contingency was communicated to Lucy by calculating the number of pennies that needed to be earned for her to meet the production requirements. After the required number of pennies was calculated, this number of openings in penny holders were left exposed and she was informed that she needed to earn that much money to purchase items in the store. If she failed to match or exceed the criterion, the pennies were removed and she was told she would need to work faster next time in order to have money.

After Lucy's production rate exceeded each criterion level for at least 3 of 4 consecutive days, the criterion level was increased again. Over 181 program days, Lucy responded successfully to 14 criterion changes and was performing well above the sheltered workshop minimum standard (see Figure 11.2). During this study, Lucy's performance reached a high of 40% of the competitive standard. However, if the amount of nonproduction time (e.g., placing pulleys in the jig and self-administering penny reinforcers) was subtracted from her total time, Lucy's assembly time was virtually equivalent to a nonhandicapped production standard.

Although the results of this longitudinal vocational training demonstration involving a person with profound mental retardation are important, several limitations need to be noted. First, this study was conducted in an experimental

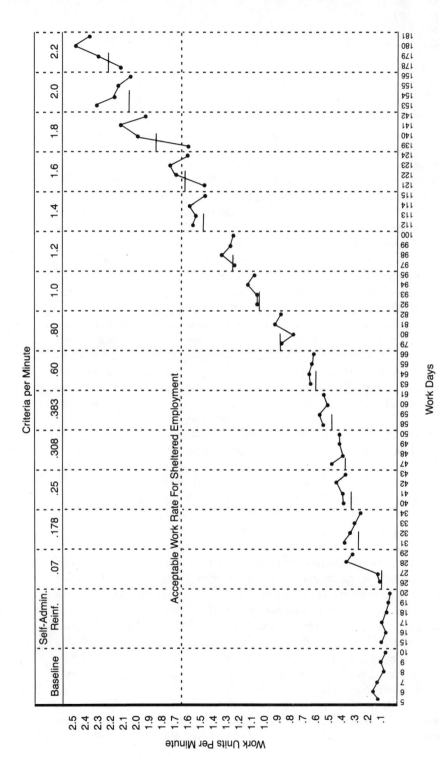

Figure 11.2. Lucy's work production rate on a drapery pulley assembly as a function of self-administered reinforcement and a changing criterion. (From Bates, P., Renzaglia, P. & Clees, T. [1980]. Improving the work performance of severely/profoundly retarded young adults: The use of a changing criterion procedural design. *Education and Training of the Mentally Retarded, 15,* 95–104; reprinted by permission.)

program and the individual's ability to generalize the findings is limited by the restricted nature of this setting. Second, the focus of this study was on workshop readiness rather than integrated community employment. Finally, the program contingencies were not faded and the long-term success of this training effort was not evaluated. It is extremely important that future research activities address the limitations of this study and contribute to the development of an empirical base for enhancing the participation of persons who are profoundly handicapped into integrated community work settings.

Despite the evidence of successful behavioral interventions, including vocational behaviors, the potential for all persons with profound handicaps to perform meaningful work in integrated settings is questionable. The extensive amount of vocational training research in special education and rehabilitation journals contains very little information regarding successful strategies for involving people with profound handicaps in community employment. Despite the fact that many of these vocational training studies cite the inclusion of persons with profound mental retardation in their titles (e.g., Bates et al., 1980; Bellamy, Peterson, & Close, 1975), very few if any of these studies involved participants with additional handicapping conditions and/or employment in integrated community settings. Ferguson and Ferguson (1986) state that:

> Professionals involved in adult services should be increasingly uncomfortable with the knowledge that despite the undeniable improvements, there are still people for whom the field has only a vague idea of what an adult life of meaningful community participation might encompass. (p. 335)

If persons with profound handicaps are to participate more effectively in integrated community employment settings, behavioral interventions and applied research must be extended to these target settings and individuals. The focus of these behavioral interventions must be expanded to include the multiple variables that influence the availability of community employment. Possible targets for such intervention include employers, coworkers, supervisors, and education and rehabilitation professionals.

Generalization Training

Efficiency in providing instruction is a major concern in training programs in the vocational area. If learners fail to generalize, they may require individualized instruction when task demands vary slightly, when work settings change, and/or when supervisory conditions are altered. In a major review of behavioral research, Stokes and Baer (1977) observed that generalization training was inadequately addressed in most studies; however, several strategies were identified that represent more active efforts to promote generalization. The concept of "general case" instruction has been introduced as a methodology for enhancing generalized responding (Becker & Engelmann, 1978). This methodology incorporates strategies identified by Stokes and Baer (1977), including training sufficient exemplars and programming common stimuli. With general case programming, teaching examples are selected on the basis of their ability to incorporate the range of stimulus and response variations associated with targeted behaviors in the natural environment. After acquiring behaviors that represent the variability in stimulus and response requirements of a particular task, learners should be able to perform novel vocational tasks for which they have not received prior training. Horner, Sprague, and Wilcox (1982) provide guidelines for adapting the general case methodology for teaching community living skills to individuals with severe handicaps. In the vocational skill area, examples of general case programming include generalized table bussing (Horner, Eberhard, & Sheehan, 1986), and generalized crimp and cut skills for assembling biaxle electronic capacitors (Horner & McDonald, 1982).

Although Horner and his colleagues (Horner et al., 1986; Horner & McDonald, 1982; Horner et al., 1982) have operationalized the general case methodology through programmatic guidelines and empirical research, the target population in most of the research in this area are individuals with moderate or severe mental retardation, not persons with profound mental retardation and/ or multiple handicaps. In a general case research study involving individuals with profound mental retardation, Pancsofar and Bates (1985) examined the effect of acquiring successive training examples on the skills involved in generalized soap dispenser operation. Three different types or response classes of soap dispensers were used as training materials in this study, with multiple variations of each type. When the individuals with profound mental retardation demonstrated the ability to operate at least two types of soap dispensers, they were able to use novel or unfamiliar soap dispensers. From a subjective perspective, it appeared that the subjects were more likely to approach novel soap dispensers after they learned that a similar task could be performed correctly in at least two different ways. Further research is needed in this area to more directly investigate learning experiences that facilitate generalized responding with this population.

If young children experience multiple opportunities for success in performing simplified vocational behaviors, they may be likely to successfully approach new tasks. Seligman (1975) suggests that a history of successful experiences is the most effective treatment for overcoming "learned helplessness," a belief that nothing one does makes a difference. Since individuals with profound handicaps are particularly vulnerable to the debilitating effects of learned helplessness, vigorous efforts need to be taken to increase experiences of control and predictability of environmental events. Vocational training should be viewed as an opportunity to enhance a person's competence through a sequence of carefully planned curriculum experiences. In conjunction with general case programming principals, systematic behavioral training, and technological innovations, the curriculum experiences enacted by future generations of persons with profound handicaps will afford this population the increased opportunity to develop skills and make meaningful vocational contributions.

Rehabilitation Engineering

The sensory deficits and physical movement limitations of many individuals require the development of adaptations to meet the unique needs of the individual and the task. Since many of these situations pose engineering technology challenges, the use of rehabilitation engineers in vocational program development is increasingly being used. Given the value of their expertise, rehabilitation engineers should be involved more frequently in job analysis for identifying job modifications, designing work stations, and developing assistive devices.

Job modifications involve adjustments in job routines and/or simplification of task demands to compensate for the worker's physical and/or sensory disabilities that may interfere with his or her performance. Work station design may include changes in the surface height of work tables, location of materials, and seating arrangements. These job modifications and work station design changes can be used in conjunction with assistive devices (e.g., hand or head switches) to facilitate involvement and meaningful vocational participation by individuals who are disabled.

Although there is tremendous potential for expanding the involvement of rehabilitation engineers into the vocational training and placement of persons with profound handicaps, virtually all demonstrations involving these resources have involved individuals with physical disabilities who were cognitively normal or who had mild mental retardation. For example, Leslie (1980) reported on the development of a head controlled switching device that enabled an employee who was physically handicapped with normal intelligence to operate a lathe. With individuals who are mildly mentally retarded and physically disabled, Biddy, Smith, and Swarts (1975) reported on the use of jigs and fixtures to increase worker safety and productivity on a wide variety of sheltered work tasks. More recently, Pietruski, Everson, Goodwyn, and Wehman (1985) described several modifications that facilitated more independent performance in an integrated community work setting by persons with physical disabilities.

As of this time, rehabilitation engineering interventions have not been reported in community work settings involving individuals with profound handicaps. The absence of such reports is disturbing, yet encouraging. The failure of people with profound handicaps to participate in community employment settings may not be the result of inherent limits posed by their disability, but may instead reflect society's failure to best use behavioral and rehabilitation engineering technology to meet this population's needs. In a discussion of technology and persons with handicaps, Withrow, Withrow, and Withrow (1986) observe that special interface means can be used to enable people to operate a computer if their only controllable motor-reponse is a blink of the eye. Rehabilitation engineering technology, in combination with behavioral interventions to improve motor control of persons with severe physical disabilities (Neilson & McLaughey, 1982; Skrotzky, Gallenstein, & Osternig, 1978), will afford new opportunities for meaningful vocational participation. It is important to realize that current projections regarding a person's ability to contribute vocationally are made in the absence of universally available exemplary curriculum practices, sophisticated behavioral training, and rehabilitation engineering practices.

SUMMARY

A number of human services reform movements involving persons with developmental disabilities have changed from being overly optimistic to taking on a conservative deviation from traditional practice. In many cases, deinstitutionalization has come to mean the movement of individuals from large state operated residential facilities to slightly smaller, but still quite large community residential facilities. Normalization has fallen short of its expectations of enforcing systemic and radical changes in human services delivery systems. Ferguson and Ferguson (1986) provide the following words of caution regarding current reform movements in vocational services: "The field must ask whether the undeniably needed reform is broad enough in vision to incorporate improvements for individuals with even the most profound and multiple disabilities" (p. 331).

This chapter attempts to articulate ways in which this vision can be expanded. First, it is important to recognize that the lack of involvement in meaningful work experience by persons with profound handicaps may be, in part, attributed to the restricted focus of interventions. Specifically, the focus on the individual's strengths and weaknesses fails to recognize that a person's ability to contribute vocationally is influenced more by opportunity, values of significant others, and support services that are available.

The focus of intervention must expand beyond the individual's behavioral deficits and incompetencies, and encompass the interpersonal culture that supports or rejects expanded vocational opportunity and community participation. Employers, coworkers, parents, and service providers need to be the focus of the inquiry. Strategies that result in employers being more willing to hire persons with disabilities and to make individualized support arrangements must be identified. Coworker support must be examined as a critical variable in the short- and long-term effectiveness of job placement. Parental involvement in transition planning and maintenance must be nurtured through close working relationships. Personnel preparation strategies must be examined to identify the best preservice and in-service training combinations, and to pinpoint the most important competencies that need to be developed.

Finally, the value of vocational training for persons with profound handicaps is best judged by the contribution that this involvement makes to the individual's quality of life. An individual's ability to partially participate in paid and nonpaid vocational situations should be respected (Baumgart et al. 1982) and arbitrary productivity or independence achievement levels should not be used to judge a person's worth. Vocational training activities can be productive for everyone, but in personally unique ways. Increased participation in integrated community work settings is an important and valued outcome of vocational training, but is not the only way in which a person contributes to his or her self-sufficiency, community, and society. Vocational training models for persons with profound handicaps should emphasize the opportunity for all people to participate in integrated work experience and to provide levels of support that nurture individual growth and development. If a person's disability prohibits participation in community employment, vocational training experiences can contribute to the individual's and others' quality of life in ways not usually used to measure program success. As a result of these experiences, the individual may be more self-sufficient within his or her household and/or have more control over circumstances that affect his or her daily routines. Also, as a result of increased opportunities for persons with profound handicaps to interact with nonhandicapped others as part of one's adult life-style, more socially responsive behaviors are being developed on the part of nonhandicapped others. Although the limits of present technology for facilitating meaningful vocational participation by all persons must be acknowledged, there appears to be much to gain and little to lose by expanding the vision of vocational involvement and pursuing the curriculum recommendations that are identified in this chapter.

REFERENCES

Andriano, T.A. (1977). The volunteer model of vocational habilitation as a component of the deinstitutionalization process. *Mental Retardation, 15*(4), 58–61.

Bates, P.E. (1986). Competitive employment in Southern Illinois: A traditional service delivery model for enhancing competitive employment outcomes for public school students. In F.R. Rusch (Ed.), *Competitive employment issues and strategies* (pp. 51 –63). Baltimore: Paul H. Brookes Publishing Co.

Bates, P., & Cuvo, A.J. (1984). Simulated and naturalistic instruction of community functioning skills with mentally retarded learners. *Association for Direct Instruction News, 7*(2), 14–16.

Bates, P., & Pancsofar, E. (1981). *Longitudinal vocational training for severely handicapped students in the public schools.* Springfield: Illinois State Board of Education.

Bates, P., & Pancsofar, E. (1985). Vocational assessment. In A. Rotatori & R. Fox (Eds.), *Assessment for regular and special education teachers* (pp. 335–360). Austin, TX: PRO-ED.

Bates, P., Renzaglia, A., & Clees, T. (1980). Improving the work performance of severely/profoundly retarded young adults: The use of a changing criterion procedural design. *Education and Training of the Mentally Retarded, 15*, 95–104.

Baumgart, D., Brown, L., Pumpian, I., Nisbet, J., Ford, A., Sweet, M., Messina, R., & Schroeder, J. (1982). Principle of partial participation and individualized adaptations in educational programs for severely handicapped students. *Journal of The Association for the Severely Handicapped, 7,* 17–27.

Becker, W.C., & Engelmann, S. (1978). Systems for basic instruction: Theory and applications. In A.C. Catania & T.A. Brigham (Eds.), *Handbook for applied behavior analysis: Social and instructional processes* (pp. 325–378).

Bellamy, G.T., Horner, R.H., & Inman, D.P. (1979). *Vocational habilitation of severely retarded adults: A direct service technology.* Baltimore: University Park Press.

Bellamy, G.T., Peterson, L., & Close, D. (1975). Habilitation of the severely and profoundly retarded: Illustrations of competence. *Education and Training of the Mentally Retarded, 10*(3), 174–185.

Bellamy, G.T., Sheehan, M.R., Horner, R.H., & Boles, S.M. (1980). Community programs for severely handicapped adults. *Journal of The Association for the Severely Handicapped, 5,* 307–324.

Bellamy, G.T., Rhodes, L.E., Wilcox, B., Albin, J.M., Mank, D.M., Boles, S.M., Horner, R.H., Collins, M., & Turner, J. (1984). Quality and equality in employment services for adults with severe disabilities. *Journal of The Association for Persons with Severe Handicaps, 9,* 270–277.

Belmore, K., & Brown, L. (1976). A job skill inventory strategy designed for severely handicapped potential workers. In L. Brown, N. Certo, K. Belmore, & T. Crowner (Eds.), *Madison's alternative for zero exclusion: Papers and programs related to public school services for secondary age severely handicapped students* (Vol. VI, part I, pp. 143–218). Madison, WI: Madison Metropolitan School District.

Biddy, R.L., Smith, D.R., & Swarts, A.E. (1975). *Examples of jig and fixture design as applied to the severely disabled functioning in a sheltered workshop.* Houston: Texas A & M University of Baylor College of Medicine, Department of Industrial Engineering and the Texas Institute for Rehabilitation and Research.

Brown, L., Pumpian, I., Baumgart, D., Van Deventer, L., Ford, A., Nisbet, J., Schroeder, J., & Grunewald, L. (1981). Longitudinal transition plans in programs for severely handicapped students. *Exceptional Children, 47*(8), 624–630.

Brown, L., Shiraga, B., York, J., Kessler, K., Strohm, B., Sweet, M., Zanella, K., VanDeventer, P., & Loomis, R. (1984). Integrated work opportunities for adults with severe handicaps: The extended training options. *Journal of The Association for Persons with Severe Handicaps, 9,* 262–269.

Federal Register, September 25, 1984, Developmental Disabilities Act of 1984, Report #98-1074, § 102(11)(F).

Ferguson, D.L., & Ferguson, P.M. (1986). The new Victors: A progressive policy analysis for work reform for people with very severe handicaps. *Mental Retardation, 24,* 331–338.

Horner, R.H., Eberhard, J.M., & Sheehan, M.R. (1986). Teaching generalized table bussing: The importance of negative teaching examples. *Behavioral Modification, 10,* 457–471.

Horner, R.H., & McDonald, R.S. (1982). A comparison of single instance and general case instruction in teaching a generalized vocational skill. *Journal of The Association for the Severely Handicapped, 7*(8), 7–20.

Horner, R.H., Sprague, J., & Wilcox, B. (1982). Constructing general case programs for community activities. In B. Wilcox & G.T. Bellamy, *Design of high school programs for severely handicapped students* (pp. 61–98). Baltimore: Paul H. Brookes Publishing Co.

Leslie, J.R. (1980). A competitive industry of severely disabled workers. In K. Mallik & E.M. Shaver (Eds.), *Unmasking abilities hidden by developmental conditions* (pp. 11–14). Washington, DC: George Washington University, Division of Rehabilitation Medicine.

Mank, D.M., Rhodes, L.E., & Bellamy, G.T. (1986). Four supported employment alternatives. In W.E. Kiernan & J.A. Stark (Eds.), *Pathways to employment for adults with development disabilities* (pp. 139–153). Baltimore: Paul H. Brookes Publishing Co.

Mithaug, D., Mar, D., & Stewart, O. (1978). *Prevocational assessment and curriculum guide.* Seattle, WA: Exceptional Education.

Neilson, P.D., & McLaughey, J. (1982). Self-regulation of spasm and spasticity in cerebral palsy. *Journal of Neurology, Neurosurgery, and Psychiatry, 45,* 320–330.

Pancsofar, E., & Bates, P. (1985). The impact of the acquisition of successive training exemplars on generalization. *Journal of The Association for the Severely Handicapped, 10*(2), 95–104.

Pietruski, W., Everson, J., Goodwyn, R., & Wehman, P. (1985). *Vocational training and curriculum for multihandicapped youth with cerebral palsy.* Richmond: Virginia Commonwealth University.

Pomerantz, D.J., & Marholin, D. (1977). Vocational habilitation: A time for change. In E. Sontag, J. Smith, & N. Certo (Eds.), *Educational programming for the severely and profoundly handicapped* (pp. 129–141). Reston, VA: Council for Exceptional Children.

Priest, J.W., & Roessler, R.T. (1983). Job analysis and workplace design resources for rehabilitation. *Rehabilitation Literature, 44,* 201–205.

Renzaglia, A., Bates P., & Hutchins, M. (1981). Vocational skills instruction for handicapped adolescents and adults. *Exceptional Education Quarterly, 2,* 61–73.

Rhodes, L.E., & Valenta, L. (1985). Industry-based supported employment: An enclave approach. *Journal of The Association for Persons with Severe Handicaps, 10,* 12–20.

Rusch, F.R. (Ed.). (1986). *Competitive employment issues and strategies.* Baltimore: Paul H. Brookes Publishing Co.

Rusch, F.R., & Mithaug, D.E. (1980). *Vocational training for mentally retarded adults: A behavior analytic approach.* Champaign, IL: Research Press.

Rusch, F., & Schutz, R. (1982). *Vocational assessment and curriculum guide.* Seattle, WA: Exceptional Education.

Seligman, M. (1975). *Helplessness: On depression, development, and death.* San Francisco: W.H. Freeman.

Skrotzky, K., Gallenstein, J., & Osternig, L. (1978). Effects of electromyographic feedback training on motor control in spastic cerebral palsy. *Physical Therapy, 58*(5), 547–551.

Stokes, T.F., & Baer, D.M. (1977). An implicit technology of generalization. *Journal of Applied Behavior Analysis, 10,* 349–367.

Supported Employment. (1987). *Rehab Brief, 10*(1), 1–4.

Turnbull, A.P., & Turnbull, H.R., III. (1985). Developing independence. *The Journal of Adolescent Health Care, 6*(2), 108–119.

Wehman, P., Renzaglia, A., & Bates, P. (1985). *Functional living skills for moderately and severely handicapped individuals.* Austin, TX: PRO-ED.

Will, M. (1985). Transition: Linking disabled youth to a productive future. *OSERS News in Print, 1*(1), 1.

Withrow, F.B., Withrow, M.S., & Withrow, D.F. (1986). Technology and the handicapped. *T.H.E. Journal, 13*(6), 65–67.

RESIDENTIAL SERVICES ⑫ FOR ADULTS WITH PROFOUND DISABILITIES

Fredda Brown, Rob Davis,
Michael Richards, and Kim Kelly

Deinstitutionalization, or the movement of people out of large public facilities, has had many intended and unintended effects upon citizens with developmental disabilities. In an evaluation of the social policy of deinstitutionalization, Willer and Intagliata (1984) indicate that one somewhat surprising result of this movement has been the shift from focusing on the residential needs of individuals with severe and profound handicaps to the needs of those individuals with less severe disabilities. This shift in focus results from a number of policy, logistic, and attitudinal factors that have supported the "selectivity" evidenced in the deinstitutionalization process. From a policy level, the concept of normalization has shifted from an issue of "rights" for citizens with mental retardation to a "prescription" for services in general, and residential placement patterns in particular (Butterfield, 1977; Willer & Intagliata, 1984).

From a logistical perspective, the issues involved in serving persons with the most profound mental retardation in the community (e.g., dealing with the lack of accessible housing and the possible need for more extensive medical services) have become apparent (Borthwick-Duffy, Eyman, & White, 1987; Cavalier & McCarver, 1981; Eyman & Borthwick, 1980). Finally, the philosophical differences among professionals in identifying the needs of and the appropriate setting in which to provide services for individuals who are profoundly disabled, continues to be debated (e.g., Ellis et al., 1981; Favell, Risley, Wolfe, Riddle, & Rasmussen, 1981; Menolascino & McGee, 1981a, 1981b).

Regardless of the rationales that underlie the form which deinstitutionalization has taken, research verifies that among those individuals left in institutional settings, a large proportion tend to be those with severe or profound mental retardation with multiply handicapping conditions (Best-Sigford, Bruininks,

295

Lakin, Hill, & Heal, 1982; Eyman & Borthwick, 1980; Scheerenberger, 1978, 1982). People within this group who are moved out of publicly operated facilities are often placed in settings that are similar to the institutional environments from which they came, in home type settings without appropriate support services, or in settings that are not considered to be "less restrictive" than the large publicly operated programs (Best-Sigford et al., 1982; Eyman & Borthwick, 1980). In addition, restricted admission policies have resulted in the very young children with severe handicaps, who were previously institutionalized, remaining with their natural family (Willer & Intagliata, 1984). The net result of this selectivity in deinstitutionalization is that persons who are profoundly mentally retarded presently make up a greater percentage of the population in institutions. Consequently, the community service delivery system has had less experience and history in designing and implementing program models to meet the unique needs of these individuals.

Although a major portion of the people who are profoundly disabled remain out of the mainstream of residential life, perhaps more significant is the fact that there is a growing number of individuals with this level of disability being served within the community array of services. For example, recent demographic studies of client characteristics and residential placement patterns report that between one-tenth and one-third of the total community-oriented placements are supporting individuals who are severely and profoundly mentally retarded (Best-Sigford et al., 1982; Bruininks, Hauber, & Kudla, 1980; Bruininks, Hill, & Thorsheim, 1982; Hauber et al., 1984). These data suggest that the community service system has absorbed some of the clientele with profound mental retardation and that the system today can be characterized as providing services to a more heterogeneous group of persons with disabilities than was the case in previous years (Borthwick-Duffy et al., 1987).

Despite the impressive flexibility of the community service system, little is known about how the needs of persons with profound disabilities are being met, or what types of residential settings and supports are the most conducive to achieving successful and meaningful placements in least restrictive settings. In addition, the expansion of the community service system, as deinstitutionalization continues, is likely to result in the need to appropriately serve citizens with more profound disabilities within the general community. Thus, it is both timely and critical to review and assess the residential program options available in the community for individuals who are profoundly disabled.

The increasing emphasis on providing residential services in community-based settings has also been attributed to various court decisions (Bradley, 1985). This, in turn, has caused states and other providers to seriously reconsider the idea that individuals with severe disabilities can only have their needs met in large institutions (Conroy, Efthimiou, & Lemanowicz, 1982). However, as described above, residential living in community settings for people with the most profound disabilities has received little attention. An extensive literature review of four major special education journals from the years 1980–1984 reported that of the 184 data-based articles that either specifically addressed people with profound disabilities or included this population within a broader range of disabilities (e.g., severe and profound, moderate through profound), none took place in an integrated home environment (Brown, Helmstetter, & Guess, 1986).

It is the premise of this chapter that all individuals, regardless of the degree of disability, can have their needs met in community environments as opposed to large institutions. This chapter addresses the types of living arrangements that are currently available for people with profound disabilities, establishes goals and criteria that may be used to evaluate the quality of community living, and provides an example of one residential program model that facilitates meaningful participation in community living environments through its staff and curriculum.

RESIDENTIAL OPTIONS

A wide variety of living options have been suggested for people with severe and profound disabilities. A person's particular living arrangement depends, to a large degree, upon the philosophy of the organization that is providing the services, the funds made available by state, federal, and other agencies, and, most importantly, the identified needs of the individual who is being served.

Perhaps the most ideal and normalized living option for young individuals with the most profound disabilities is to maintain and support that individual at home with his or her own family. This can be accomplished through the provision of an in-home instructor, if needed, for some portion of the day. This type of model is significantly different from homebound instruction in that the individual would still be involved in a community-based school or vocational program and the instructor would work in the home only during those hours when the individual would normally be at home. Furthermore, the role of the instructor is not only to teach the client, but also to teach the family how to help their child to learn. In addition to the instructor, other services, including adequate amounts of respite care for the family, need to be arranged according to the individual's needs. The benefits of such an arrangement are obvious but only succeed if the family is committed to keeping that individual at home.

In the absence of this commitment, it is still possible to provide a family environment through a specialized foster care model (Freeman, 1978). In using this model, the individual would be placed with a couple who possess the education and training to cope with the individual's needs. Additional support through in-home instructors and respite care could also be provided. As in all cases, the appropriateness of such a placement would depend upon a number of factors including the age of the individual and whether the people that are involved in the placement process felt that the individual's needs could best be met in such a placement.

The problems found in large institutions and the effects that they have on their residents have been studied and researched for many years (Balla, Butterfield, & Ziegler, 1974; Blatt, Bogdan, Biklen, & Taylor, 1977; Goffman, 1961; McCormick, Balla, & Ziegler, 1975). Even to the uninformed observer, there are striking differences between living environments in a large institution and a small community facility where three to six people reside. Many types of group living options exist for older individuals. In such places, the principle of normalization and the necessity for neighborhood acceptance of community living for people with profound disabilities require small community residences. The concept of normalized community living options entails several guiding principles—the most important of which is that any community residence must "fit in" with its neighborhood. Most importantly, the size of the residence cannot overwhelm its surroundings. In other words, in a residential neighborhood of single family homes, any facility should not be larger or serve more individuals than a typical single family and in most cases this would mean no more than six people.

Establishing ICFs/MR

As was mentioned earlier, the type of community living arrangement depends upon the philosophy of the organization and the monies allocated by the various funding agencies. However, even within a given type of living arrangement, there can be immense variations. As Taylor, McCord, and Searl (1981) point out, Medicaid money for community Intermediate Care Facilities for the Mentally Retarded (ICFs/MR) has resulted in facilities as large as 100 beds or as small as six. The authors make a convincing argument that the large ICFs/MR are, in essence, institutions that are neither normal nor community appropriate.

More recently, the trend has been toward much smaller ICFs/MR. For example, in Connecticut, the Department of Mental Retardation has assisted in the development of privately operated community ICFs/MR as few as four people with the average facility serving six people. With the process of deinstitutionalization well underway in this state, individuals with profound handicaps and severe behavior problems are increasingly having their needs met in the community. The ICFs/MR model has been particularly appropriate to the extent that its funding level allows for the intensive staff ratios required by these individuals with the most challenging behavior and enables ancillary services to provide active, quality treatment.

Providing Sufficient Staff

One critical component that is instrumental for successfully meeting the residential needs of individuals with disabilities is to have sufficient staff available on any given shift to take care of routine and crisis needs. In an ICF/MR the staff-to-client ratio for individuals with severe or profound disabilities is 1:2 or 2:3. Thus, one advantage of a six-person facility is that the staff ratio is intensive enough to provide the additional support required during a behavioral incident and active treatment, and not just custodial care. Therefore, it should be noted that those individuals whose behavioral or physical needs may at times require a 3:1 or 4:1 staff-to-client ratio will in all probability do best in a six-bed intensively staffed arrangement. This is not to say that these individuals cannot be served in smaller community living options. However, all parties involved in the development of a small unit (e.g., a three-person facility) for individuals with intensive staff needs must address the substantially higher per diem costs that result.

The tendency to place a group of individuals with the same level of disability into one facility should be resisted. There is sometimes a push to homogeneously group together several behaviorally challenging clients in order to reduce the higher cost that results from intensive staff patterns. This strategy can be disastrous in that three individuals, each of whom may need three or four staff to be available during an incident, can cause the staff to become "burnt out" more quickly than in a living arrangement where clients with less intensive needs are balanced with those who require more attention. The likelihood of staff "burn out" is also increased when individuals with profound mental retardation and multiple handicaps are grouped together.

Utilizing Available Local Housing

The ICF/MR model is only one type of living arrangement available to persons with the most profound disabilities. Local housing availability influences what can be developed. For example, in urban areas, the use of condominiums and apartments to provide housing for two or three individuals is becoming increasingly popular. If carefully planned and supported by the proper resources, this type of community facility can provide a normalized environment that will allow the individual to take increasing control over his or her life as adaptive skills are acquired without having to move him or her to a less restrictive environment. Staff patterns can be arranged to meet the needs of the person, so that through time, the environment itself becomes less restrictive with a reduction of staff intensity, and by not moving the individual. The success of this type of living arrangement hinges on proper planning and support. However, those individuals whose behaviors pose a threat to others are better served in less confined environments than city apartments or condominiums. As must be the case in all community living arrangements for people with the most severe disabilities, the rights and needs of the client must be carefully weighed and balanced with the rights of the neighbors to the quiet and safe enjoyment of their own homes. No one's best interests will be served if a highly aggressive or destructive client is placed in an environment that exposes the neighbors, or the client, to unnecessary risk.

Because of their availability, three-bedroom homes offer another excellent housing option for three or four individuals. These houses can be found in both residential neighborhoods and in more rural areas. With such availability, there is usually little difficulty in locating a house that best suits the individuals. Because of their size, they fit in easily with surrounding neighborhoods and offer the potential for perhaps the most normalized group living situation. Again, staff patterns can be adjusted over time so that the less restrictive environment is created without having to move the client, requiring them to relearn acquired skills and to adjust to a new home and neighborhood.

Duplexes offer another housing alternative that can be extremely flexible. Clients requiring intensive teaching and staffing can live on one side while clients needing only occasional supervision and assistance can live on the other side. As a result, staff can be used interchangeably to provide the occasional supervision or additional back-up when needed. This arrangement can also allow for the grouping of heterogeneous client populations that reduce the likelihood of staff "burn-out" (previously discussed) and, of course, increase opportunities for more appropriate models.

As should be obvious by now, any type of community living arrangement can be found and adapted to meet the needs of individuals with the most profound disabilities and challenging behaviors. Once those organizations providing services move away from the traditional community housing arrangements, such as large group homes, and creatively explore other living options, more individuals will be able to have their needs met in the community. This will require extensive planning and the cooperation and commitment of state and other funding agencies.

GOALS AND CRITERIA FOR RESIDENTIAL SERVICES

The dearth of community-based residential settings for people with profound disabilities prohibits the establishment of an empirically derived set of realistic goals and criteria to judge the efficacy of a home in providing an environment that facilitates growth, while simultaneously respecting the individual choices of that home's residents. In the absence of an established data-base to assist in the development of realistic goals of community-based residential facilities, one is left applying standards and philosophies that are derived from experience with other populations, most of which also are not data-based (Brown et al., 1986).

As the age of accountability advances, the need and desire to measure an individual's progress in meeting his or her goals becomes prevalent. Obviously, the first step is the establishment of a valid set of criteria against which success is measured. For the reasons discussed above (and those discussed in Chapters 3 and 4, this volume), this becomes a most difficult task since, as one variable is measured, there become apparent other variables that should have or could have been measured as well. This issue relates to the collateral effects of service delivery, effects that are predicted and sought (Horner, 1980; Voeltz, Wuerch, & Bockhaut, 1982), and others that unexpectedly occur and are usually described informally and anecdotally in research papers. However, it is these unmeasured behavioral outcomes that often represent the changes in the resident's quality of life. This section describes a variety of goals and criteria for residential services for people with profound disabilities.

Increasing Traditional Curriculum Areas

Increases in traditional curriculum areas can be measured by the acquisition of skills in language, fine motor, gross motor, social, and self-help areas. Some programs may judge their success by the percentage of skills mastered by the residents in each domain; that is, the more targeted skills acquired, the better the program. Although these accomplishments may be meaningful and encourage participation in a wider variety of activities, when they are the only measures of successful programming, the probable outcome is isolation of skills and practice within nonfunctional activities. This is especially true for people with profound disabilities, since an increase in skill acquisition is likely to reflect only partial acquisition of an activity. The skills practiced may contain little social validity and represent only prerequisites to other more functional skills. This could prohibit the person from acquiring skills that may be useful during his or her present activities. If the validity of skills were to be judged by the standard of age-appropriateness, then there would be an inverse correlation between the person's age and the likelihood of finding nonhandicapped peers learning prerequisite skills. However, instruction of these skills may serve the purpose of establishing a reinforcing relationship between the resident and the instructor.

Increasing Participation in the Community and at Home

A community-based residence only offers a physical structure in which individuals with disabilities can live, unless care is taken to increase the frequency and quality of participation in the community. From the measurement standpoint, there are many possible levels that may be evaluated. One of these levels is the frequency of activities that take place in the community (e.g., number of trips to the grocery store or to recreational facilities). Although at first glance this type of measurement may appear to be void of any standard of quality participation in the specific activity, it may indeed be appropriate for some clients at different phases of adjustment in their new residence. Clients who come from large institutional settings have had little or no opportunity for community participation. For these residents, it may be appropriate to arrange frequent community activities, with the goal being to determine which activities are preferred. However, with many clients who have profound disabilities, this must occur simultaneously with staff learning how an individual expresses his or her preferences (see Chapter 8, this volume).

Following this phase of frequent community visits or simultaneous to it (depending on the individual), staff may find that the generalization of specific skills (e.g., language, fine motor, social skills) in more structured learning situations (e.g., at home, in school, at work) could become a concern. For this reason, staff may want to establish more general "community" skills and routines for their students such as handing money to a cashier or increasing mobility by going through automatic doors.

One point of conflict for many professional staff members in regards to the aforementioned approach of increasing community activities is the act of measuring behavior in the community. That is, in some community situations the intrusiveness of the measurement process must be weighed against the goal of fitting the individual into the community. For example, one is reminded of a tourist in a big city who buys new clothes to look like a native but invariably purchases ones that only emphasize his or her tourist status. Similarly, an instructor carrying a clipboard and reinforcers, and observing and recording behavior, will do little to encourage the community-member status of the resident.

Another point of conflict to this approach reveals that the narrowness of measurement systems may exclude many important dependent variables that are too difficult to measure or predict. For example, a task analysis for purchasing a piece of fruit at a convenience store may be designed to include such components as being able to: move in the store, find the fruit section, choose one fruit, bring the fruit to the cashier, and pay for the item. The client may be averaging 20% on the task analysis this week, as compared to 10% last week; however, this is not the accomplishment about which all of the staff are bragging. Instead, the staff may note that, upon coming home with the pear that the client selected, the individual sat for 20 minutes examining this fruit that was never seen before in its natural noncanned state, and was found smiling, laughing, and twirling it. Staff felt that the young woman in this example was experiencing and expressing a new form of enjoyment. This enjoyment, to them, far outweighed the accomplishment of handing the money to the cashier with only a partial physical prompt.

Participating in Household Management   To the greatest extent possible, people who live in the home should participate in the management and completion of household routines. Staff must begin to feel that they are there to assist the residents in running the house, rather than getting the residents to partially participate as staff conduct the household routines. That is, instead of a staff person saying, "I'll try to think of a way to have Ed participate while I make dinner," the staff person should say, "I'll help Ed make dinner." Although on the surface there appears to be little difference in the two phrases, in implementation and staff perception of participation, there is a great difference. As staff attend to various household needs, this small difference becomes important since incidental teaching opportunities arise during noninstructional time.

Reducing Behaviors that Interfere with Participation

Whether or not to target an excess behavior for reduction is a complex issue. Intervention options include conducting direct intervention (e.g., differential reinforcement of other behavior [DRO], differential reinforcement of incompatible behavior [DRI], extinction), monitoring the collateral effects of the new environment (e.g., routines, choice, schedules), or viewing the client's actions as an acceptable part of his or her behavioral repertoire (e.g., the self-stimulatory behavior of finger-flicking is a highly preferred activity and does not interfere with active programming). Many factors must be considered when making the decision to reduce a client's excess behavior (c.f. Donnellan, Mirenda, Mesaros, & Fassbender, 1984; Evans & Meyer, 1985; Gast & Wolery, 1987; Gaylord-Ross, 1980), and it is crucial that all team members are included in the process. Staff members must ultimately weigh the right of the person to choose to engage in certain behaviors, the safety of the client and others in the environment, and the right of the neighbors to a certain life-style and community environment before attempting to reduce a behavior.

Increasing Enjoyment of Residential Life

The area that is in the most need of a collaborative effort to operationalize variables or classes of variables that may represent quality of life factors for each individual is that of enjoyment of residential life. The importance of this effort has been emphasized by many authors (Brown, Evans, Weed, & Owen, 1987; Guess, Benson, & Siegel-Causey, 1985). If the concepts of the "criterion of ultimate functioning" and age-appropriate parallel are applied (Brown et al., 1979; Brown, Nietupski, & Hamre-Nietupski, 1976), then different questions arise than with a school-age population. The following are a few of these questions: At what point in adult life do people leave the learner role and expect to rest on past accomplishments? At what point is formal education considered to be in the past, and when should learning become informal and attributed to leisure experiences, social experiences, and the wisdom of age? Although there is always more to learn, whether referring to a person's profession, new skills, or life in general, nonhandicapped adults choose to continue participation in these challenges to varying degrees. At what point, if ever, do educators say that it is not age-appropriate to engage in formal instruction? Of course one may think that it is appropriate at any age to learn to communicate with others or to gain independence in toileting, but what emphasis should be placed on these as goals? Should they be presented as task analysis to master and demonstrate progress in life? What are priorities for an adult who has little daily living skills but who has had an adequate educational experience? Reminiscent of this issue is a question raised at a workshop by an employee of a large institution. The question referred to an 80-year-old woman with severe mental retardation and who clearly (at least to this staff person) indicated that she wanted to sit in her rocking chair, rock, and manipulate small objects; she clearly indicated refusal to go to "day programs," especially when it was rainy or snowy. Of course, if the day program were more meaningful and if she had a variety of options from which to select, she might be very pleased to attend. But it is conceivable that even with an improved day program, she still may clearly indicate rejection of work activities, as is likely the case with most of her nonhandicapped age peers.

The crucial variable is the validity of the goals and objectives targeted for an individual. When possible, the goals and objectives should be representative of what the client chooses or indicates as important and meaningful, and not solely derived from a set of educational practices and philosophies developed on people who are typically less handicapped and younger. Is there a point in a person's life when he or she says that after 20 years of more or less adequate instruction in daily living, household, and other skills, that these skills should no longer be identified as formal goals and objectives? The challenge then becomes how to incorporate these skills into meaningful routines and how to identify those skills that will contribute to that person's quality of life.

ADMINISTRATIVE CONSIDERATIONS

Physical Setting

The New Haven Project of the Institute of Professional Practice (IPP) provides residential services in ICFs/MR community-based homes in Connecticut for persons ranging in disability from mildly to profoundly disabled. In addition, the majority of residents have severe behavior problems and/or multiple handicaps. While the abilities and needs of these individuals differ greatly in each residence, it is the philosophy of IPP that all persons, regardless of their disabilities, have the right to live in small community-based homes and are entitled to vocational and residential teaching programs that are individualized to meet their specific needs.

While there are many characteristics and features generic to facilities for persons with developmental and physical disabilities (especially where compliance with regulatory requirements is an issue), residences must be tailored to fit the residents' individual needs. If it is the belief that environmental factors affect the way people learn and behave, then it is imperative that those persons who are responsible for the design and construction of facilities for individuals with profound disabilities do so with regard to both functionality and aesthetic quality. Its appearance is a factor that is vitally important if community integration and acceptance are to be achieved. Program directors, clinicians, therapists and instructors should all participate in the planning stages for the community service homes in order to ensure that they will best meet the needs of their residents. Following are some basic guidelines in designing facilities for persons with profound and multiple disabilities that have been utilized by the New Haven Project:

1. Private bedrooms for each resident, sufficient in size to accommodate any adaptive equipment that may be required.
2. Functional adaptations of tubs, showers, appliances, and furniture needed to facilitate participation by persons with mobility, visual, or hearing impairments, while maintaining the home-like qualities of the residence.
3. Facility vehicles just large enough to accommodate the mobility needs of the residents, but devoid of all markings that may label the passengers (e.g., "retarded," "handicapped").
4. Ramps, accessible entrances, and landscaping designed to fully meet the needs of the residents, while being sensitive to the neighbors' rights and wishes.

Staff Considerations

A major factor in the development of small community-based residences for individuals with profound disabilities is the selection, training, and scheduling of direct care and management staff. Residences that primarily serve persons who are profoundly disabled, medically fragile, or physically handicapped will require higher ratios of staff. These staff members will need increased training to enable them to meet the physical as well as instructional needs of the residents.

There are a number of reasons why someone with profound disabilities may require more intensive staff ratios than those individuals with less severe disabilities. First, persons coming out of large institutional settings typically lack any prior exposure to even the most basic functional household routines or community experience. Because the person may also lack the skill to self-select and independently participate even partially in leisure activities, it is more difficult for staff to leave him or her unattended for even short periods of time to work with other individuals and to feel that the unattended resident is not being neglected.

Second, the resident's level of cognitive and/or physical disability may make it difficult or impossible for him or her to complete most tasks independently, or even partially, thereby requiring almost constant staff presence to maintain meaningful participation in the functional activity. This is especially true when residents are encouraged to participate in a broader range of home- and community-based activities. Furthermore, if a resident may be able to ultimately complete an activity independently, the amount of time and staff supervision required to teach or monitor that task may be greater than for someone with less severe disabilities.

Third, in addition to the direct care and instructional responsibilities required of residential staff, there are many services that they must perform that are not conducted by their institutional counterparts. Small community-based homes do not have the therapeutic and medical services that are available in larger segregated settings. Given this lack of on-site ancillary caregivers, as well as the desirability of a transdisciplinary approach to delivering therapeutic services in a functional and integrated manner, the need for well-trained staff becomes apparent. Therefore, in-house managers and direct care staff must be trained, whenever possible, in the areas of supervision of self-medication, mobility training, augmentative communication systems, and integration of occupational and physical therapy objectives into functional routines.

As was mentioned earlier in this chapter, a resident staff ratio of 1:2 or even 2:3 is required to ensure quality, proactive programming for persons with profound disabilities. It is imperative to have direct care staff in sufficient numbers to provide for the level of instruction that is necessary to increase the opportunities for participation in activities across a variety of skill and recreational domains. Since it is most educationally sound to teach skills at the time when they are most likely to be used, it is important to have sufficient staff available to instruct and assist the residents during all waking hours of the day. With lesser staff ratio, residents and instructors are unable to follow schedules that are based upon normalized routines, including full or partial participation in those routines. The shortage also affects the residents' opportunities for choice and individualized community-based instruction, where group instruction is neither possible nor desirable.

Staff Training

Although most agencies that provide residential services employ an administrative and clinical staff that provide support and assistance in a number of facilities, it is equally important to ensure that the facility staff are trained and empowered to make managerial and clinical decisions on a daily basis. If the in-house staff has a greater input into the design, implementation, and review of the residents' programs, they are more likely to assume ownership of those programs and to take a vested interest in their success. Since program managers and instructors often have varied educational and practical backgrounds, as well as a broad scope of assigned responsibilities, it is necessary to design a comprehensive and longitudinal training curriculum that will address the various levels of training that is needed. Minimally, there are three interrelated and overlapping phases of staff development and training: preservice and in-service trainings, weekly staff meetings, and in situ supervision and training.

Preservice or In-Service Training Training is provided for all staff both as an introduction to working with people with profound disabilities in residential settings and as a continued training effort at regularly scheduled intervals after employment begins. When possible, this level of training is provided to staff prior to their instructional responsibilities. This is easily accomplished when staff are hired before the residence opens. However, as a result of staff turnover, this is not always possible. Training is then offered as soon as possible after their employment begins. As can be seen from Table 12.1, some of the in-service training that is offered to staff provides a thorough foundation in providing generic residential services and using applied behavior analysis techniques, while others are designed to meet the needs of the specific population for the facility in which they will be working. Such in-service training is somewhat limited in scope and is usually taught in isolated settings. However, it does provide a framework for teaching more applied and client-specific teaching strategies in the next two phases of training.

Weekly Staff Meetings Staff training also involves the analysis of instructional programs at weekly staff meetings that are held at the residence. Since the residential instructors play an integral part in the assessment, design, and implementation processes, they are given the responsibility of presenting specific instructional and behavioral data, leading discussions on the evaluation of those data, and designing strategy changes as needed. To assist the instructor in analyzing the data, as well as documenting the analysis of the programs, staff are provided with either a Weekly or Monthly Review Form. Figure 12.1 is an example of a Monthly Review Form for the review of instructional programs.

Table 12.1. Required in-services for Connecticut ICFs/MR

Medical

Safe administration and handling of medicines (D)
First aid (D, I)
Infection control (I)
Signs and symptoms (I)
Medical emergencies (A)
Cardiopulmonary resuscitation (CPR) (A)

Therapeutic services

Nutritional services (D, I)
Oral hygiene (D, I)
Occupational therapy (I)
Physical therapy (I)
Speech and communication (I)
Recreation (I)
Social services (I)

Administrative/house management

Overview of agency philosophy (A)
Human rights and abuse reporting (I)
Agency policies and procedures (D)
Fire safety and disaster training (D, I)
Supervisory training (I)

Clinical

Program development and implementation (D, I)
Personal relationships and sexuality (I)
Behavior management (A)
Teaching and supervising self-medication programs (I)
Passive restraint techniques (A)

D = Required by the Department of Mental Retardation & Agency.
I = Required by Intermediate Care Facilities & Agency.
A = Required by Agency only.

MONTHLY PROGRAM REVIEW AND PROGRESS NOTES

Resident: _____ Instructors: _____

Program/phase: _____ Date of review: _____

Program Summary

Descriptions	Program Trend			
	Acceleration	Deceleration	Fluctuation	Maintenance
Program Plan:				
Current Program:				

Current Phase (last 2 weeks): ____% Prior Phase (two weeks): ____%
       (circle one)   (circle one)

Possible Program Revisions/Comments on Progress (circle one):

1. _____

   _____

2. _____

   _____

3. _____

   _____

Selected Program Revision (if needed): # ____

1a. Describe program change exactly as it will appear on computer:

   _____

   _____

   _____

  b. Initial when change has been entered: (____) Date: ___/___/___

2a. Describe necessary changes on task analysis: _____

   _____

   _____

  b. Initial when changes have been recorded on task analysis: (____)
    Date: ___/___/___

Date changes to be implemented: ___/___/___
Date initiated: ___/___/___

Reviewed by QMRP: _____ Date: ___/___/___

Figure 12.1. Monthly Review Form used to summarize and analyze progress on instructional programs.

Behavioral programs are reviewed using similar forms on a weekly basis. These forms summarize the data, indicate the frequency of program implementation, record staff ideas for possible program changes, and identify any graphic or computer changes that must follow. These program evaluations are excellent opportunities to discuss the application of theory to practice. For example, it is much easier for staff to grasp the concept of differential reinforcement or re-direction when they can relate these strategies to specific residents and behavioral issues that are currently ongoing in the residential facility.

In Situ Training Another phase of the training package involves the supervision and training of the residential instructors during programming time. Through direct observation, the management team evaluates a number of variables that are difficult to measure through analysis of data alone. These observations include variables such as the quality of teaching interactions with residents, consistency of program implementation, frequency of incidental teaching opportunities, and data collection procedures. The supervision of direct care staff is not designed to be punitive in nature and is approached as an educative training tool used to evaluate and improve upon their teaching skills. Opportunities for postobservation discussions, as well as follow-up training and evaluation, are included in the training process.

ASSESSMENT AND SELECTION OF TARGET BEHAVIORS

While the selection process for targeting behaviors for instruction is vitally important for persons of all functioning levels and disabilities, it becomes even more crucial for individuals with profound disabilities. Some of the factors in designing appropriate curricula that contribute to the special needs of this population include: speed of skill acquisition, lack of previous individualized educational or habilitative services; increased direct staff assistance due to accompanying physical disabilities, the need for development of functional alternatives and adaptive equipment, and expressive or receptive communication deficits. Given these variables, it is imperative that assessment and teaching strategies be developed that will best aid those with profound disabilities to functionally access their environment, to increase their ability to make choices, and to participate to the greatest extent possible in normalized routines.

A variety of assessment tools should be used to determine the current needs and functioning levels of individuals who are targeted for residential placement and to develop individualized functional routines in an effort to meet those needs. These assessments may be classified into two categories: preadmission assessments and postadmission assessments.

Preadmission Assessments

Preadmission assessment information allows a receiving agency to obtain baseline information about a referred client and to best prepare for that person's admission to his or her new residence. If more emphasis is placed on gathering reliable and pertinent information regarding the person's abilities, preferences, dislikes, and behavioral characteristics, the transition and chance of a successful placement is likely to be smoother. Information may be gathered from norm-referenced tests, review of interdisciplinary reports and assessments, staff interviews, parent or guardian interviews, and direct observation of the individual in his or her residential and day environments.

Norm-referenced tests, such as the American Association on Mental Deficiency (AAMD) Adaptive Behavior Scales (Lambert, Windmiller, Cole, & Figueroa, 1975), although not sufficient as the only initial assessment, are useful for a number of reasons. As a preliminary tool, they: 1) provide the receiving agency with a gross measure of the incoming individual's abilities and maladaptive behaviors in order to develop interim strategies for addressing possible behavioral problems; 2) offer staff some idea as to what to expect of the client physically, behaviorally, and cognitively; 3) assist with staff training prior to the person's move into the house; and 4) furnish valuable information when the individualized curriculum is developed. Also, since this assessment is designed to be administered in an interview format, discussions often ensue between the interviewer and the interviewee that may expand upon topics only superficially covered by the instrument.

In reviewing ancillary and therapeutic reports and evaluations, it is helpful if the sending agency provides reports that are current, thorough, and relevant. A determination should be made of each of the evaluations received as to the timeliness of the report and to the validity and functionality of the recommendations given. Reviews and/or additional assessments by the appropriate service providers should then be prioritized and scheduled for each evaluation that is found to be deficient.

Some of the most useful information gathered about a client prior to admission comes from direct discussions with the persons who are responsible for the client's care and instruction in his or her current environment. While other assessments offer gross measures of the client's abilities, a direct interview provides very specific information about the client's characteristics and preferences that will enable the new residence to create an environment that is most conducive to his or her transition and creation of a meaningful individualized curriculum. Figure 12.2 is an example of a questionnaire that is focused on eliciting information from parents and can be used either in an interview format or completed independently if the parents or guardians are not available for a meeting.

Observations of the client by the staff of the receiving agency prior to admission in both the day and residential settings is an important part of the assessment process. This allows staff to verify some of the information that was received (to a limited degree), as well as to observe and question behaviors that may not have been evident in the records or that came up in previous conversa-

Parent Input Questionnaire

Parent/guardian/advocate: _____

Client: _____

Date: _____

The purpose of this questionnaire is to get your input on the development of goals and objectives for your son or daughter. Your feedback will help us to design the best possible program for your child. Our goal is to develop a program that will reflect your concerns and preferences and that will help your son or daughter adapt to his or her new home and become a more participating and independent member of our community.

Please answer any of the following questions that you can. Some of the questions may be difficult for you to answer if your child has not lived at home with you recently, but please answer as many questions as possible.

Personal Management

1. What do you consider to be your child's special strengths in taking care of him- or herself (e.g., eats independently, can put on most of his or her clothes without help, washes own hands)?

2. Of the above personal management activities, are there any that your child especially likes to do?

3. Are there any specific personal management responsibilities in which your child does not like to participate?

4. What kinds of personal management skills do you think we should be working on with your child?

Household Responsibilities

1. Please list any household responsibilities in which your child participates (e.g., clearing or setting the table, cleaning his or her room, taking out the garbage).

2. Which of the above responsibilities does your child seem to enjoy?

3. Which of the above responsibilities does your child seem to dislike?

(continued)

Parent Input Questionnaire
(continued)

4. What kinds of household responsibilities do you think we should be working on with your child?

Leisure

1. What types of leisure activities do you and your family do at *home* (e.g., watch TV, play cards)?

2. In which of the above activities has your child shown some interest?

3. In which of the above home activities would you like your child to participate that he or she does not at the present time?

4. In what types of *community* activities do you and your family engage (e.g., going to the movies, picnics, shopping)?

5. In which of the above activities has your child shown some interest?

6. In which of the above community activities would you like your child to participate that he or she does not at the present time?

Social

1. What do you consider to be your child's special social strengths (e.g., cooperative, friendly, smiles a lot, polite)?

2. What do you consider to be the most important social skills that we could work on with your child (e.g., interacting with others, participating in activities without tantruming)?

(continued)

Parent Input Questionnaire
(continued)

Vocational

1. In what types of jobs do you think your child might be able to participate now or in the future (e.g., assembly work, janitorial work, restaurant work, office work)?

2. What types of work-related skills would you predict that your child would need to work on (e.g., getting along with coworkers, waiting on line for lunch, letting the supervisor know when a problem arises)?

Comments

Please provide any additional information that may assist us in developing your child's program.

Figure 12.2. Parent Input Questionnaire to be used in an interview format or to be completed independently.

tions with staff or parents. Additionally, it allows the client to become familiar with the staff who will be working with him or her in their new environment. With clients who, in the past, may have had very dramatic or life-threatening reactions to environmental changes (e.g., stops eating, displays severe tantrums), sessions may be systematically and intensely scheduled just prior to admission. In addition to observation during these sessions, staff can begin interacting with the client and even assuming some instructional and caregiving responsibilities.

The information gathered through preadmission assessments, while important in obtaining an overview of an individual's strengths, preferences, and needs, has to be used with caution. This is especially true when a person with profound disabilities moves from a large institutional setting into a small community-based residence. Opportunities for increased choice, environmental differences, increased demands, new teaching strategies, and staff expectations all may have a major effect on an individual's behavior, thus invalidating much of the data collected during the preadmission period. The individual may react to these new variables in ways never predicted by the referring agency. Additionally, the person may not have had the opportunity to participate in many of the skill areas in which they may be participating in the new environment (e.g., food preparation, laundry, shopping), resulting in test scores that are deflated and not necessarily representative of the person's participation in those activities once in the new residence.

Postadmission Assessments

Criterion-Referenced Assessment Criterion-referenced tests measure an individual's functioning level as it relates to a predetermined criterion level (Browder, 1987; Brown, 1987; Gaylord-Ross & Holvoet, 1985). These assessments may be individualized to determine the variety of skills that may be necessary for both current and future functioning within domains relevant to community, residential, and vocational/educational settings. These assessments could then be used to provide a framework for more refined environmental analysis or inventory as described by Brown and his colleagues (1979).

While norm-referenced scales of adaptive behavior measure global skills and test for independence in using these skills, the criterion-referenced test may either task or component analyze the individual's skills to measure for partial independence (Gaylord-Ross & Holvoet, 1985). The criterion-referenced test will also assess additional critical skills that may be necessary for more independent functioning. In addition, these assessments may be adapted to account for an individual's intellectual, communication, or physical disabilities to a degree not permissable on standardized tests. As such, criterion-referenced assessments are more likely to yield information useful for program planning.

Criterion-referenced assessments are most effectively accomplished by using the following guidelines:

1. Assess skills in the settings in which they naturally occur.
2. Assess skills at the times of day at which they naturally occur.
3. Use materials that reflect those needed in real-life situations.
4. Use natural cues and consequences to elicit behaviors.
5. Assess a sufficient range of skills that reflect performance in the natural environment.

Assessing Excess Behaviors Although a residential facility should not solely focus its instructional attention on excess behaviors, it is important to identify and measure these behaviors and, through certain decision-making strategies, conclude which excess behaviors, if any, require direct intervention. As Gast and Wolery (1987) point out, a behavior management model must "emphasize an ecobehavioral approach to modifying a behavior problem. That is, the model should present intervention alternatives that are based on reinforcement, environmental, and curricular manipulations," and "it should be educational in that it addresses deceleration of the maladaptive behavior while concurrently teaching functional/adaptive replacement behaviors" (p. 304). The New Haven Project uses two strategies to assist in the complex process of deciding which behaviors will be targeted for direct behavior intervention and which will be formally or informally monitored to see the collateral effects of the enriched environment.

The Interim Schedule and Behavior Observation Form (see Figure 12.3) is designed to reflect typical routines that occur throughout the day. Staff use this general form for the period of time before a more individualized schedule for the resident is designed, based upon the goals and objectives defined by the interdisciplinary team. Although it does not provide a precise measure of the resident's behaviors, since staff record excess behaviors that may occur within a routine, it does allow the possibility of determining a relationship of excess behaviors and the time of day or type of activity. Thus, this form is very useful in preparing the child's programming. It also gives the staff a more objective picture of the frequency with which behaviors occur, thus providing information on choosing a specific intervention option.

The Client Excess Behavior Rating Checklist (see Figure 12.4) addresses qualitative aspects of an individual's excess behaviors (Donnellan et al., 1984; Evans & Meyer, 1985) that are to be considered in the identification of behaviors to be targeted for intervention. Because the checklist requires subjective judgments by the staff, it is completed by two staff people independently. Staff are asked to complete the checklist 2 to 3 weeks following the person's admission into the house. The scale includes a rating of frequency of occurrence, intensity of the behavior, and topographical descriptions of the behaviors. Staff are then asked to judge whether or not the behavior interferes with the activities of the client or with others in the environment and what they believe is the intent or function of each of the excess behaviors.

In studying variables such as interference with others and intent, staff are forced to consider the values that are used when identifying behaviors for reduction. For example, even though a staff member may judge the self-stimulatory behavior of finger-flicking as occurring frequently, he or she may feel that the behavior does not interfere with others and the behavior does not seem to occur when the person is directed to tasks or during interactions. The decision may be that finger-flicking need not be addressed directly and that it will be monitored to assess the impact of the new residential program on the excess behavior. Another behavior, such as severe self-injurious behavior, may occur only infrequently, but may be of such intensity that a decision may be made to plan both direct intervention and skill-building programs to correct the behavior. Staff may indicate on this checklist that the intent of the behavior is to avoid having to do a certain task. The team will also, at this point, refer to the Interim Schedule and Behavioral Observation Form and note, for example, that the self-injurious behavior seems to occur during household tasks. By looking at the intent of excess behaviors and information from the Interim Schedule and Behavioral Observation Form, educative alternatives and approaches for reducing those behaviors can be explored (e.g., introducing choice into household tasks, teaching alternative communication responses). Any behavior identified

Interim Schedule and Behavior Observation

Client: _____   Date: _____

Time	Planned activity	Actual activity	Participated in activity?	Behaviors SS	SIB	AGO	AGP	Initials
8:00 a.m.	Wake up/self-med program		Y N					
8:15 a.m.	Bathroom routine		Y N					
9:15 a.m.	Breakfast prep		Y N					
9:30 a.m.	Breakfast		Y N					
10:00 a.m.	Dressing		Y N					
10:30 a.m.	Room maintenance		Y N					
11:00 a.m.	Bathroom routine		Y N					
11:15 a.m.	In-house leisure by self		Y N					
11:45 a.m.	Lunch preparation		Y N					
12:00 p.m.	Lunch		Y N					
12:30 p.m.	Bathroom routines		Y N					
12:45 p.m.	Community outing		Y N					

Time	Activity		
4:00 p.m.	Return home/Bathroom routine	Y	N
4:30 p.m.	In-house: Leisure with others	Y	N
5:15 p.m.	Dinner preparation	Y	N
5:30 p.m.	Handwashing	Y	N
5:45 p.m.	Dinner	Y	N
6:15 p.m.	Dinner cleanup/Household maintenance	Y	N
6:45 p.m.	Bathroom	Y	N
7:00 p.m.	In-house: Leisure with others or community outing	Y	
7:45 p.m.	Bath/shower routine, toothbrushing	Y	N
8:00 p.m.	Self-med program	Y	N
8:15 p.m.	Snack preparation	Y	N
8:30 p.m.	Bathroom	Y	N
9:00 p.m.	In-house: Leisure activity	Y	N
9:30 p.m.	Bedtime	Y	N

Figure 12.3. Interim Schedule and Behavior Observation Form used prior to the individualized program development and during transition into the new residence (SS, self-stimulatory; SIB, self-injurious behavior; AGO, aggression to objects; AGP, aggression to people).

Client Excess Behavior Rating Checklist

Client: _____ Date: _____ / _____ / _____

Name of person/position completing sheet: _____

Category	Occurrence				Intensity low to high	Interfere with client's activity	Interferes with others
	None	Occasionally	Frequently	Continuously			
1. Self-stimulation					1 2 3 4 5	Y N	Y N
2. Self-injurious					1 2 3 4 5	Y N	Y N
3. Aggressiveness with persons					1 2 3 4 5	Y N	Y N
4. Aggressiveness with objects					1 2 3 4 5	Y N	Y N
5. Inappropriate contact					1 2 3 4 5	Y N	Y N
6. Tantrum					1 2 3 4 5	Y N	Y N
7. Inappropriate vocal./verbal.					1 2 3 4 5	Y N	Y N
8. Other					1 2 3 4 5	Y N	Y N

Description of excess behaviors: Please describe the topography of the behaviors that occur in each of the categories listed above. Next to each description, please select a Category of Intent code that you feel best describes the purpose of the excess behavior.

Category	Behavior	Code*
1. Self-stimulation		——
		——
2. Self-injurious		——
		——
3. Aggressiveness with persons		——
		——
4. Aggressiveness with objects		——
		——
5. Inappropriate contact		——
		——
6. Tantrum		——
		——
7. Inappropriate vocal./verbal.		——
		——
8. Other		——
		——

*Category of intent code: A = Attention seeking, B = Escape/avoidance, C = Assistance, D = Stimulation, E = Frustration, F = Ritual thwarted, G = Other _____ .

Date reviewed by team: _____ / _____ / _____

Future analysis needed on the following behaviors: _____

Figure 12.4. The Client Excess Behavior Rating Checklist is used as an initial evaluation of qualitative aspects of a resident's behaviors.

on the Client Excess Behavior Rating Checklist as needing some type of intervention is followed up with more systematic and reliable data collection.

PROGRAM IMPLEMENTATION

Program Foundations

Selection of target behaviors is only the first step in providing people with profound disabilities a context for meaningful participation in their homes. Because many of the target behaviors may be very basic or critical skills, it is only too convenient to teach these skills in isolated contexts since they may not apparently relate to functional contexts. If programs are not related to real home environments and needs, then being in a house in the community offers little more than a physical relocation. The curriculum in the New Haven Project is based upon three other models that have been developed since the early 1980s. These models include: the Individualized Curriculum Sequence (ICS) (Holvoet, Guess, Mulligan, & Brown, 1980; Guess & Helmstetter, 1986), the concept of "routines" (Donnellan & Neel, 1986; Neel et al., 1983), and the Component Model of Functional Life Routines (CMFLR) (Brown et al., 1987).

ICS   The ICS focuses on sequencing two to six skills into a cluster, in an effort to develop a natural relationship among them. This model is based upon two premises: related skills can be learned concurrently, and skills can be learned best in a distributed trial format (Mulligan, Guess, Holvoet, & Brown, 1980). For example, rather than teaching a person to grasp a particular object at the same time each day, discriminate between objects used at one time of the day, and functional objects used at another time of the day, the instructor should cluster the skills together so that the person would first discriminate between objects, grasp that object, and then use it. This sequence would ideally take place with objects that are meaningful to the person (e.g., eating utensils, leisure items) and at times when these activities most naturally occur.

Concept of Routines   The concept of routines provides a structure for the organization of a day. Of course, a series of routines could be designed that, at best, represents nonfunctional activities arranged sequentially. However, Neel and his colleagues (1983) defined a routine as a sequence of behaviors that begins with a natural cue and ends with a critical effect (Donnellan & Neel, 1986; Neel et al., 1983). For example, the behaviors that are needed when a client goes shopping include entering the store, finding the items to be purchased, and paying for them. Designing routines becomes more challenging for people with profound disabilities because their participation in the normal rhythm of the day is often very discrepant from those who show greater activity participation. This may be true for a number of reasons: 1) some of the routines in which a person with a profound disability engages may be different (e.g., whirlpool, postural drainage); 2) the time spent actively participating in the routine may be shorter in duration, leaving a great deal of time when the instructor is actually doing some portion of the task (e.g., a client may begin a leisure program by participating in 2 minutes of active leisure in a 15 minute time period); 3) if a routine is indeed functional, the client's participation in the routine may not be sufficient enough to accomplish the critical effect of the routine, leaving the instructor responsible for the functional outcome of the routine (e.g., a client can participate in preparing dinner, but the critical effect of the routine is that there must be an edible dinner ready for consumption); and 4) some routines may take more time to complete than they do for their non-handicapped peers (e.g., toileting, dressing, showering). Establishing a meaningful series of routines for the client to accomplish throughout the day becomes crucial since the rhythm of the home, the contexts in which the residents learn new skills, and the meaning of living in that home all depend on this schedule.

CMFLR   Perhaps the greatest challenge, however, is to ensure that the participation in the routines established in the house are meaningful to the people who live there. The CMFLR focuses on the way in which a person partially participates in a routine (Brown et al., 1987; Evans, Brown, Weed, Spry, & Owen, 1987). Many times professionals will break down functional activities into smaller and smaller components until the person can achieve some success. However, the components derived from the traditional task analytic approach may, at some point, become so far removed from the intent or function of the activity that participation in the activity loses its meaning. The CMFLR delineates several types of participation in functional activities that may facilitate the quality of participation in an activity. Skills such as initiating the activity, choosing the activity or some element of the activity, locating the needed materials, and monitoring the quality of the activity are suggested in addition to the core physical components. This becomes crucial for a person with severe physical impairments since participation may be impossible on the physical core level, but may be more likely on other dimensions.

Schedules

Schedules provide the backbone for the organization of the house, and serve several functions, including:

1. Provides staff with a clear picture of what is expected of them
2. Allows supervisors a mechanism to evaluate staff accountability for program implementation
3. Provides clients with a predictable day
4. Allows coordination of scheduling among the residents of the home
5. Allows identification of possible trends in behavior
6. Establishes the context for learning and the rhythm of the house

For a person whose participation in routines and activities is fairly major, the routine itself may become the target behavior. For example, "preparing dinner" is a routine that may be broken down into component parts such as initiating dinner preparation, getting out the menu, finding all of the items needed for a recipe, and setting the timer after preparation is complete and the meal is cooking. Each of these components may be a feasible target for the person who is participating in the activity. However, for a person who is more profoundly disabled, the level of participation in these components may be so minimal that they are not appropriate target behaviors. Instead, these routines become contexts for the acquisition of more basic skills and become the vehicle for distributed practice throughout the day. The Activities Schedule (Figure 12.5) and accompanying Routine sheet represent an extension and adaptation of the ICS (Guess & Helmstetter, 1986; Holvoet et al., 1980) to a community-based residential setting.

Figure 12.5 is a sample Activities Schedule that was developed for Mondays, Wednesdays, and Fridays for a nonambulatory client named Evan, who has been diagnosed as having profound mental retardation. Schedules for other days of the week are similar; however, minor differences do occur (e.g., laundry is done three times a week, community outings are planned twice a week). There are three basic steps to the development of a schedule. These steps include: identifying the sequence of routines by time, listing target behaviors, and applying target behaviors to contexts.

Identifying the Sequence of Routines by Time Because of the aforementioned reasons, routine identification can be a challenging task. Several strategies can facilitate the development of a specific sequence of routines. Routines that should be listed first are those that must occur at a regular time. These can be identified as those routines that need to be: 1) coordinated with one or more of the housemates because they occur at the same time (e.g., mealtimes), 2) coordinated with other housemates because of limited materials or resources (e.g., showering), 3) prescheduled at very specific times of the day (e.g., medications, toileting), and 4) conducted to enable the person to participate in the rest of the day (e.g., waking-up, getting dressed).

These routines should be listed by time down the side of the matrix, considering the approximate duration of each routine. Someone who is ambulatory and who can use the bathroom independently is likely to need much less time for toileting than is a person who is nonambulatory, cannot remove clothing, and needs assistance in transferring from a wheelchair to the toilet. After the above four types of routines are listed throughout the day, there will be a number of open slots to fill with enriching types of routines. They can be scheduled as those routines that: 1) need to be scheduled with others to facilitate socialization (e.g., sharing leisure time, community outings), 2) need to be coordinated with others because of limited materials (e.g., washing machine, leisure materials to be used alone), 3) facilitate participation in communal household management (e.g., vacuuming the living room, preparing dinner, going grocery shopping), and 4) facilitate participation in personal management (e.g., vacuuming and dusting own bedroom, preparing own snack, washing clothes).

It should be remembered that these routines are simply providing the context for the acquisition or deceleration of the target behaviors. Depending on the individual, the routines themselves may or may not be the target for acquisition.

Listing Target Behaviors   The second step in developing a schedule is to delineate the selected target behaviors across the top. A total of 20 target behaviors were selected for Evan, covering various skill-building domains as well as two excess behaviors. These target behaviors need not be listed in any particular order, other than perhaps grouped by domain, since the actual order of the behaviors will change and the specific behaviors that will be addressed, will vary according to the specific routine.

Applying Target Behaviors to Contexts   The third step in schedule development determines the contexts or activities in which the target behaviors will be practiced. The staff member simply goes down the row of one target behavior and determines if it could be functionally applied to each activity listed in the left column. For example, Figure 12.5 shows that the target behavior of "choice" (i.e., defined for Evan as scanning two alternatives and then touching one of them) is practiced during dressing, breakfast, leaving for day program, during snacktimes, while engaging in leisure activities with others in the house, during dinner, and while engaging in leisure activities by himself.

Once this procedure is done for all of the target behaviors, it is easy for the staff to evaluate the density of the schedule. Figure 12.5 shows that some of the target behaviors (e.g., wheelchair mobility) are practiced frequently throughout the day, while others are either not scheduled at all on a given day (e.g., laundry on Monday), or are done so on an infrequent basis throughout the day (e.g., toothbrushing). Staff often decide that the infrequent scheduling of desirable activities is appropriate; however, various trends in acquisition may lead the staff to try to schedule more opportunities for learning these activities.

Various types of behavior checks (Holvoet et al., 1980) are incorporated into each identified activity. Evan has two behaviors that are being monitored: "hands out of mouth" and "inappropriate throwing." The "hands out of mouth" behavior is a nondiscrete and sometimes continuous behavior and is being sampled within each activity, providing a percentage of intervals measure. Although certainly not the most refined measure, the sampling is less burdensome for the staff to measure than is a duration measure. This sampling also provides valuable information about the behavior's possible relationship to specific routines. "Inappropriate throwing" is measured by frequency. It is not a very high frequency behavior and is, therefore, a manageable measurement for the staff to accurately employ. Again, although the frequencies in each activity are totaled separately at the end of the day, more specific analyses are possible that

M W F EP _/_/_	1 Peer interact sign	2 Peer interact pass	3 Choice	4 Initiate routine	5 Hands out of mouth	6 Inappropriate throwing	7 Tooth-brush	8 Fork use	9 Washer	10 Dryer
6:00 A.M. Wake-up bathroom					_/_	_/X				
6:30 A.M. Dressing			Choice _/_		_/_	_/X				
7:00 A.M. Bed making					_/_	_/X				
7:15 A.M. Breakfast	"Hi" _/_		Food _/_		_/_	_/X		_/_		
7:45 A.M. Brush teeth					_/_	_/X	_/_			
8:00 A.M. Leave day program	"Bye" _/_		Coat _/_		_/_	_/X				
4:00 P.M. Return toilet	"Hi" _/_				_/_	_/X				
4:15 P.M. Snack	"Hi" _/_		Snack _/_	Scoot _/_	_/_	_/X				
4:30 P.M. Leisure peers	"Hi" _/_	_/_	Peer _/_		_/_	_/X				
5:15 P.M. Toilet					_/_	_/X				
5:45 P.M. Dinner	"Hi" _/_	_/_	Food _/_	Scoot _/_	_/_	_/X		_/_		
6:30 P.M. Laundry washing					_/_	_/X			_/_	
7:00 P.M. Leisure self			Activity _/_		_/_	_/X				
7:30 P.M. Laundry dryer					_/_	_/X				_/_
8:00 P.M. Bath				Scoot _/_	_/_	_/X	_/_			
9:00 P.M. Bed					_/_	_/X				
Totals	_/_	_/_	_/_	_/_	_/_	_/X	_/_	_/_	_/_	_/_

Figure 12.5. A sample Activities Schedule that reflects target behaviors and their relationship to daily routines. (This example was developed by Margaret St. Clair and Mark Kaelber; adapted from Guess, D., & Helmstetter, E. [1986]. Skill cluster instruction and the individualized curriculum sequencing model.

324

11 T-shirt off	12 Drinking slowly	13 Pouring	14 Sign 'toilet'	15 Wheel- chair use	16 Active self ranging	17 Flush toilet	18 Clapping attention	19 Transfer to couch	20 Transfer to chair
			_/_	_/_		_/_			
				_/_	_/_				
	_/_	_/_							
				_/_					
				_/_					
			_/_	_/_		_/_			
	_/_	_/_					_/_		
				_/_					
			_/_	_/_		_/_			
	_/_	_/_					_/_		
				_/_					
				_/_	_/_				
				_/_					
_/_			_/_		_/_	_/_		_/_	_/_
				_/_					
_/_	_/_	_/_	_/_	_/_	_/_	_/_	_/_	_/_	_/_

In R.H. Horner, L.H. Meyer, & H.D.B. Fredericks [Eds.], *Education of learners with severe handicaps: Exemplary service strategies* [pp. 221–248]. Baltimore: Paul H. Brookes Publishing Co.)

may reflect a relationship between the targeted behavior and the specific routines. This analysis can be conducted on each of the targeted behaviors to determine if acquisition is related to only specific routines or whether it is occurring more equally throughout all routines.

Routine Sheets

Routine sheets (see Fig. 12.6 for an example) are the "scripts" that staff will follow when implementing instructional programs and activities. They precisely describe the order of implementation of each of the target behaviors. There is generally one routine sheet for each activity listed down the left side of the matrix (Figure 12.5). Routine sheets are composed of target behaviors, as well as other naturally occurring behaviors, sequentially arranged in an order that makes sense for a specific time of day and in a particular environment.

Figure 12.6 is the Routine Sheet for the "wake-up" routine. It starts with a behavior that the staff should demonstrate (i.e., sign/say "good morning" to Evan), thus providing a cue to the staff and not allowing this excellent opportunity for incidental teaching to be lost. The "Xs" in the scoring column indicate that this is not a target behavior and that data need not be recorded even though Evan is informally prompted to return the greeting. The next behavior on the routine sheet is another one in which staff will encourage Evan to participate. This activity involves transferring him from his bed to his wheelchair. This also is not scored. It is emphasized to staff that participation in nonscoring activities is as important as the formal instructional programs. The third behavior listed on the routine sheet is "wheelchair mobility." To reduce the data requirements, staff record the first three trials of practice, as indicated in the three spaces for recording; however, the instructional strategy is continued for as long as it takes to reach the destination.

The prompting system to be used with each target behavior appears in the scoring column, and the prompt levels at which Evan is to be reinforced is indicated by the underlined number. Also on this routine sheet is a code describing the reasons that a program may not have been implemented and is recorded by the staff. This information is then analyzed and solutions are developed in an effort to increase program implementation. This information is also useful in determining the relationship of certain variables (e.g., toileting accidents, seizures, behavior problems) to a specific time or activity.

Staff assist Evan, when necessary, to participate in all scheduled activities. Although initial selection of target behaviors and the design of the activities reflect Evan's preferences and incorporate "choice," there are many times, and it is hoped that these times will increase, that Evan appears to demonstrate clear indication that he would prefer to engage in a different activity or perhaps no activity. A choice, based upon awareness of the alternatives versus one made without awareness, is sometimes a difficult distinction to make. Staff are faced with difficult decisions as to whether to "strongly encourage" a client

Routine Sheet

Client's name: Evan   Week of: ___/___/___   to   ___/___/___

Routine 1/Wake-up/Bathroom   number/task: ___   Time: 6:00, MTWThF, 9a, SSA

If a program is not run, please indicate reason by placing appropriate code letter in the scoring box. For nonscored programs, indicate whether the client performed the action (Y) or did not perform action (N).

Codes:
A = Aggression
B = Insufficient time
C = Physical/medical problem
D = Insufficient resources/staff
E = Insufficient resources/materials
F = Client refuses

Verbal cue	Learner response	Scoring	Date/initials
Say/sign, "good morning"	Say/sign "good morning"	XXXXX	/ / / / / / / / / / / / / / / /
Move into your chair	Transfers from bed to chair	XXXXX	/ / / / / / / / / / / / / / / /
	Hands out of mouth	Y N	/ / / / / / / /
Go to the bathroom	Wheels chair with both hands to bathroom	543 21	/ / / / / / / / / / / / / / / /
		543 21	/ / / / / / / /
		543 21	/ / / / / / / /
Sit on toilet	Transfers from chair to toilet	XXXXX	/ / / / / / / / / / / / / / / /
What are you doing?	Sign "toilet*"	5 1	/ / / / / / / / / / / / / / / /
Flush the toilet	1. Reach for handle	5432 1	/ / / / / / / /
	2. Push handle down	5432 1	/ / / / / / / /
	3. Release handle	5432 1	/ / / / / / / /
Move into your chair	Transfers from chair to toilet	XXXXXXX	/ / / / / / / / / / / / / / / /
Wash your hands	Washes hands	XXXXXXX	/ / / / / / / /
	Inappropriate throwing	tally _____	/ / / / / / / / / / / / / / / /
Totals	Wheelchair mobility Sign "toilet" Toilet Inappropriate throwing	___/15 ___/5 ___/15 ___/X	/ /

Comments: *Place Evan's hand into the proper configuration for signing "toilet" and if he maintains the sign for 3 seconds, score as a "5"; if not, score as a "1."

Figure 12.6. A sample of a Routine Sheet that reflects the wake-up and bathroom routines of a resident named Evan.

to participate in a scheduled activity or to strongly encourage the client to follow through with his or her possible initiation. Was the client's refusal an issue of "laziness" or was he indicating a preference to engage in another activity? Of course, the answer to this question may be obvious if the client begins to ambulate to another activity, or can reliably communicate his or her interest; however, many clients have neither skill, and only careful analysis and testing of the behaviors and staff knowledge of the client allows the instructors to make this determination. Even if staff determine that the refusal is one of "laziness," they must consider the client's right to refuse, to avoid, or to do nothing (see Chapter 3 for a discussion of these issues). It is crucial that staff be aware of these issues and discuss possible problems with the client's "choices" at staff meetings.

Scoring

All formal instructional programs are scored using the routine sheets during, or as soon as possible following, the instructional program. At the end of the routine sheet, the instructor totals the scores at the bottom. These score totals are then transferred onto the Activities Schedule. The schedules are then totalled, yielding a composite score of each target behavior for the day. The graphs that consist of the day's totals for each target behavior are then analyzed on a monthly basis. If staff feel that progress is attributable to only certain routines, the instructor must analyze the more refined data that is found on the schedules.

SUMMARY

This chapter reviews a variety of living arrangements that are currently available for adults with profound disabilities. It identifies some goals and criteria that may be used to evaluate the quality of community living. A description of one residential program model is provided that incorporates currently suggested "best practices" for individuals with severe and profound disabilities and describes its specific implementation with adults with profound disabilities.

It is the premise of this chapter that all individuals, regardless of the degree of disability, can have their needs met in community environments as opposed to large institutional settings. Research has shown that it is feasible for individuals with severe and profound disabilities to live in community settings (Bellamy & Horner, 1987); however, research on such living options needs to be conducted. This will not be an easy task as community living arrangements, by their very nature, limit the extent to which an individual can exercise tight experimental control over a plethora of potentially confounding variables. The more normalized the environment, the less conducive it is to experimental analysis and control. The challenge to researchers is to develop methods of analyzing the different living environments in such a way that those that provide services can benefit from the research and to most optimally match each individual to the living environment.

REFERENCES

Balla, D., Butterfield, E., & Ziegler, E. (1974). Effects of institutionalization on retarded children: A longitudinal cross-institutional investigation. *American Journal of Mental Deficiency, 78,* 530–549.

Bellamy, T.G., & Horner, R.H. (1987). Beyond high school: Residential and employment options after graduation. In M. Snell (Ed.), *Systematic instruction of persons with severe handicaps* (pp. 491–510). Columbus, OH: Charles E. Merrill.

Best-Sigford, B., Bruininks, R., Lakin, K., Hill, B., & Heal, L. (1982). Resident release patterns in a national sample of public residential facilities. *American Journal of Mental Deficiency, 87,* 130–140.

Blatt, B., Bogdan, R., Biklen, D., & Taylor, S. (1977). From institution to community: A conversion model. In E. Sontag, J. Smith, & N. Certo (Eds.), *Educational programming for the severely and profoundly handicapped* (pp. 40–52). Reston, VA: Council for Exceptional Children.

Borthwick-Duffy, S., Eyman, R., & White, J. (1987). Client characteristics and residential placement patterns. *American Journal of Mental Deficiency, 92,* 24–30.

Bradley, V.J. (1985). Implementation of court and consent decrees: Some current lesions. In R.H. Bruininks & K.C. Lakin (Eds.), *Living and learning in the least restrictive environment* (pp. 81–96). Baltimore: Paul H. Brookes Publishing Co.

Browder, D.M. (1987). *Assessment of individuals with severe handicaps: An applied behavior approach to life skills assessment.* Baltimore: Paul H. Brookes Publishing Co.

Brown, F. (1987). Meaningful assessment of people with severe and profound handicaps. In M. Snell (Ed.), *Systematic instruction of persons with severe handicaps* (pp. 39–63). Columbus, OH: Charles E. Merrill.

Brown, F., Evans, I.M., Weed, K., & Owen, V. (1987). Delineating functional competencies: A component model. *Journal of The Association for Persons with Severe Handicaps, 12*(2), 117–124.

Brown, F., Helmstetter, E., & Guess, D. (1986). *Current best practices with students with profound disabilities: Are there any?* Unpublished manuscript, Institute of Professional Practice, New Haven, CT.

Brown, L., Branston, M.B., Hamre-Nietupski, S., Pumpian, I., Certo, N., & Gruenewald, L.A. (1979). A strategy for developing chronological age appropriate and functional curricular content for severely handicapped adolescents and young adults. *Journal of Special Education, 13,* 81–90.

Brown, L., Nietupski, J., & Hamre-Nietupski, S. (1976). Criterion of ultimate functioning. In M.A. Thomas (Ed.), *Hey, don't forget about me* (pp. 2–15), Reston, VA: Council for Exceptional Children.

Bruininks, R., Hauber, F., & Kudla, M. (1980). National survey of community residential facilities: A profile of facilities and residents in 1977. *American Journal of Mental Deficiency, 84,* 470–478.

Bruininks, R., Hill, B., & Thorsheim, M. (1982). Deinstitutionalization and foster care for mentally retarded people. *Health and Social Work, 7,* 198–205.

Butterfield, E. (1977). Institutionalization and its alternatives for mentally retarded people in the United States. *International Journal of Mental Health, 6,* 21–34.

Cavalier, A., & McCarver, R. (1981). Wyatt v. Stickney and mentally retarded individuals. *Mental Retardation, 19,* 209–214.

Close, D. (1977). Community living for severely and profoundly retarded adults: A group home study. *Education and Training of the Mentally Retarded, 12,* 256–262.

Conroy, J., Efthimiou, J., & Lemanowicz, J. (1982). A matched comparison of the developmental growth of institutionalized and deinstitutionalized mentally retarded clients. *American Journal of Mental Deficiency, 86*(6), 581–587.

Donnellan, A.M., Mirenda, P.L., Mesaros, R.A., & Fassbender, L.L. (1984). Analyzing the communicative functions of aberrant behavior. *Journal of The Association for Persons with Severe Handicaps, 9*(3), 201–212.

Donnellan, A.M., & Neel, R.S. (1986). New directions in educating students with autism. In R.H. Horner, L.H. Meyer, & H.D.B. Fredericks (Eds.), *Education of learners with severe handicaps: Exemplary service strategies* (pp. 99–126). Baltimore: Paul H. Brookes Publishing Co.

Ellis, M., Balla, D., Estes, O., Warren, S., Meyers, C., Hollis, J., Isaacson, R., Pal, R., & Siegel, D. (1981). Common sense in the habilitation of mentally retarded persons: A reply to Menolascino and McGee. *Mental Retardation, 19,* 209–214.

Evans, I.M., Brown, F., Weed, K.A., Spry, K.M., & Owen, V.E. (1987). The assessment of functional competencies: A behavioral approach to the evaluation of programs for children with disabilities. In R.J. Prinz (Ed.), *Advances in behavioral assessment of children and families* (pp. 93–121). Greenwich, CT: JAI Press.

Evans, I.M., & Meyer, L.H. (1985). *An educative approach to behavior problems: A practical decision model for interventions with severely handicapped learners.* Baltimore: Paul H. Brookes Publishing Co.

Eyman, R., & Borthwick, S. (1980). Patterns of care for mentally retarded persons. *Mental Retardation, 19,* 63–66.

Favell, J., Risley, T., Wolfe, M., Riddle, J., & Rasmussen, P. (1981). The limits of habilitation: How can we identify them and how can we change them? *Analysis and Intervention in Developmental Disabilities, 1,* 37–44.

Freeman, H. (1978). Foster home care for mentally retarded children: Can it work? *Child Welfare, 57,* 113–121.

Gast, D., & Wolery, M. (1987). Severe maladaptive behaviors. In M. Snell (Ed.), *Systematic instruction of persons with severe handicaps* (pp. 300–333). Columbus, OH: Charles E. Merrill.

Gaylord-Ross, R. (1980). A decision model for the treatment of aberrant behavior in applied settings. In W. Sailor, B. Wilcox, & L. Brown (Eds.), *Methods of instruction for severely handicapped students* (pp. 135–158). Baltimore: Paul H. Brookes Publishing Co.

Gaylord-Ross, R.J., & Holvoet, J.F. (1985). *Strategies for educating students with severe handicaps.* Boston: Little, Brown.

Goffman, E. (1961). *Asylums.* New York: Anchor Books.

Guess, D., Benson, H.A., & Siegel-Causey, E. (1985). Concepts and issues related to choice-making and autonomy among persons with severe disabilities. *Journal of The Association for Persons with Severe Handicaps, 10*(2), 79–86.

Guess, D., & Helmstetter, E. (1986). Skill cluster instruction and the individualized curriculum sequencing model. In R.H. Horner, L.H. Meyer, & H.D.B. Fredericks (Eds.), *Education of learners with severe handicaps: Exemplary service strategies* (pp. 221–248). Baltimore: Paul H. Brookes Publishing Co.

Hauber, F., Bruininks, R., Hill, B., Lakin, K., Scheerenberger, R., & White, C. (1984). National census of residential facilities: A 1982 profile of faciliites and residents. *American Journal of Mental Deficiency, 89,* 236–245.

Holvoet, J., Guess, D., Mulligan, M., & Brown, F. (1980). The individualized curriculum sequencing model (II): A teaching strategy for severely handicapped students. *Journal of The Association for the Severely Handicapped, 5,* 337–351.

Horner, R.D. (1980). The effects of an environmental "enrichment" program on the behavior of institutionalized profoundly retarded children. *Journal of Applied Behavior Analysis, 13,* 473–491.

Horner, R.H., Meyer, L.H., & Fredericks, H.D.B. (Eds.). (1986). *Education of learn-*

ers with severe handicaps: Exemplary service strategies. Baltimore: Paul H. Brookes Publishing Co.

Lambert, N., Windmiller, M., Cole, L., & Figueroa, R. (1975). AAMD adaptive behavior scale, public school revision (rev. ed.). Washington, DC: American Association on Mental Deficiency.

McCormick, M., Balla, D., & Ziegler, E. (1975). Resident-care practices in institutions for the retarded. American Journal of Mental Deficiency, 14(1), 1–17.

Menolascino, F., & McGee, J. (1981a). The new institutions: Last ditch arguments. Mental Retardation, 19, 215–220.

Menolascino, F., & McGee, J., (1981b). Rejoinder to the Partlow Committee. Mental Retardation, 19, 227–229.

Mulligan, M., Guess, D., Holvoet, J., & Brown, F. (1980). The individualized curriculum sequencing model (I): Implications from research on massed, distributed, or spaced trial training. Journal of The Association for the Severely Handicapped, 5, 325–336.

Neel, R.S., Billingsley, F.F., McCarty, F., Symonds, D., Lambert, C., Lewis-Smith, N., & Hanashiro, R. (1983). Teaching autistic children: A functional curriculum approach: The IMPACT curriculum. Seattle: University of Washington.

Scheerenberger, R. (1978). Public residential services for the mentally retarded. In N. Ellis & N. Bray (Eds.), International review of research in mental retardation (Vol. 12). New York: Academic Press.

Scheerenberger, R. (1982). Public residential services, 1981: Status and trends. Mental Retardation, 20, 210–215.

Taylor, S.J., McCord, W., & Searl, S.J. (1981). Medicaid dollars and community homes: The community ICF/MR controversy. Journal of The Association for the Severely Handicapped, 6, 59–64.

Voeltz, L.M., Wuerch, B.B., & Bockhaut, C.H. (1982). Social validation of leisure activities training with severely handicapped youth. Journal of The Association for the Severely Handicapped, 7(4), 3–13.

Willer, B., & Intagliata, J. (1984). An overview of the social policy of deinstitutionalization. In N. Ellis & N. Bray (Eds.), International review of research in mental retardation (Vol. 12). New York: Academic Press.

INDEX